THE FAST

THE HISTORY, SCIENCE, PHILOSOPHY, AND PROMISE OF DOING WITHOUT

JOHN OAKES

AVID READER PRESS

New York   London   Toronto   Sydney   New Delhi

AVID READER PRESS
An Imprint of Simon & Schuster, LLC
1230 Avenue of the Americas
New York, NY 10020

First Avid Reader Press hardcover edition February 2024

AVID READER PRESS and colophon are trademarks of Simon & Schuster, LLC

Simon & Schuster: Celebrating 100 Years of Publishing in 2024

For information about special discounts for bulk purchases, please contact
Simon & Schuster Special Sales at 1-866-506-1949
or business@simonandschuster.com.

The Simon & Schuster Speakers Bureau can bring authors to your live event.
For more information or to book an event, contact the Simon & Schuster Speakers
Bureau at 1-866-248-3049 or visit our website at www.simonspeakers.com.

Interior design by Joy O'Meara

Manufactured in the United States of America

1   3   5   7   9   10   8   6   4   2

Library of Congress Cataloging-in-Publication Data
Names: Oakes, John G. H., author.
Title: The fast : the history, science, philosophy, and promise
of doing without / John Oakes.
Identifiers: LCCN 2023044307 (print) | LCCN 2023044308 (ebook) |
ISBN 9781668017418 (hardcover) | ISBN 9781668017425 (trade paperback) |
ISBN 9781668017432 (ebook)
Subjects: LCSH: Fasting—History. | Fasting—Religious aspects. |
Fasting—Health aspects.
Classification: LCC RM226 .O25 2024 (print) | LCC RM226 (ebook) |
DDC 613.2/5—dc23/eng/20231106
LC record available at https://lccn.loc.gov/2023044307
LC ebook record available at https://lccn.loc.gov/2023044308

ISBN 978-1-6680-1741-8
ISBN 978-1-6680-1743-2 (ebook)

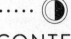

CONTENTS

Introduction vii

DAY 1, SUNDAY
"Spaces Between":
A Visit to the Quietest Place on Earth
1

DAY 2, MONDAY
Ascetic Roots 1:
The Greeks, Buddha, and Their Legacies
23

DAY 3, TUESDAY
The Marvelous Machine:
What Happens to Our Body When We Fast
43

DAY 4, WEDNESDAY
Ascetic Roots 2:
The Abrahamic Traditions
75

DAY 5, THURSDAY
The River of Kings:
Fasting as Protest
110

DAY 6, FRIDAY
Fasting, Frauds, and Faddism
156

DAY 7, SATURDAY
Self-Cancellation
189

Epilogue   205

Acknowledgments   211

Appendices:
A Sampling of Famous Fasters   215

Selected Books Related to Fasting   217

Notes   221

Bibliography   269

Index   291

Image Credits   300

Introduction

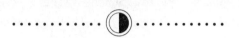

In the spring of my sixtieth year, in the aftermath of a series of national and global tragedies unprecedented in my lifetime, some of which are ongoing, and in a period that seemed to me to hold out real hope for a better future, I decided to stop eating for seven days. That is how, two days in, I found myself in the unlikely position of examining with intense interest a single, solitary lemon sitting in a basket on the kitchen table.

Undertaking a prolonged fast, or even a partial fast, is an unspectacular achievement. There are no trophies to be had, no beasts or peaks to be conquered. There is no Olympic medal celebrating self-deprivation. Fasting involves doing less, but doing less in a radical way. It adds by subtracting. It doesn't transform the world, or even your body for very long. All that happens is that your perspective on what comprises daily life and what is necessary to sustain it is shaken up. If you are fortunate, those thoughts stay with you.

I am not much of an athlete: I have always liked the *idea* of hiking, swimming, stretching, etc., but when it comes down to it, I am not big on pain. I like to sleep late, and I like to eat. I don't own a weight scale. But a prolonged fast—a voluntary refusal of nourishment—seemed to me an attempt to reset the most immediate and fundamental boundaries any of us know: the lines that separate our physical bodies from the vast, chaotic universe in which we find ourselves.

We fast all the time, even when we are not conscious of doing so. A fast manifests the idea of holding back. The flip side of a fast is similarly always with us: call it splurging, self-indulgence, or a variant of "self-care." To fast or not to fast in all its forms, that is the measure of our existence. Even a good gambler is a fasting expert, going all in, seeing the bet, or folding, as the philosopher, activist, and faster Simone Weil observed: he "is capable of watching and fasting, almost like a saint, he has his premonition." Fasting is not just about food; it involves *doing without* in the broadest sense. And the process must be voluntary. Hunger and famines can be created, but even if a fast is decreed by religious or civil authorities, it requires personal and private commitment. Its nature is anti-authoritarian.

Fasting is paradoxical: a culture-spanning spiritual exercise that plays a key role in body-shaming; a unifying practice that acknowledges, even heightens, the mind/body divide. According to some practitioners, fasting is a means to empowerment and self-advancement; according to some contemporary critics, it results from "self-hatred and desperation." But a desire for transformation requires rejecting a present state in favor of a better one. Despair only occurs when there is no hope of improvement, and fasting expresses hope.

If food is our body's fuel, then undertaking a long-term fast is an attempt to go slow. Even more, it marks an effort to reset. Unless she decides to starve herself until life is extinguished, the long-term faster is someone who upsets her daily routine by purging her interior and feasting on rich, infinite nothingness.

In the midst of the physical changes I underwent during my own fast, I began wondering about the underpinnings of the experience, both biological and philosophical. I started casually researching the subject, and learned about fasting's connections to satyagraha and ketosis, Achilles and dogs, the number forty, king penguins, Mark Twain, and hunger strikes. And I got acquainted with fasting's dark side: anorexia mirabilis ("holy anorexia"), and the eating disorder anorexia nervosa, which is essentially fasting without end. It became clear that fasting can be a tool either for self-affirmation or for self-dissolution, and that sometimes those goals coincide. I wanted to learn more.

Refusing to eat as a matter of conscience is not so much anti-materialist as it is anti-consumption, a renunciation that began several thousand years ago with the first ascetics. For the ascetic, the act challenges the presumption that physical well-being is our only goal while we live. Subsequent elements of self-denial—and specifically self-starvation—can be found in just about all major religions and most folk religions as well. In the present day, fasting-as-protest, otherwise known as a hunger strike, is done on a regular basis all over the world for just about every cause imaginable. These are not self-destructive impulses: they are nonviolent affirmations of dissent.

In the pages that follow, I explore some of these concepts, and attempt to explain as well the complex sequence of biological phenomena that occur when the human body is forced to draw on its own reserves for sustenance. I know I have not managed to exhaust the subject. For example, I specifically elected to forgo in-depth discussion of the many "fasting girls" of the nineteenth century and earlier because they have been thoroughly discussed elsewhere. Nevertheless, I hope what I present in this book can provide an overview of the history, consequences, and implications of fasting, and particularly fasting beyond food.

While there is plenty of evidence to suggest certain of fasting's benefits, and much to praise in the spiritual exercise of the practice, the last word isn't in on what it does for your body. Cure-all claims of fasting are anecdotal and should be viewed with suspicion. However, there is enough confirmed research on how fasting *can* benefit you—and on its history as a crucial element of many formative philosophies—to keep us happily occupied.

....

Fasting requires assessment (how much do I ingest) and then reassessment (I choose not to ingest). It is a rejection of passivity, an assertion of the power of choice, a reconsideration of priorities, and a defiance of authority. For some, such as Gandhi, it provided an extended moment to focus the mind before an important decision. Notable fasters include Moses, Buddha, Jesus, Gandhi, the suffragist Doris Stevens, the civil rights activist Eroseanna Robinson, Cesar Chavez, the IRA's Bobby Sands, India's "Iron Lady" Irom Chanu Sharmila, and a long, continually lengthening list of others who have drawn on its power over the ages and across borders and cultures. It was a tool of which gods availed themselves: the Norse god Odin fasted for nine days and nine nights as part of his successful quest to acquire the power of the runes.

When implemented as a hunger strike, fasting signals purity of purpose. It signifies that the faster is sincere and allied with a higher moral power (or believes she is). In the fall of 2021, the young climate activists of the Sunrise Movement reaffirmed fasting's relevance when they engaged in hunger strikes in front of the White House. In the same period, New York City cabdrivers called for a mass hunger strike to call attention to their crippling debt. "It's dangerous and it's drastic," Bhairavi Desai, executive director of the New York Taxi Workers Alliance, said at the time. "And I tell you, we've been pushed to that edge." The taxi drivers fasted for fifteen days before winning their case, causing city officials to renegotiate the amount due to lenders. The Sunrise strikers didn't immediately win their cause—the environmental initiatives they were battling for didn't clear Congress at that time, although they were resurrected months later—but they demonstrated the intensity and clarity of their purpose to a broad public and, of course, received plenty of media coverage as a result. "As a person I'm really small, and before, that might have made me feel ineffective," said Kidus Girma, one of the hunger strikers. "But now I see that a lot of small people add up to something big, and I feel big in my smallness." Fasting is a demand to be seen and to be heard. It provides a clear answer to the question: "How dedicated are you to your cause?"

"I'm always aware of being a flea near these giants and of my perceived inability to put convincing arguments on the table," said Stella Jean, a prominent Haitian-Italian designer who undertook a hunger strike in protest at the racism of the fashion industry in February 2023. "I had nothing else left to barter with." At its most basic, a fast is a refusal to plug one's mouth with food. But that act can also be a call of sorts. In ancient Ireland, people were "fasted against" or "fasted upon," as they still are to this day in India. In these cases, fasting becomes a means to leverage power. It opens a portal to a spiritual realm, whose powers can be summoned to aid the faster and to right wrongs (more about this in chapter 5). Throughout recorded history, the weapon of fasting has been adapted according to social need. From premedieval times, it has often signaled a ritual challenge, a drive for independence, becoming a threat to officialdom. It has just as often become a means for self-arbitration, making it a conduit to moral or spiritual power without an intermediary. And it has more recently been associated with tortured attempts to fit cultural ideals, particularly (although not exclusively) among young women.

Many people around the world see a fast as a form of prayer with a strong element of worldly activism—an extra punch. And until the twentieth century, fasting was inseparable from the spiritual well-being of Americans. At numerous points before the turn of the last century, various presidents regularly called for national fasting days in response to moments of crisis. Today, a call for a national fast would be perceived as extreme, smacking of self-hatred and/or theocracy. But perhaps it is time to reconsider that view.

....

For anyone who embarks on a fast—whether for moral, political, or health-related reasons—the process marks a break in the consumerist narrative, a small but potent rebellion against the inflexible demarcation of our days formed by the steady lockstep march of breakfast, lunch, and dinner. Indoctrination for this regimen begins before we are self-aware. Beginning in the late nineteenth century, instead of feeding infants when they were hungry, breastfeeding mothers were instructed to follow feeding schedules "as rigid as railway timetables." To a large degree, our meals define our lives.

The faster refuses such direction. The act of fasting is symptomatic of a Bartleby-like decision to refuse reasonable behavior. It won't stop routine, but impedes it for a bit, signifying a shift and a determined unwillingness to follow standard operating procedure. In its striving toward self-improvement, the fast evokes both St. Paul ("Work out your own salvation with fear and trembling") and the last words of Buddha ("Decay is inherent in all component things. Work out your salvation with diligence"). Fasting signals precedence of mind over matter, demanding careful assessment of the most normal of acts. And because it takes place over an extended period, fasting demands some measure of commitment.

In another sense, fasting allows for room in our bodies, for the inclusion of something new, and for the acceptance of emptiness. It cultivates the presence of an absence. After a time, this absence of food (food that in the normal course of things is first a necessity, then a comfort, then a luxury) enables us to focus on other, less material things. Fasting reveals itself as an exploration of borders and barriers. As Weil understood, with reference to Plato's concept of *metaxu* ("between" spaces), barriers imply connection: "Two prisoners whose cells adjoin communicate by knocking on the wall. The wall is the thing which separates them but it is also their means of communication. . . . Every separation is a link." The meditative experience induced by long-term fasting links humans who seek to focus on what is relevant and essential the world over and across millennia. Fasting's effects are replicated in the Hasidic process of *hitbodedut*, or "self-seclusion"—a search for inner stillness, a fast from the presence of others—as it is in the more common meditation espoused by Buddhist and Hindu teachings. In Arabic, the modern word for fasting is etymologically associated with "standing still." In English, volume XVI of the *Oxford English Dictionary* connects "starve" and "stare"—both are credited with possible origins in *starren*, Old High German for "to be rigid." Like staring and starving, fasting involves stillness. If you are "steadfast," you resist. You are strong and you endure.

Is fasting reserved for a select few? I am not particularly fit, as suggested earlier. Anyone in reasonably good shape can go on a fast. There is nothing to boast about here (besides—as St. Jerome says—boasting about fasting is reprehensible). But as fasting comes back into the mainstream discourse, both as part of a focus on well-being and as a reaction to consumerism, it's worth reconsidering its value and its roots. Fasting reminds us of the virtues of paring back, of not consuming all that we can. There are few more timely messages.

Is it a mark of privilege to fast? Once, it would have been impossible to associate fasting with self-indulgence, but now it has become entwined with self-obsession. Many see fasting as a signifier of luxury, a paradoxical indication of excess. You can only surrender what you already have, as the Greek philosopher Diogenes of Sinope is reported to have observed two millennia ago.

Fasting can be a great unifier, an instant leveler that connects us purely by virtue of being an act accessible to all. This shared experience is another reason that fasting has been adopted by religions and political movements all over the world. Notably, places marked by devastating famine are also often home to ancient fasting traditions. Cultures most commonly associated with fasting include those of Ireland, India, and Ethiopia, where devout Coptic Christians fast intermittently up to 210 days a year. This is not to suggest that the world does not suffer from hunger. In the words of philosophers and fasting advocates Eva Lerat and Sébastien Charbonnier, "malnutrition and starvation are scourges largely orchestrated by our society of overconsumption and profit, and our thinking cannot in any way allow us to minimize the suffering and damage that this entails." In a society where, by some measures, the largest single component of landfills is food waste and where one-third of all food is lost or wasted, focusing for a time on what we consume versus what we need to consume seems like a perennially beneficial exercise.

The choice to fast is more easily made if you know there will again be food on the other side of the experience. But to my mind, fasting is a sign of strength rather than privilege—a subtle difference, to be sure. A decision to put a hold on eating doesn't necessarily indicate a surfeit of food. It only means the choice has been made not to eat. That decision is what I intend to explore.

Somewhere in his *Book of Five Rings*, the seventeenth-century swordsman Miyamoto Musashi writes that an effective warrior moves like a stream that flows over and around rocks. Although I am no warrior, to me, a self-imposed fast—even one that is not followed to the point of no return—is not dissimilar. It is a graceful way to confront immutable circumstance amid the constant battle of existence that sweeps us along. Although it is a distant cousin to suicide in that it is self-abnegation—a willful step away from continuing as things have been and turning one's face toward finality—limited fasting is closer to what the French call the "little death" of post-orgasm. It is a resetting of consciousness. Given time, the effects largely dissipate: it's more like a haircut (which is also a flirtation with instruments that could be deadly) than a permanent makeover.

Wellness and weight-loss culture often seem bound up in vanity. Susan Sontag wrote that to think only of oneself is to think of death. Self-obsession means a relentless focus on the decay our bodies inevitably undergo. And while, of course, we all need self-care, the wellness movement's connection with buying things means it requires dependence on materiality that looks suspiciously like an outgrowth of capitalism. The standard interpretation of the modern mantra "Be kind to yourself" is to stuff yourself and go out and buy things. A prolonged fast, on the other hand, lacks any gimmickry. Fasting demands only your own agency, and it strangely requires the temporary abandonment of what we think we need. It inverts self-obsession, as though the act itself were some kind of Klein bottle—that weirdly impossible object lesson in physics where the outside is inside and vice versa.

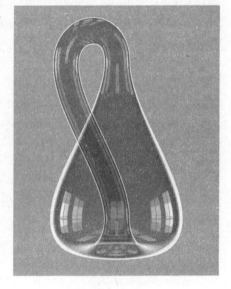

A Klein bottle.

By turning our gaze inward, focusing on the most mundane physical acts over a set period, fasting enables its practitioners to approach, if not achieve, self-erasure—and at the same time, achieve self-empowerment, in an affirmation of the right and ability to self-direction. Even if you fast together with a partner, the act sets you apart. No one else, nothing else is required. There is nothing to exchange but ideas. Not everyone is equipped to benefit from the fasting experience. But fasting's principles, and what it sparks and what it confronts, are worth everyone's consideration.

....

I had been looking for a personal exorcism. I wanted a profound cleansing, a decortication so thorough that it would reach down to my very cells and force them to renew. I didn't delude myself thinking the process would be curative or permanent or that it would change the world. I simply wanted to shuck my then current mental state in favor of something else, anything else, even if only for a few days.

In March, as the long, cold winter started to give way to signs of spring, I thought to undertake a fast. Not just a day or two—that seemed routine, familiar to anyone who'd observed Lent (Christianity), Ramadan (Islam), Yom Kippur (Judaism), Uposatha (Buddhism), or Ekadashi (Hinduism). But a time long enough to go beyond normal limits, to explore eyebrow-raising territory without inflicting self-harm. And I also wasn't sure how long I could endure. A few days wouldn't make the point. A week felt just about right: seven days of real abstinence seemed a statement of some sort, even if it was a statement of significance only to myself. As climbing a mountain is a way for some people to take stock of physical being, a prolonged fast was my attempt to assert a perhaps illusory control over my most immediate surroundings: my own fleshy landscape.

I proposed the fast to my spouse. She agreed, surprised that a commitment to cutting back had come from me. About thirty years ago we had done just such a fast together, in very different circumstances: back then, no national crisis was at hand. We thought of that earlier fast as a test of endurance, as a purging good for the soul. I didn't remember much about the experience, but I did recall how I felt weak but empowered at its end. That sounded good. I felt enervated as it was and could do with some empowerment.

Although fasting is at its core a private, personal exercise, a partner on the journey seemed crucial, as much for encouragement as for monitoring fidelity to the goal. Alone, I didn't think I could complete a week without food. After all, it is a major decision to skip a meal, much less a day's, much less a week's worth of food. But I knew that it was possible for us to do and likely even healthy. Sheltering in place though we were, I felt as though we were about to embark on a brave adventure.

"There's hidden sweetness in the stomach's emptiness."

—Rumi (trans. Coleman Barks)

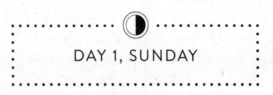

"Spaces Between":
A Visit to the Quietest Place on Earth

We have agreed on ground rules: we aren't aspiring ascetics, so we have decided we can drink as much water, tea, coffee, and vegetable broth as we want, but no solids. Nothing containing processed sugar. That seems doable. You must work to approach the negative: abstinence requires a commitment. But the beginning is as easy as falling out of an airplane. I just let go, and the world continues without me. I woke up, didn't eat. Fixed myself a cup of tea. Some stomach pangs, but no other issues. My immediate goal was *not* to do something, which is rattling. Normally I wake up, get dressed and so on, prepare breakfast and then eat it, clean up after. Steps to a day. But, of course, there are still things to do, just different ones. I seize a bowl of almonds and hustle it out of sight, handling it as if it were radioactive. In the afternoon I suddenly feel wistful about the non-presence of food, letting go of preparing meals and eating them, as though I'm on the deck of an ocean liner pulling away from its berth, watching the city recede, the expanse growing between us. Nothing to do but lean on the railing, wait, and watch. I've given myself a gift of time, a space in the day. How much time we spend preparing, cooking, and cleaning up after ourselves! But if I've rejected the business of eating, I've taken up the business of fasting, and it *is* an effort. It feels as though the day stretches out to infinity. Yet I've only added about three hours, give or take, to do whatever I choose: work, leisure, or errands. I sit and sip tea, staring off into space. I'm busy fasting. The prospect of a week, of just over ten thousand minutes, seems so long right now. We picked a week to balance between the minimal (a day) and the excessive (a month). And it seems attainable. I keep checking my watch. The seconds tick by. Am I building toward something or chipping away at something? In either case, what is it? We don't exist in stasis in a void. "We are what we eat," wrote Brillat-Savarin. But in eating nothing, I feel more substantive than ever. My normal perspective is so limited. I feel like someone gasping in amazement at the night sky: Everything seems new, unexplored. But it's always been there, all around us, waiting.

To all appearances, emptiness and humans do not go well together. Fullness is equated with happiness: a full stomach, a full bank account. To be empty is to be drained. A fundamental antipathy between the void and the human condition exists on both an internal and an external level, and that extends to speech. Remaining still (not necessarily through meditation) and fasting (not necessarily by not eating) are closely related. In fact, remaining still is movement fasting and/or speech fasting.

When I decided to explore fasting, like most of us I focused on its relation to food. It immediately became apparent that the real impact of the presence or absence of food was its use as a metaphor. The equation seems straightforward: you don't eat, you starve. But that is the beginning of an internal discussion on the power of absence, and that led me to think about fasting in other forms. Something I have rarely practiced, fasting from speech, caught my interest.

If you've ever been stuck in an elevator with someone for an extended period, you'll know that to begin a conversation is obligatory. To refrain from talking to another person when you're in unexpectedly close proximity for more than a few minutes is just about impossible, particularly in a potentially perilous situation. It wouldn't be sensible, it wouldn't be polite, it would be perceived as hostile and strange. Silence threatens because it evokes nonexistence. Beyond silence, withheld speech challenges established structures, which require constant affirmation. All those parades and endless speechifying—the bunting, hymns, and anthems—are not just about spectacle and egos. They create an ethereal edifice without which the establishment crumbles. In recent years, Russian and Chinese dissenters facing imprisonment or worse have waved blank sheets of paper. During the third week of the 2022 invasion of Ukraine, police in Nizhny Novgorod, Yekaterinburg, and Rostov-on-Don arrested anti-war activists who held up such signs. Protesters held empty signs and sheets of paper in Hong Kong in 2020 and in Beijing, Shanghai, and other cities in 2022. If critical words are forbidden, there is nothing to say. And yet saying nothing becomes unacceptable, and an empty sign instantly conveys the substance of an absence. It makes a world of difference to *choose* this silence: to refrain from engagement is radically different from being prevented from engaging.

....

One of the quietest places on earth is in the middle of the United States in Minneapolis, in the anechoic chamber at Orfield Labs, an acoustical consulting laboratory. At one point, it held the Guinness record for the quietest place on the planet. The room has a sound level of *negative* thirteen decibels. By comparison, normal hearing starts at zero decibels. As decibels are measured on a logarithmic scale, each increase or decrease of ten indicates a corresponding exponential tenfold change. The sound of breathing is about ten decibels, and the rustle of leaves is about ten times as loud, twenty decibels.

The room in Minneapolis is so thoroughly sound absorbent that if someone turns away while speaking to you, the high frequencies are stripped out of the voice. Sound waves can't travel around their head. Your balance is thrown off due to the inability of your senses to calibrate the evenness of the floors and the distance of the walls.

When the chamber was first set up in 1995, an English tabloid claimed that no one could spend more than forty-five minutes in the room alone. "That is not what I told them," says Steve Orfield, the owner of the lab. From New York, I try to explain my interest in visiting his laboratory. My intention is to explore the connection between fasting and his an-echoic chamber. It quickly becomes apparent that Orfield is receptive to the idea. Orfield sees himself as a chronicler of the conflict between the conscious and the unconscious. He brings up the idea of perceptual fasting, the lack of all stimuli. "You experience all sensations at once," he says. "The only real way to talk about silence is to talk about silence in every modality. Stop thinking about noise as acoustics and start thinking about noise as everything sensory. What happens when people become minimally exposed to their world?" Orfield feels that all sensations have an engineering side and a sensory side. "All humans have is perception," Orfield tells me. "Nothing else makes sense to our world. Outside of our human perception all we have are dreams."

For an engineer, Orfield has an atypically spiritual view of the chamber. He claims that it sends people on a kind of souped-up path to meditation, which he calls "transcendent." He has a gnomic, sage-like air. "You can feel what's going on, you can know what's going on, but you can no longer express what's going on, in the words of Joseph Campbell," Orfield says. With a near-absence of complexity—of any true signaling—our brain lacks reference points.

The room was built to test the sound levels of various commercial products, and it still is used to test, say, people's responses to the sound level of a certain dishwasher. As word of its existence has leaked out, Orfield has had so many inquiries that he eventually opened it up to tours. Silence is a rare and valuable commodity, even as it challenges us. He tells me that the longest anyone has stayed in the room is two hours. In an arbitrary bit of goal setting, I opt to match the record. It seems hubris to try to outdo this span. It is an odd sort of record in any case—a kind of resolute nonachievement.

Orfield is indignant about the loss of his lab's status in the record books. In 2015, the top accolades for silence went to Building 87 at Microsoft's Redmond campus, which claimed negative 20.6 decibels. Orfield says that he was told "in confidence" by an unnamed technician involved in the record switch that the Microsoft measurement was a one-time spike, whereas Orfield's anechoic chamber sustained its negative reading over a period of ten minutes. I'm happy to side with the little guy.

....

A "moment of silence" in the day marks a memorial. It is a solemn grave-stone in the quotidian bustle. "Silence is suspect," writes communication theorist Roy Christopher. It is a choice, like fasting from food. Our own silence is bearable, but the extended silence of a mass of people is a heavy weight that seems inexplicable and even terrifying. It is the sense of something pending, of time frozen, of an unnatural state. Hell is not others, as Sartre told us—hell is being deprived of others. Dogs, cats, and virtual analysts can almost fill the need, but what we really live for is the active assessment of our fellow humans.

Unfairly or not, for some the discussion over silence has become a question of gentrification. In "Let Brooklyn Be Loud," an article in the *Atlantic*, Xochitl Gonzalez opined that "living is loud and messy, but residing? Residing is silent business." Gonzalez went on to argue that making noise is a cultural and political decision, connecting it with youth, diversity, and general rebellion against stultifying authority. But authority is loud and overbearing, and the individual . . . at least less so.

When we're together our instinct is to make noise. We instinctively shrink away from doing nothing. According to one study at the University of Virginia, "most people seem to prefer to be doing something rather than nothing, even if that something is negative." A good number of that 2014 study's participants (67 percent of the men and 25 percent of the women) preferred physical pain to merely sitting unmolested for fifteen minutes. "What is striking," wrote the scientists, "is that simply being alone with their own thoughts for fifteen minutes was apparently so aversive that it drove many participants to self-administer an electric shock that they had earlier said they would pay to avoid." The researchers found that it was not a matter of people thinking negative thoughts about themselves or their personal situations: the problem seemed to be more that the subjects discovered they had to be both "'script-writer' and an 'experiencer'; that is, they had to choose a topic to think about ('I'll focus on my upcoming summer vacation'), decide what would happen ('Okay, I've arrived at the beach, I guess I'll lie in the sun for a bit before going for a swim'), and then mentally experience those actions." Taking complete responsibility for our actions can be an overwhelming burden. And focusing on nothing, or attempting to do so, apparently rarely occurs to us. It takes effort and conscious decision-making to be still.

And yet the basic need for stillness seems to be a matter of quantifiable well-being. A recent article in *New Scientist* detailed how sensory deprivation sessions—which of course involve near-absolute silence—decrease "activity in the default mode network (DMN), a collection of brain regions that are active when the brain is at rest or not involved in a particular task." As with so much else involving fasting, these results are counterintuitive. Why would activity in this area of the brain, which comes to life precisely when we are resting, *drop* when sensory input is tamped down? "Rumination, stress and anxiety"—basically what characterizes most of the bustling humans I know—overwhelm the mind's communication network. High levels of activity in the DMN are associated with schizophrenia and "negative, self-referential information" that results in depression. With a limited period of self-enforced near absence, such as intense meditation, "internal mind chatter" diminishes, allowing the nervous system to reset.

It is easy to place loudness on the side of rebels. Noise distracts and disrupts. But so can silence, and silence carries a mystery, power, and permanence that noise can never match, for all its physicality. Silence is not nothing. The universe may have started with a bang, but stillness is the real hard work of ongoing creation. It is also a threat to the establishment. "To rest in a DreamSpace is a red brick through the glass window of capitalism," writes Tricia Hersey of the Nap Ministry in *Rest Is Resistance: A Manifesto*. "I want our intentional rest to scream at oppression on a bullhorn, then emerge soft and full." Unlike noise, silence is a cohesive unit. It's why we say the silence is "broken" when noise intrudes. Silence descends, like a blanket. It seems to me that living can also be quiet, and that the cultural debate over noise has more to do with perceptions of power—of needing to be heard. What is labeled "noise" and what is essential to living depends on who is doing the defining. Just as someone has a right to speak her mind, she also has a right to be quiet, and to experience quiet. This argument has been going on for a long time: the elder Babylonian gods had their contemplation disrupted by the noisy younger Babylonian gods, who in turn were irritated beyond measure by their raucous creations, the humans, and so determined to rid the earth of their presence. The result was the Flood, "roaring like a bull, the clouds bellowing, the winds howling. . . ."

Ultimately, noise and silence are connected. Just as creation needs absence, noise and silence come full circle and meet. Roy Christopher observes: "A constant sound can seem like a kind of silence, receding into the background of your consciousness until it stops abruptly, leaving true silence, or until it is accompanied by a louder sound, splitting the heard world in two. Hearing, in a cognitive sense, is less about being able to detect sounds than it is being able to tell the difference between these vibrations."

....

Orfield Labs is a low, ivy-covered building on a silent side street. The building was once the home of Studio 80, one of the great recording studios of the Midwest. Bob Dylan recorded part of the album *Blood on the Tracks* here, and Prince and Cat Stevens also recorded in the studio. The 1980 disco classic "Funkytown" by Lipps Inc. was crafted in its studios. It's on the National Register of Historic Places. Now it is best known for its prodigious output of silence, thanks to the anechoic chamber that Orfield arranged to have transported to his laboratory in the late 1980s from Chicago, where it had formerly been used in research by the Sunbeam Corporation, a manufacturer of household appliances ("Lighter . . . higher . . . finer textured cakes!").

Upon entering the concrete, bunker-like building, a visitor is greeted with an artwork that says "White Silence Is Violence." "Here's the adventurer," Orfield says when we first meet. I smile wanly. He escorts me to the anechoic chamber, which is located deep within the laboratory in a specially constructed extension of the original building. The bunker-within-a-bunker is windowless, not quite bare, but bizarre, unlike any room I've seen before. It doesn't seem large, about eight by ten by twelve feet, but appearances deceive: the thickness of its walls, floor, and ceiling comes close to doubling its interior volume. Three tractor trailers were required to move the heavy walls and door, insulation, springs, and related padding from its original home. The walls are punctuated by thick foam wedges made from fiberglass, placed there to trap sound waves. A plain metal desk chair sits at the center; bare bulbs hang from the ceiling. Wooden particleboard suspended on airline cables serves as the floor. It bounces slightly as I walk across it, as though I'm traversing a stiff trampoline. The combined effect is destabilizing in the extreme. From its name on down, the anechoic chamber recalls the setting for a horror movie. It's not a "room": it's a portal to something else.

Mike Role, the pony-tailed laboratory manager, shows me how to open the massive, three-foot-thick door, "in case you panic." Why would I panic? He tells me he plans to turn off the lights—not something I'd considered. It will be as complete a sensory fast as I can imagine, and for two hours. I practice opening the metal-lined door, which requires bracing myself against the floor and pulling with both hands. I focus on remembering the exit's position relative to the chair so that when the moment of panic comes, before the dark thoroughly digests me, I can shoot straight for the door. I settle myself in the chair with a small notebook on my lap and a pen in my hand, and then Role says, "See you in a couple of hours." He swings the door shut (it makes no sound that I can hear) and the lights go out.

At first there is a big smile on my face. At last, I am traveling on the highway to emptiness, a "going from something towards nothing." My second thought is that I won't make it. I've seen too many scary movies, and I fear hallucinating. A phantom hand on my shoulder, something brushing against my leg. What if I get a cramp? It is pitch-black, so black I can't see my hand an inch from my face, so black there is no difference between eyes open and eyes closed. After a few minutes, the numbers on my watch start to glow faintly—something I'd never before noticed that they did—and I remove it from my wrist and place it face down on the floor. Silence and darkness weigh on me.

I feel a light pressure blanketing my body. The air itself seems heavier. Of course, there is no pressure—we experience sound pressure as loudness, and there is none, less than none. What I perceive is what my mind tells me I should be perceiving: that pressure is increasing. In the dark, I kick off my shoes. They make an oddly muffled sound as they hit the wooden floor, as though they were very far away. There is no sound other than what I bring to the story. The iconoclastic composer, poet, and mycologist John Cage, who also spent time in an anechoic chamber, wrote that sounds occur whether or not we purposefully create them, but it is only in conscious silence that we discover our connection to everything around us. That's my goal. But at first I can't sit still. I fidget, I whisper to myself; the words die, as though smothered by the heavy silence.

Cage, whose anarchic inclinations reverberate throughout his work, felt that humans were addicted to "controlling" sound, and that giving up that control opens us to new paths of processing information, perhaps even comprehension. Rejecting control means embracing creativity, and it is only through creativity that the world, or a portion of the world, can be deciphered. "What we require is silence; but what silence requires is that I go on talking." It is only through sound that we measure silence. Often, when I'm waiting at a New York City street corner for the light to change, shoulder to shoulder with other silent, stock-still pedestrians, who are also engulfed by the flow of traffic—the honking of horns and the roar of cars, trucks, and buses—I remark to myself on the absolute stillness of the people around me, all of us standing motionless, staring straight ahead as though frozen in place. The light changes and we spring to life, charging across the intersection.

Now I take several deep breaths, in through my nose, out through my mouth. The "box": five seconds in, hold for five, out for five, rest, repeat. The oxygen courses through my body and I start to relax, undergoing what Orfield calls "perceptual adaptation." I consider analogies—not lying in bed at night, that's too physical an experience, with light and noises from the street percolating in and the sensation of sheets covering me—but here I can imagine sitting on a chair at the bottom of the sea, miles down. Except with oxygen. The HVAC is turned off, but Role has assured me I won't suffocate.

In the dark, without any mechanism for gauging the passage of time, I am unmoored. I push off from the sea bottom, and, as I once did, I swim deep under the ocean's surface to where the ground drops away. I am suspended over a dark, bottomless abyss, and see only shades of darkness in every direction and hear the sound of my own breathing. Floating through the void. I wave my arms, trying to stir the dark as though it were water. I separate my scattered thoughts by heavy lines on the paper and trace the indentations with my finger. I scrawl blindly in my notebook: *Waiting to stop waiting. Impatience is my problem. As I see less, I perceive more clearly.* It's all about measurement: how much I hear, how little; how much I consume, how little. The monotony of no measure provided by fasting is a barrier-erasing gift. How much I need to eat, how much I think I need to eat. *How much running makes you a runner?* How little I notice. Much later I come across this apposite quote by W. G. Sebald in *The Rings of Saturn*, where he muses on the writing of the seventeenth-century essayist Thomas Browne: "The greater the distance, the clearer the view: one sees the tiniest of details with the utmost clarity. It is as if one were looking through a reversed opera glass and through a microscope at the same time. And yet, says Browne, all knowledge is enveloped in darkness. What we perceive are no more than isolated lights in the abyss of ignorance, in the shadow-filled edifice of the world."

Something and nothing need each other, as Cage observes. Mystics through the ages have sought to free themselves of material stuffing and to stuff themselves instead with the holiness of indescribable nothingness. Cage cites Meister Eckhart, the thirteenth-century German mystic, quoting a somewhat copulocentric meditation at the end of "Lecture on Something": "Earth has no escape from heaven: flee she up or flee she down, heaven still invades her, energizing her, fructifying her, whether for her weal or for her woe." "Heaven" lies before us all, whether we want it or not, Eckhart seems to say. And with absence, something new arrives.

Hunger de-genders us. It not only takes us out of our social contexts, it can transform our bodies; and that may not amount to de-gendering so much as re-gendering. Literary scholar Maud Ellmann cites Wole Soyinka's account, writing on his fifth week of a hunger strike in a Nigerian prison: "'I made a strange discovery this morning,' he reports. 'I'm pregnant.' His lower belly, he explains, has swollen up as if he had 'secreted a large egg just beneath the skin' to fill the corresponding chasm in his trousers." This curious passage lends heft to psychoanalyst Julia Kristeva's assertion of appropriated motherhood by Christian mystics such as Eckhart, St. Bernard, and St. Augustine, all of whom are associated with fasting (although both Eckhart and Augustine make the case for moderation). Kristeva argues that the mystics "assimilated" Mary to Christ, and in effect appropriated the Immaculate Conception by filling themselves with devotion to Jesus, becoming his "lover." They placed worship of the Virgin Mary and its "beliefs with pagan roots" at the heart of Christianity, sometimes in opposition to the official dogma of the Church.

Strength, growth, creativity are derived from absence, but too much isolation destabilizes us. Loners are oddities, or wild philosophers (like Cage), whose pronouncements are alternately absurd and frightening. We are social animals, and derive our sense of worth from interactions with others: Aristotle reminds us that "We hold that a friend is one of the greatest goods and that friendlessness and isolation are most dreadful." Without the support of other humans—struts to bolster us against the vacuity of existence—we become unbalanced. Exile is a basic punishment founded on biological hardwiring. To chastise misbehavior, we send children to stand alone facing a corner, to ponder horrible misdeeds, but more than that to signal a temporary banishment from human society.

What is key to the fasting process is asserting our agency. Stripped of our volition, missing that crucial act of decision-making, the empowering fast-from-others becomes destructive, and we undergo a rapid decline. A UK study involving more than 460,000 participants found that if an elderly person lives alone, chances of dementia dramatically increase. Gray matter volume—the outermost layer of the brain, which contains a high concentration of neuronal cells—falls. In prison, solitary confinement is universally recognized as extreme punishment. Prisoners kept in solitary for any amount of time have a higher rate of recidivism than ones kept in the general population. Upon release, they also have consistently higher rates of overdoses, homicide, and suicide. In 2020, the United Nations' special rapporteur on torture called for a global ban on solitary confinement longer than two weeks. Even shorter periods can be devastating.

And in the vast social experiment that accompanied the COVID era, when more people were required to confine themselves to their immediate living space than at any time in history, drug overdoses reached record highs, as did teen suicides. Humans are typical social creatures in not only thriving on companionship, but needing it to stay sane: in some places, it is illegal to own only one guinea pig, and many research laboratories mandate a minimum number of mice for an experiment—not to increase statistical reliability, but so the mice don't lose their little minds. To be conscious is to be conscious in relation to something else, and our consciousness is defined by these interactions.

Collectively or individually, humans are agents of change. We don't often sit still. Our inclination is anti-entropic—to do something, to exercise, to slim down, to educate ourselves. That puts us in opposition with the guiding principle of the universe, as theoretical physicist Carlo Rovelli explains in *The Order of Time* and elsewhere. Rovelli suggests that things do not proceed on fullness, but on emptiness. Fullness is the anomaly. We believe that we are proceeding to a summit, but all along we are winding down together with everything else. This is not necessarily a cause for mourning: it is simply the way of things. But recognition of entropy can also impart clarity, even insight. It is only through the dissolution of structures that new ones can arise. Stoics and quantum physicists agree when they tell us that death, emptiness, and the passage of time should not be the source of paralyzing fear and instead need to be appreciated and understood to the degree that we are able to muster understanding.

Is it presumptuous to associate being alive with relentless activity? What if stillness—a lack of activity and a lack of *processing*—are just as necessary to life, inspiring us to new, more productive ways of being and thinking, even as we are contained within a failing system? I am brought to mind of the "spaces between the joints" of the *Zhuangzi*, the third century BCE Chinese text essential to Daoism, an antecedent to Zen Buddhism. The heroes of the *Zhuangzi* are not noble warriors or fierce prophets assailing moral decadence. Nor are they hermits. They are often modest but tremendously skilled craftspeople, at once inward-looking and drawing profound lessons from the environment in which they live.

The so-called inner chapters of the *Zhuangzi*, which scholars have labeled the most ancient text—over the centuries, it was added to by succeeding poets—appear to have been written by an otherwise un-heralded philosopher, Master Zhuang, a minor official of the lacquer garden (lacquer in ancient China being tapped from trees of the species *Toxicodendron vernicifluum* to coat objects with a fine glaze). The *Zhuangzi* comprises a series of anecdotes and apothegms that in its whole is anti-bureaucratic, deeply poetic, and often slyly humorous. And it is in some respects subversive; it extolls the "use of uselessness" and criticizes traditional notions of worth.

In many ways, the *Zhuangzi* articulates arguments for fasting, particu-larly "heart fasting," or "fasting of the mind." Even its consistent references to Confucius as a source of authority for its anecdotes are a mark of its radical nature, because the book's message counters Confucian ideals of practicality and ways of accumulating knowledge. In chapter 4, "In the World of Men," Yan Hui—who was a favorite disciple of Confucius, according to the historical record—approaches the master, asking for advice. He is planning to travel to the palace of an intemperate ruler to attempt to steer him away from bad policies. Confucius counsels against doing so. After analyzing his disciple's various strategies and predicting their disastrous consequences, he tells Yan Hui that he should make a visit to the ruler, but to be an effective adviser, he must fast beforehand. Yan Hui responds that his family is poor, and he hasn't drunk wine or eaten anything substantial for months, so a fast is not called for. Confucius explains: "That is the fasting one does before a sacrifice, not the fasting of the mind. . . . Don't listen with your ears, listen with your mind. No, don't listen with your mind, but listen with your spirit. Listening stops with the ears, the mind stops with recognition, but spirit is empty and waits for all things. The Way gathers in emptiness alone. Emptiness is the fasting of the mind." Yan Hui then says that before he had heard from his master he was certain of his identity, but now "there is no more Hui." Confucius at last appears to approve of his disciple's conclusion: it is only with a suppression of self, a "fasting of the mind," that wisdom may be attained and then shared. "You have heard of the knowledge that knows, but you have never heard of the knowledge that does not know."

The anecdote of Cook Ding and Lord Wenhui from chapter 3, "The Secret of Caring for Life," also provides spiritual food for the faster. Lord Wenhui marvels at Cook Ding's ox-cutting skills, and the cook replies:

> I've had this knife of mine for nineteen years and I've cut up thousands of oxen with it, and yet the blade is as good as though it had just come from the grindstone. There are spaces between the joints, and the blade of the knife has really no thickness. If you insert what has no thickness into such spaces, then there's plenty of room—more than enough for the blade to play about in. That's why after nineteen years, the blade of my knife is still as good as when it first came from the grindstone.

The cook inhabits "the space between," the place where the blade meets no resistance and thus has no wear after years of use. Entropy has no domain there, and yet it is the place of creation and productivity.

Like Plato's *metaxu* or the notion of *tzimtzum*—first put forth by the sixteenth-century Kabbalist scholar Isaac Luria—the space between is sacred because of its purity. Luria posits that once God had created the earth, he withdrew, and it was his very withdrawal—his absence—that made room for an alternative: the imperfection that is our world. (This concept of a "clockmaker God," who created, then stepped away from the world, was taken up by the Deists, of whom Thomas Paine and Benjamin Franklin were prominent advocates.) It is only by stepping back, by withholding Perfection, that God allows life with all of its inconsistencies and finities to flourish.

....

Sound . . . There it is. A faint rushing noise that I am later told is the blood flowing through my veins. I turn my head, and the bones in my neck grind audibly. I make a face, a grin, a grimace, and I *hear* the crinkle and crackle of skin. I hear a rustling, as though of wrapping paper: it is the sound of my eyelids opening and closing. In here, butterflies would thunder through the air. I roll my eyes in their sockets, but to my slight disappointment I can't hear them shift; that's a level beyond. There is a universe of tiny sounds I've been missing, that I'll always miss. *Solitude and silence are our destinations.* But there is no such thing as silence. Cage again. We can't turn off our listening. In *Zero Decibels*, the writer George Michelsen Foy hypothesizes that this constant "on" mode is an evolutionary legacy of our distant ancestors' water-bound days: "We listen like fish, as if everything in our soundscape, potentially at least, were a matter of life and death. We listen so hard, in fact, that our brain no longer allows for the possibility of silence."

I gingerly lower myself to the wood floor. I stretch out and try to embrace the darkness, to let it overtake me. I open my eyes wide and stare . . . at nothing. I have no sense of how long I've been here—ten minutes? twenty?—but I feel comfort beyond comfort. I've gone beyond settling in, and am content in my shell of nonengagement. Not thinking about myself and my relation to the world is freeing. After what seems much too short a time, Role soundlessly pushes open the door. Steve Orfield is there as well in the doorway, and greets me. Two hours, gone in a flash. I am truly amazed: I was just getting going. I emerge into the maelstrom of sensations.

The contrast is not what I anticipated. I'd thought that leaving the chamber after two hours in its near-total dark and silence would be a shock, like waking up after a bad night's sleep, like climbing out of a grave, and that I would stumble around while my zombie brain tried to get up to speed. I am mildly surprised at how calm, collected, and alert I feel. I am absolutely refreshed. I don't feel sleepy at all. Orfield has witnessed this reaction many times before. But while relatively brief periods spent in isolation seem to soothe the harried soul, longer periods derail us, sometimes permanently.

Orfield debriefs me in his wood-paneled, 1980s-cool office, complete with thick carpeting. "Most of our lives, we live in pattern behavior, not as conscious observers," Orfield says. He explains that it is impossible to absorb and analyze even a fraction of what we sense—we perceive a very small portion of what's going on around us. To protect ourselves from the bombardment of sensations, we've developed a thick shield of automatic behavior: automaticity. That covers complicated, common maneuvers like knitting or reading, but it also extends to things like breathing or the feel of a cotton shirt on our skin. The process of learning is the process of applying perception, but it is also automaticity: losing awareness of some sensations and embracing others.

The French philosophers Eva Lerat and Sébastien Charbonnier recently observed, as part of a book-length rumination on fasting, that the more one is performative, the less one is conscious; and the less one is conscious, the less one is creative. They cite the work of Australian researcher Allan Snyder, director of the University of Sydney's Centre for the Mind, who has shown that once the brain recognizes that a certain experience is repeated, it speedily automates its own functions and the body's reactions to that experience. Once automatization is put into place, the brain favors these information-processing highways over inventiveness. By contrast, after barely five minutes of a log-out from certain parts of the brain—via "transcranial magnetic stimulation"—a person can once again become capable of appreciating the novelty of a repetitive situation and can therefore invent new solutions for how to react to them. What does this have to do with fasting? Fasting allows us to log out of our automated behavior and to consider familiar situations with a fresh perspective.

Without leaving room for emptiness, we never grow. To converse in a language, you need to memorize the vocabulary, but you also need to be able to respond to a question with minimal hesitation. The same holds true for the language of stillness. I don't speak it; I don't really understand it. I think all I can do, or anyone can do, is observe it from afar, as though it's an island ringed by towering cliffs, unapproachable from our little storm-tossed boats.

The idea that "silence is violence" may indeed be true in the presence of moral outrages. We're reminded not to be "divisive," but this reprimand can be a method to quash dissent. Noise, however, is often both the by-product of violence and even its root cause, as studies show. For example, in 2022, Danish noise researchers at Aarhus University examined towns around Frankfurt Airport. They found that a 4.1 decibel increase in noise pollution "causes a 6.6% increase" in violent crime.

And, of course, prolonged exposure to noise is bad for your health: hypertension, hearing loss, and even diabetes can result. Levels of cortisol—a stress hormone that also stimulates eating—soar in loud environments. Over time, as the body's baseline cortisol level increases, a slew of problems result. Blood sugar and blood pressure levels rise, and the immune system is weakened. Numerous studies draw a direct line between cardiovascular dangers and traffic noise: too much noise is bad for the heart. In 2011, for example, the World Health Organization reported that "at least one million healthy life years are lost every year from traffic-related noise in the western European countries, including the EU Member States." Their researchers found that excessive noise was second only to air pollution as an environmental problem, increasing the risk of cardiovascular disorders and high blood pressure. As the U.S. Army has long known, being assailed by loud noise is a weapon that devastates concentration and leaves little evidence on its victims. It was used on prisoners in Guantánamo Bay and elsewhere, and regularly employed by U.S. forces in Iraq and Afghanistan as a means of subjugation. Ruhal Ahmed, a former Guantánamo Bay detainee who was forced to endure extended bouts of extreme, pounding noise, said: "You're in agony. . . . It makes you feel like you are going mad." (Ahmed was released without charges in 2004.) As one journalist present during Russian shelling in the Donbas region of Ukraine put it, the sound of the firepower was as terrifying as the explosions themselves, and effective over a greater range: "As the volume increases, so do the chaos, misery, death, and fear. You cannot experience such fatal noise without instinctively grasping its purpose, which is to brutalize psychically as well as physically—to demoralize and stupefy." Throughout the report of the U.S. Senate Select Committee on Intelligence on the CIA's use of torture in the post-9/11 years—once designated "TOP SECRET NOFORN" ("NOFORN" is military-speak for "not releasable to foreign nationals," presumably meaning the facts are so embarrassing as to be a national security issue)—blaring music is documented as being conjoined with bright lights or no lights, isolation, and dietary manipulation "to enhance a sense of helplessness." Unpredictable noise drains us of our volition. One of the brain's jobs is to discern patterns in the jumble of things in which we are immersed, and when faced with chaos that overwhelms, it closes in on itself and starts to shut down. On the flip side, controlled, limited sessions of silence have been shown to improve healing. They can lower blood pressure and appear to stimulate brain growth. "Fortune and blessing gather where there is stillness," says the *Zhuangzi*.

Silence doesn't imply aloneness. Even bouts of silence are most effective within a community. The key is moderation, as any Stoic, Confucian, or Epicurean could tell you, and as later practitioners of asceticism came to appreciate. At the height of the Renaissance, Ignatius Loyola, the founder of the Jesuits, reportedly spent seven hours a day in silent prayer. During meals he never spoke, although it was not strictly forbidden in the rules of the order he founded. Instead, he listened to whatever was said, and presumably meditated on the food, which sustained his body and mind. Focus, and consequently perception, requires absence. When we reject automaticity, we move from pattern behavior to vigilance, and we then start processing how we perceive things. "In order to make a signal clear, you either up the signal or dampen the background," says Orfield. "Everything is about signal-to-noise ratio, whether it's sound or sight. Everything is about how much contrast is in the background. In the chamber you were getting rid of cognitive complexity and taking inventory of what you already have."

The Jesuits were great admirers of asceticism, as long as it was Christian-based: in 1601, the Jesuit Luis de Guzmán published his two-volume *Historia de las misiones de los religiosos de la Compañía de Jesús en India, China y Japón*. In it he documents the *yamabushi* ("worshippers of the mountains"). These were ascetic, self-isolating monks, followers of the syncretic religion Shugendō, a crossover religion mixing Buddhism, Taoism, and Shintoism that emerged in the mountains of central Japan roughly 1,200 years ago. The yamabushi seem to have had much in common with the desert saints revered in early Christianity. They lived with few possessions, fasted extensively, and pushed themselves to extreme physical limits, devoting themselves to meditation, studying, and guiding pilgrims to mountain temples. In Guzmán's eyes, however, they were "entirely devoted to the service of Satan." In the same areas of Japan, particularly devout Buddhist ascetics practiced *sokushinbutsu* ("Buddha in the living body"), which involved fasting to the point of death to achieve enlightenment, striving to become a Buddha without having to undergo reincarnation. In the process, they aimed to become a self-mummified corpse. Twenty such revered corpses are scattered throughout Japan (subsequent investigations of *sokushinbutsu* in the 1960s revealed that "mummification took place by artificial means, rather than occurring naturally"). To this day, Japanese followers of Tendai Buddhism keep the related practice of *kaihōgyō* alive, a one-thousand-day-long period of harsh ascetic training that includes nine consecutive days of fasting from food, liquids, and sleep known as *doiri*. Since the nineteenth century, only fifty people are known to have successfully completed the trial.

In the later chapters of the *Zhuangzi*, prescriptions for earthly enlightenment are more specific. The scholarly consensus is that, in Talmudic fashion, they were added to the book long after Master Zhuang by anonymous writers, but they retain much of the poetic (and political) impact of the earlier segments. A passage in chapter 19, "Mastering Life," begins with a carver of bell stands who is being praised for his extraordinary skill. The bell-stand carver explicitly connects fasting to the mastery of his craft. He explains:

> When I am going to make a bell stand, I never let it wear out my energy. I always fast in order to still my mind. When I have fasted for three days, I no longer have any thought of congratulations or rewards, of titles or stipends. When I have fasted for five days, I no longer have any thought of praise or blame, of skill or clumsiness. And when I have fasted for seven days, I am so still that I forget I have four limbs and a form and body. By that time, the ruler and his court no longer exist for me. My skill is concentrated and all outside distractions fade away. After that, I go into the mountain forest and examine the Heavenly nature of the trees. If I find one of superlative form, and I can see a bell stand there, I put my hand to the job of carving; if not, I let it go. This way I am simply matching up "Heaven" with "Heaven."

Notably, the wood-carver's fasting does not remove his consciousness to another realm. It opens a door, allowing him to retrieve something transcendent and bring it into this world. By asserting the irrelevance of worldly cares in the form of the court and honors, by freeing him from the limiting demands of his ego, and finally by allowing him to shuck his corporeal self, fasting allows the wood-carver to approach selflessness and the sublime. With the serenity brought about by fasting, he can "match up" the divine pulse he perceives in the trees with the divine pulse of his innate creative power and unite these forces in the present, in the form of his craft. His dip into the pool of self-improvement ("in order to still" his mind) results in clarity, a truer relationship with his environment that enables him to pull a bit of heaven to earth. Like Michelangelo, who famously wrote that he had only to free a statue from the marble that encased it, our carver "finds" a bell stand. He releases it into the world: he does not create it alone; he taps into an otherworldly energy. The woodcarver here recounts the transformation of an ordinary person into an instrument of grace. Like Cook Ding, once the artist frees himself from spurious demands and accepted doctrine (as "Confucius" enjoins Yan Hui to do), he becomes purely reactive to his environment and is able to access the "spaces between."

....

In 1615, the Jesuit Heribert Rosweyde translated a collection of sayings (known as "apophthegmata") of the fourth century CE "Desert Fathers" from a mid-sixth-century Latin collection that was in turn translated from a now-lost Greek source. Leaving aside for the moment the sexualization of desert asceticism, *The Sayings of the Fathers* has a number of striking parallels to the *Zhuangzi* in terms of both format and content. It regularly features a sage who admonishes "an old man" who is otherwise convinced of his rectitude. For example: "They said of one old man that he ate no bread and drank little water for fifty years. And he said: 'I have destroyed lust and greed and vanity.'" But Abba Abraham questions the old man, and concludes he has killed neither lust, nor greed, nor vanity, but only "imprisoned" them. The "passions are alive: only in some measure holy men have got them chained." Another in the long procession of pious old men muses that he "should shut [him]self in his cell, see no one, and eat every other day." Abba Ammon explains that it wouldn't profit him. "Stay in your cell, and eat a little every day, keeping always in your heart the words of . . . the Gospel, and you can be saved." Extreme measures, even if well-intentioned, rarely do us any good.

Fasting can be a tool to help us contemplate our situation. It is precisely because an embrace of emptiness is going against our nature that so many of us, contrary and fidgety beings that we are, are tempted to do just that. There is no better way to explore the power of one's mind than to deny the body's imperative. Body-based distractions are welcome, soothing, and necessary. But the core truth of our lives as brief biological flashes, and correspondingly of even a rock as nothing more than "an extended event" in Rovelli's awe-inspiring image, is lost when we are worrying about social interactions, our next meal, or the buzz of traffic.

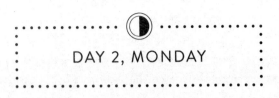

Ascetic Roots 1:
The Greeks, Buddha, and Their Legacies

Slept well last night—certainly no worse, and probably better, than usual. Actually feel better today. I dreamed I held a head of lettuce in my hand, took one lone leaf and stuffed it in my mouth, then remembered the fast—in the dream—and rushed to spit it out. I feel I'm moving from being obsessed with the physical absence of food—being hungry—to thinking about what being hungry means. Only two days. Did morning exercises, no apparent change in endurance. Drank a couple mugs of tea. Stomach growling in afternoon, but just making a bit of noise, not uncomfortable. C. caught me staring blankly into space, something she says I don't normally do. It occurs to me I am dissipating. In physics, dissipation is what happens when energy is lost through conversion to heat. We participate in this process from the moment we are born, and by not refueling I am cooling down more rapidly: going from hot (full) to cool, both metaphorically and literally. I am not only stepping back from human society, I am stepping back from interaction with the world. Digesting food heats us up. Fasting is entropic, relying as it does on absence. A. cooked a delicious-smelling lunch of soba noodles and scallions. I made a point of chatting with her as she ate. My mouth didn't water from longing for a bite and I was perfectly fine, able to focus on the conversation. Wonder if sense of smell is heightened. Certain scents (lemon, toothpaste, coffee, chocolate) are piercing. The lone lemon sitting in a basket on our table calls out to my olfactory senses as though it were a Klaxon. From a sociobiological POV, the increasing intensity of sensation makes sense: my poor body is trying to alert my mind to the proximity of sustenance. Pleased not to find myself longing for a bite (not that I'd have minded). Biked a mile or so to the eye doctor and back. There was little traffic in the streets, although one driver did manage to swerve perilously close. He had to make a real effort to do so, almost as though he were targeting me. Home, lot of gum chewing. Perhaps a bit edgy. By end of day I have nothing left in me to offer the NYC sewer system. Wouldn't mind a glass of wine to soothe the nerves.

> *"Nothing is enough for the person to whom*
> *what is enough is (too) little."*
>
> — Epicurus, *Vatican Sayings*

Making a conscious decision to abstain—to turn away from the mundane—allows us to determine our boundaries. As children, we hold our breath underwater for as long as we can. When we surface, the first intake of air is a little victory. The source of our exultation comes from recognition that we have successfully defied the most basic biological process. In the same way, we inwardly cheer our mastery over our bodies when we manage to do something as spectacular as climb a mountain or as subtle as sitting perfectly still for five minutes.

Fasting is often interpreted as abstinence from food: asceticism, in essence the practice of living lean, involves both abstinence and fasting. While you certainly don't have to be an ascetic to fast, fasting is an ascetic practice. "Asceticism" takes its root from the ancient Greek *askēsis*, which comes from the verb meaning "to work," "to train," or "to honor." The origins of the word are connected with effort, with decision-making. It is voluntary, like fasting. You can't accidentally become an ascetic. To strip down requires a commitment, an active determination to redirect yourself. Fasting was the most visible commitment of such piety, but it was not necessarily an indicator of passivity. In the *Iliad*, the champion Achilles rejects the food and drink urged on him by stomach-driven Odysseus in favor of "slaughter and blood and the rattle in the throats of the dying." The fast of Achilles after the death of his companion Patroclus is a furious sacrifice to the gods, one made out of sorrow and introspection, a turning away from worldly concerns. Some scholars have said that this marks Achilles as extreme, but that may be reflective of modern prejudice against fasting. To me, his enthusiasm for carnage seems better evidence of extremism.

By denying physical pleasures, the cleansing fast becomes preparation for the purity of battle, a step toward a heroic ideal. Similarly, in eleventh-century Japan, the Buddhist monk Osho prepared himself for self-immolation by "eating only pine needles and drinking rainwater." This was the quiet prelude to a fiery finale that linked the realms of the enlightened and the samsaric (the cycle of birth, death, and rebirth).

A desire to approach the incorruptible lies at the core of asceticism. It presumes a connection between body, intellect, and the possibility of betterment. In this light, a fast is akin to a prayer. It is a positive action, not a retreat from the world so much as it is a turn toward the metaphysical, a shift from presence to transcendence that also can demand that the divine's attention be drawn back to this world. (In its intellectual retreat from the physical, metaphysics itself suggests a kind of fasting.) Asceticism requires, at its most basic level, a conscious application of the will to abstain from luxuries, but also from common comforts or physical necessities such as food, drink, sex, and even sleep. A sacrifice is an offering made holy, a privation by the self. Only a commitment on that level approaches the ascetic. This privation takes place on two levels, one social and the other personal.

In the West, asceticism has its formal origins in 2,500-year-old Greek philosophy. Modern conferences and "celebrity ascetics" demonstrate the enduring appeal. Asceticism has evolved over time—there was no first ascetic; it is a characteristic, a tradition, rather than a formal school. There were undoubtedly Stone Age ascetics: the presence of luxuries in the form of a little extra food, or a seashell necklace, suggests not only their intermittency but also the possibility of voluntarily refusing them. There is no "one size fits all" asceticism, but its intellectual rationale is associated first with Pythagoras, who is said to have fasted for forty days before his admittance to the Theban "school of mysteries." He subsequently recommended fasting to his followers. Socrates and Herodotus were also advocates.

The Greeks saw the divine manifested in each person as the mind of spirit, which is *true*. To free the divine was virtuous. The idea that the senses are a distraction gained currency with the teachings of Parmenides, a pre-Socratic philosopher who is generally thought to be the founder of ontology. Parmenides held that whatever is apparent—that is, what we perceive with our senses—is less perfect than what is beyond the senses. This concept of corruption by matter, its intrinsic inferiority in opposition to the purity of the metaphysical, shaped much of Western thought.

Early ascetics sought an alternative to the corporeal prison. The most immediate way to do this was to deny the body its pleasures as part of the effort to turn inward and therefore beyond. The most direct way to do *that* was to restrict the body's intake of food. Lust and gluttony are partners. Sensuality begins with the mouth, after all; seductive words and sweet kisses. And while you can't have sex without food for fuel, you can enjoy a good meal without sex. To strike at the core of licentiousness, it made sense to strictly control intake.

Pythagoras is typically held up as the first great exemplar of asceticism. Seven hundred years after his death, scholars in the late Roman period cited his vegetarianism as evidence of his ascetic, and therefore principled, lifestyle. The biographer of Pythagoras, Porphyry, wrote in *On Abstinence from Eating Animals* (*De abstinentia ab esu animalium*) that "the most beautiful part of justice consists in piety to the gods, and this is principally acquired through abstinence. . . ." Porphyry himself was later cited as an inspiration for early Christian ascetics. Why should abstinence be associated with piety? In the ancient world, it was held that digestive processes generated heat (true) that served to kindle sexual desire (not so true). Eating less, or even nothing, "cooled" you and made you more receptive to what is holy, a theme that was later picked up and expanded upon by the philosopher of medicine Galen in the second century CE. At the most practical level, in times of famine, abstaining from sustenance would have meant more for the rest of the community. In the short run, a fast means you are less distracted, more ready to hunt, defend, or attack. Extended, a fast transforms itself into a kind of unmooring, and is associated with a hermetic, saintly lifestyle. As fasting works to disconnect us from the physical, it reconnects us to what makes us human: our thinking selves.

In ancient texts, the Pythagoreans are described variously as eschewing wine, eating nothing "animate," restricting their diet to bread and water—and having a strict prohibition against fava beans. It may be safe to assume that some of the information that has been passed down over the millennia is the work of anti-Pythagorean propagandists, but Pythagoras pretty clearly laid the groundwork for modern Western asceticism. By tradition, Pythagoras is associated with the Pythagorean theorem. His name is also connected to a strange teaching device that continues to fascinate, and is used either as an object lesson in the perils of greediness or as a practical joke: the Pythagorean cup, also known as the Cup of Tantalus or the Cup of Justice. The cup appears to be normal, except for a nub or protrusion that rises from its base to about halfway below the cup's lip. A channel inside the nub runs from the cup's bottom, up through the nub, and opens inside at the base of the nub, forming a loop. Fill the cup below the protrusion's summit, and all is well. Fill it above the top of the protrusion, and because of a siphon effect, the entire contents of the cup drain through its bottom. The sequence seems to defy logic. It very clearly conveys the principle that there is a silent, unforgiving judge who assesses all that we do. Everything has its limit: only moderation precents depletion and waste.

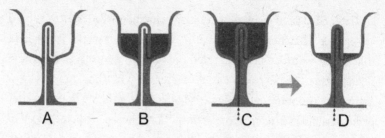

The Pythagorean Cup.

A few decades after the death of Pythagoras, in the fifth century BCE, a wealthy young prince in what is now Nepal was reevaluating his life choices. On the cusp of assuming his father's throne after having his first and only child, Siddhartha (meaning "He who achieves his aim") Gautama, a member of the warrior caste, drew on many ascetic Hindu traditions and decided to renounce his princely status. In his search for enlightenment he gave up everything: riches, pleasures, duties, and relationships. He became the Shakyamuni Buddha (Shakyamuni meaning "sage of the Shakyas" and Buddha meaning "Enlightened One").

He fasted to an extreme degree, eating but a grain of sesame a day, withering to the bones. He stayed naked out in the elements, sat in freezing rivers in winter, and meditated in summer in the blazing sun surrounded by four fires. He sat sleepless in contorted postures. He did not speak for years. His only companions were others just as isolated and self-afflicting.

By exploring his physical limits, Buddha embraced the extreme asceticism current at that time, the lifestyle and commitment of the hermetic *shramanas* (wanderers). The wanderers followed the teachings that the Upanishad sages had established beginning in 700 BCE to achieve unity between Brahman (the Universal Soul) and Atman (the Individual Soul). But after Buddha had fasted for forty-nine days, incidentally proving he could best the saints of the Old Testament, he turned away from extreme asceticism. As Buddha is consistently portrayed as doing, he opted for a rational solution: he decided that wasting away was not useful, and instead created a third way, a middle path between hierarchical social strictures and the rule-free, asocial tradition of hermetic life. Buddha concluded that enlightenment did not come from following orders, doctrine, or hierarchy, but by actively embracing a complete lack of identity. Humanity was only prevented from salvation by the social and cultural baggage with which it burdened itself. To free the self, Buddha advocated ethics, discipline, and training—*samādhi*—which led to wisdom beyond wisdom, a step on the path to divine insight, or *prajnā*.

The earliest Buddhist images, known as "aniconic," from the Gandhāran period (the first to third century CE) evoke Buddha through images such as an empty throne, a parasol, a tree, or a footprint. His first followers worshiped the absence, the ultimate emptiness that Buddha contemplated, and strove not to focus on the man-as-body. Buddha himself became the embodiment of a Simone Weil–like "between" being—but not supreme, because that term is not applicable (hence a possible interpretation of the famous Zen koan "If you meet the Buddha on the road, kill him": if you think you've attained enlightenment, it still eludes you). The "goal"—although again that word is inadequate—is to move beyond silence.

"God has no hand, he needs no organ," wrote philosopher Jacques Derrida in 1967 in a particularly beautiful and uncharacteristically accessible passage in his book *Of Grammatology*. "Organic differentiation" is humanity's misfortune. "Here the silent movement does not even replace an elocution. God has no need of a mouth to speak, nor of articulating the voice." Derrida treats interpretation and writing as acts of destruction. They cultivate ruin, but also creation, because of their evasion of meaning. This recalls Simone Weil's longing for "decreation" and also suggests a connection to physics and Werner Heisenberg's notorious uncertainty principle, now applied to the act of contemplation: if language deforms a concept, so, too, the act of considering something deforms it. Fasting is itself a process of translation and transformation, but one that reverts to its origins.

In a stunning break with Vedic Hindu tradition, Buddhism rejects the notion of a creator deity. But Buddha also built on Hindu traditions in his doctrine of Brahmavihārā, in essence the idea that compassion and equanimity are pathways to enlightenment. The oldest of the Buddhist schools, Theravāda, holds that there is no ultimate god, no transcendent state to achieve, no soul to save. Some contemporary monks and nuns following this school incorporate fasting into their daily discipline and eat one meal a day. For the Theravāda Buddhist, the desire for transcendence is interpreted as deluded, earthbound longing. Longing itself is delusionary. More emphatically than his predecessors or contemporaries, Buddha rejected materiality as well as obsessions with the past.

In describing the human struggle to perceive reality accurately, Buddha drew on the Hindu concept of maya, which means "illusion" in Sanskrit (Maya was also the name of Buddha's mother). In many Hindu traditions, we swim daily through the sea of maya, the dream of Brahma, the god of creation (distinct from Brahman, the omnipresent universal soul). Brahma dreams the universe into being and his dream is maintained by Vishnu, the preserver. Because of maya, we fail to perceive the world as a single entity.

Legend has it that Buddha's first followers were five fasting ascetics in the classic Hindu tradition of the Upanishad sages. Life for these Brahmins was divided into four successive stages: study (*brahamacarya*), home (*grhastha*), seclusion in the wilderness (*vanaprastha*), and renunciation (*sannyāsi*). Buddha's innovation was that study should be unrestricted and continue beyond one's student days: *brahamacarya* begins any time one renounces the world.

It took patience and study to abandon human convention. As Buddha's followers gained in number, he set up ascetic communities comprised of both men and women, who were instructed to beg the community for sustenance and who would in return instruct civilians on the path to wisdom. Seven hundred years before such traditions took root in either the West or the East, Buddha established a monastic ascetic tradition in India. Although he had by then rejected extreme fasting, partial and frequent abstention was still very much a part of Buddha's doctrine. He expected sexual continence, poverty, non-killing, and non-pretension to spiritual attainment from his most ardent followers, the monks and nuns whose behavior was highly regulated. These devotees were instructed in humbling disciplines, such as directing their gaze to the ground one cartwheel diameter ahead as they went to beg for food.

In the middle of the third century BCE, Emperor Ashoka, a Buddhist convert, sent nine Buddhist emissaries from his capital in what is now eastern India to various of his demesnes and trading partners. They traveled to places such as Greece, Syria, the Himalayas, Thailand, and Sri Lanka. Consequently, Buddhist ascetic practices and principles can be found in most of the world's religions, including Judaism, Christianity, and Islam. For example, Buddhist doctrines may be discerned in the Christian Orthodox Hesychast movement that has its origins in Syrian desert monasteries from the second half of the first millennium and that flourished in the fourteenth-century Byzantine church. Derived from the Greek word for "divine peace" or "stillness," adherents of Hesychasm seek to transcend the ego through meditation and fasting. Hesychasts even employ specific Buddhist practices of breath control and focusing on the navel as a means of concentrating during meditation. Such methods "restrain to some extent the wanderings of the imagination," wrote the fourteenth-century archbishop of Thessalonica Gregory Palamas. The Hesychasts were derided as *omphalopsychoi*, "people with souls in their navels." Although its followers were once denounced as heretics, Hesychasm persists in Christian Orthodox monasteries to this day.

One particularly fascinating instance of such syncretism deserves special mention: in medieval times, one of the most popular Christian parables was the legend of Barlaam and Josaphat. Described as "a cultural phenomenon second to none at the time," at least three different versions of the story circulated in thirteenth-century Europe. The parable of a righteous prince, Josaphat, who forsakes his throne and goes through extreme deprivations, fasting from the privileges of rank and refusing food before accepting Christian salvation via the teachings of the wise Barlaam, is a close approximation of Buddha's life story, even to the point of being set in northern India. Its origins were first discovered by nineteenth-century linguists, who traced how the Arabic "Būδāsaf" (for "bodhisattva"—someone who has attained nirvana, but remains on Earth to help show others the path) became "Yūδāsaf" and then was translated into Georgian as "Iodasaph," and then finally, when a translator decided that a name closer to the biblical "Jehoshaphat" was better suited to a Christian tale, became "Josaphat." For a thousand years, St. Josaphat was revered as an ideal manifestation of a good Christian, with a feast day celebrated on November 27. Ironically, Jesuit missionaries took the story to Japan in 1549. There they printed the first Japanese book with moveable type in 1591, a compendium of lives of the saints which includes the Barlaam and Josaphat story, in effect transporting Buddha to a Buddhist land in order to convert Buddhists to Christianity. Buddha would have laughed.

....

In about 400 BCE, Socrates's student Plato further emphasized the mind/ body split. Plato's appreciation of the transcendental, and its relevance to those trapped in the material world, endures. For Plato, what we put inside our minds brings us closer to a pure truth than what we stuff inside our bellies; more than that, the body gets in the way of truth: "While the soul is infected with the evils of the body, our desire will not be satisfied."

> For the body is a source of endless trouble to us by reason of the mere requirement of food; and is liable also to diseases which overtake and impede us in the search after true being: it fills us full of loves, and lusts, and fears, and fancies of all kinds, and endless foolery, and in fact, as men say, takes away from us the power of thinking at all. Whence come wars, and fightings, and factions? Whence but from the body and the lusts of the body?

Plato's mistrust of the body is consistent. Although he is sometimes blamed for the fear and hatred of physicality of early Christianity, his mistrust does not extend to self-torture, or to suffering that does not lead to mental or physical advancement. Plato disdained conspicuous consumption and admired virtue, dicta that later inspired the Cynics.

Many of the Socratic virtues of self-control were put on display in Aristophanes's instructive comedy *Lysistrata* (411 BCE), which hinges on the violence and animal desires of its men and the intelligence and determination of its women, who withhold sex in order to lead the male characters to more reasonable paths of behavior. Withholding sex is distinct from simply not having sex in the same way that fasting from food differs from experiencing a famine: the *potential* of sex hovers over all discussions. The women's sex-fasting, presumably fictional, is prompted by their desire to end a real war that lasted twenty-six years, the Peloponnesian War between Athens and Sparta. The organized sex strikers prove the power of abstinence from intercourse and the power of absence, according themselves strength and influence, where they had little of either under Athenian law (women in classical Athens were excluded from government and had no political rights). In what is ostensibly a comedy of reversals, but, of course, is also a lesson in morals, "manly virtues"—restraint, rationality, strategic thinking—become the province of the fasting women, who by disrupting the normal course of things return society to stability and harmony.

One of the first Cynics was another student of Socrates, Antisthenes. According to the bits of testimony that have come down to us (principally from the historian and soldier Xenophon, a contemporary of Antisthenes, and from Diogenes Laërtius, a Roman historian who wrote a millennium later), Antisthenes—who may not have identified himself with any school other than the Socratic—admired Socrates's "hardiness" and "impassivity" and supposedly said he would prefer madness to pleasure. Antisthenes disdained comfort to the degree that he felt luxury was a curse: "To someone praising luxury, he said, 'May your enemies' children live in luxury.'" About the same time as Antisthenes was active, the Confucian *Analects* provide the same message in less warlike terms: "To take joy in extravagance, to find joy in desultory wandering, and to take joy in feasting—these things injure." Luxury, by definition the acquisition or consumption of something unnecessary, debilitates. Both Confucius and Antisthenes agree: it brings about physical and moral weakness because it increases humanity's distance from virtue. Excess ties us to the earth. Like the Christian hermits of the Egyptian desert, the wandering Parivrajaka and Shaivists of India, the yamabushi of Japan, and Buddhist ascetics throughout Asia, the Cynics valued physical toughness. Unlike these later self-isolating holy men and women, they did not reject family and social life. A virtuous life was one lived within society, improving on it and oneself.

Antisthenes taught in the Cynosarges ("white dog"), a gymnasium within a sanctuary of Hercules, and his nickname was "Haplocyon" ("single dog"). Cynicism, the school he is credited with founding, was sometimes known as the "Army of the Dog" (*kynikos* means "doglike"). If Diogenes Laërtius is to be believed, Antisthenes, if not the first ascetic, was one of the first to place asceticism as a core virtue, making it more important than social conventions and even more important than the laws of the polis. Somewhat confusingly, Antisthenes's followers chose the hero Hercules as their spiritual patron—a demigod venerated for his brutish strength, multiple slayings and labors, but who was very much a creature of duty . . . not unlike a ferocious guard dog. Single-minded devotion and simple living are common to both ascetics and dogs. Diogenes Laërtius couldn't resist inserting a short poem to the memory of Antisthenes in his *Lives of Eminent Philosophers*:

> So much the natural dog in life, Antisthenes,
> You lacerated the heart with words and not with teeth.
> But you died of consumption. Perhaps one might say,
> What of it? We must surely have a guide to Hades.

Antisthenes taught Diogenes of Sinope, who in turn became the most influential philosopher of the Cynics, and reportedly was doggedly devoted to his spiritual master. If Antisthenes played with idiosyncratic behavior, Diogenes the Cynic embraced it wholeheartedly, and lived as a stray in the streets, ranting at the citizens. It's easy to imagine Diogenes in a modern context: he'd be locked up in prison or a mental institution. Even at the time, Plato referred to Diogenes as a "Socrates gone mad."

Diogenes assaulted what he saw as the pretensions of society so ferociously that the intensity of his convictions still shocks us millennia later. Bitterly opposed to Plato's abstractions and anti-materialism—he must have detested the Platonic notion of a "philosopher king"—Diogenes was famous for tirades against self-indulgence (although, by all accounts, Plato was not exactly decadent). His extremist views on the necessity of asceticism resonate to this day and have arguably tainted asceticism ever since. His convictions manifested themselves in asocial behavior, and he had what might be called a conflicted approach to carnality: he reportedly masturbated in public, urinated on those who annoyed him, and lived in a large tub or wine jar in the *metroon* ("mother's building"), also known as the temple of the Mother of the Gods. When questioned about his self-abuse, he supposedly replied that he only wished that all his yearnings could be satisfied with as little trouble. His absolutist approach was as off-putting to ancient Athenians as it hopefully is now to us, but because these early ascetics rejected society and its comforts, they considered themselves better able to criticize it.

The Stoics, a group more relatable to tender twenty-first-century sensibilities, arose fast on the heels of the Cynics. Zeno of Citium, whose school's location at the Stoa Poikile (the "colored porch") in the ancient Agora of Athens gave its name to the movement, rose to prominence in the early third century BCE. Zeno's obsession was self-mastery, by which he meant overcoming desire— a purposeful recalibration of his predecessors' emphasis on living a natural life. While the Stoics drew on some of the principles of Cynicism, in particular its principle that people should live according to nature, they represented a still-durable tempering of the fierce Cynic commitment to remaking society. If the Cynics can be likened to the Jacobins of the French Revolution—revolutionaries who wanted to tear down society in order to rebuild it—the Stoics might represent the Thermidorian Reaction, the conservative response to radical restructuring. They were keen on hierarchy and, like the other schools, fasted from luxury. Zeno is supposed to have confined himself to eating bread, honey, and water. The Stoics reasonably believed that there are things under our control and things that are not, and that care for one's individual self should precede care for others. For the Stoics, pleasure had its place, but their idea of pleasure was closer to what Plato in book 9 of *The Republic* refers to as "pleasure": meaning pleasure of the rational part of the spirit, as opposed to the sensual or emotional part. If there is one guiding principle that unites the teachings of ancient Stoics, it is that only the thoughts and actions within one's immediate circle of control merit uncompromising contemplation.

The antithesis of asceticism is hedonism, a philosophy that places its emphasis on the preeminence of physical sensations and owes more to the pre-Socratic philosophers than to the Platonic ethos. Surprisingly, the fasting tradition may owe more to the hedonists than it does to the Stoics. In ancient Greece, the hedonists were best represented in the school founded by Epicurus, who began his school slightly before that of Zeno, in the third century BCE. The common understanding of "epicurean" is very far from its origins.

Rejecting what he saw as the vulgarity and extremism of the Cynics and the exclusivity of the Platonists and Aristotelians, Epicurus (yet another vegetarian) advocated modest pleasures as a way to achieve fulfillment. He was a *moral* hedonist, someone who argued that our physical boundaries, particularly our sensations of pleasure and pain, are life's guideposts. Per Epicurus, we are free agents and can use our senses to choose appropriate behavior. Sensations must not be ignored; they are manifestations of natural, and therefore divine, law. Pleasure is appropriate and pain is not. Pleasure promises serenity and stability; pain is a violation of what is natural because it signals destruction. Such a devotion to pleasure and a conviction that all sensations are "true"— hedonism—does not necessarily translate to wanton self-indulgence; according to both contemporaneous accounts and Epicurus's own surviving letters, Epicurus lived austerely and exhorted his followers to do the same, all in an attempt to achieve moral and emotional equanimity and to avoid bodily suffering. Sensations, he argued, are all we have and all that can be relied upon. Suffering arose not only from physical pain, but also from longing for what one didn't have or couldn't have. Therefore simple, frugal habits would lead to a life filled with the least suffering and the greatest pleasure. Diogenes Laërtius reports that Epicurus is said to have been content with bread and water, and to have once requested a little cheese be sent to him so that he could really live it up. In short, he was an exemplary faster.

For the Epicurean, desire comes in three flavors: natural and necessary, natural and unnecessary, and unnatural and unnecessary. Together with the Stoics, the Epicureans felt that morality was rooted in the natural order, and that intelligence and reason provided connection to truth. But unlike the Stoics—who believed in a divine presence—the Epicureans only trusted what could be perceived by the senses. Tranquility, or ataraxia, required a Buddha-like acceptance of the facts of nature, along with the avoidance of overindulgence, anger, and passionate advocacy. Life itself was a matter of determining the minimum of what one needed for pleasure, and death was merely the state of becoming "untroubled." Pleasure was divided into two main classes: the kinetic (coming from a good deed) and the katastematic, a word derived from the Greek for "standing still": the state of suspension, of existing free from change. And the body's pleasure gauge lay in the stomach. In *The Learned Banqueters*, a second century CE collection by Athenaeus of Naucratis purporting to chronicle the exchanges at a series of dinner parties, Epicurus is quoted as saying, "The origin and root of everything good is the pleasure derived from our belly, and whatever is wise or exceptional is to be measured by that standard." Pleasure came from judicious management, not from overstuffing.

In a departure from the Platonic school, Epicurus was a committed atomist in the tradition of Democritus. He argued that the movement of indestructible atoms in the void, not the whims of gods, determine what happens, and free will is created by unpredictable atomic "swerves." Our world came into being because of the interaction between atoms that shift in both determined and random ways. It followed that creation exists without a creator. This led Epicurus to the distinctly modern conclusion that our planet is but one of many floating in the cosmic void. Desire itself, he felt, was a void, a void that seeks to be fulfilled and thus to eliminate its own existence. At the same time, desire seeks to perpetuate itself, which leads to a soul-splitting paradox. As Sartre wrote: "man stands by his desires fiercely."

The pervasive sense that humanity and individuals were not uniquely endowed with special qualities, that each one of us is an atomic agglomeration, led Epicurus at the age of thirty-four to open his school to all comers. Unusual if not unique among Greek philosophers, for the better part of the following four decades Epicurus welcomed foreigners, women, concubines, and enslaved people, the untutored as well as the learned, to what he called the Garden. He shared with Buddha the conviction that his philosophy could be adopted by anyone and everyone. The school itself was located in an Athenian garden, instead of on a porch or in a gymnasium. Above the gates of the Garden were inscribed the words "Stranger, this is a good place to stay, for here the highest good is pleasure." This openness was in marked contrast to the inscription purportedly engraved above Plato's Academy, that only those well-versed in mathematics might enter. For Epicurus, any artificial or preexisting social definitions were to be shunned in favor of a strict focus on the reality and truth of the senses.

Like most worthwhile endeavors, fasting has paradoxical attributes. While it goes against animalistic instincts (eating), by stripping away distraction it temporarily forces us to focus on nothing more than our bodies and what we have in our bodies. That refocus leads us to contemplate the state of *not having*. Recognizing our physical limitations becomes a democratizing, humanizing experience that affirms our shared vulnerability and our susceptibility to the most mundane aspects of the natural environment. The Epicureans held that none of us are special and all of us are special: we are all combinations of the same astounding, eternally shifting atomic construction. Purposefully or not, when we muse that we contain a small part of the universe within our skin, we take an Epicurean approach; so, too, do present-day astrophysicists exploring the phenomenon of nucleosynthesis, the making of elements inside stars, a tiny portion of which ends up inside each human being.

While they relied on sensations as natural guideposts to morality, the Epicureans disdained physical excess. Epicurus felt that "diminishment" could be a precursor, or companion, to a different, more subtle strength and creativity. This stepping-back gave rise to the criticism of the Stoic Epictetus, who (if we believe Diogenes Laërtius) accused Epicureans of being "unmanly." Roman orators similarly associated Epicurus with *mollitia*, a word variously translated as "softness," "effeminacy," and "diminishment." To Romans such as Cicero, *mollitia* threatened social well-being because "the appetites of the effeminate were uncontrollable." Epicurus gave as good as he got: he engaged in spirited attacks even on his own teachers, the most prominent of whom he condemned as a "'lung-fish,' an 'illiterate,' a 'deceiver,' and, oddly enough, a 'prostitute.'" At least the last two epithets, noted one scholar, "may be mere statements of fact."

Anti-Epicurean criticism gained in volume with the rise of Christianity, whose early adherents singled out Epicurus from other ancient philosophers for maintaining that death ends all—that there is no afterlife—and that the world has always existed, that divine powers had not magically formed us and our environment from nothing. The Epicurean emphasis on the truth of sensations became twisted as an obsession with pleasures of the flesh, and "hedonist" became a sobriquet for someone who is debauched (the "débauché" is literally someone who strays from duty)—the opposite extreme of what the Epicureans admired.

Throughout the Middle Ages, Epicurus and devotees such as Lucretius were labeled heretics. Dante relegated Epicurus, along with his followers, to the Sixth Circle of Hell, trapped in flaming tombs for eternity. Epicurean principles only began to be resurrected with the coming of humanists such as Thomas More who, in his 1516 treatise *Utopia*, extolled the pleasure of the pursuit of knowledge. The so-called "Prince of Humanism," the Dutch priest Desiderius Erasmus also sympathized with the Epicureans in his writings. He did so most particularly in his 1533 colloquy "Epicureus." Erasmus admired the Epicurean emphasis on the equilibrium brought about by living free from worldly concerns and by avoiding personal excess. Later, Thomas Hobbes drew on Epicurus for *Leviathan* (1651), but for most Catholic as well as Puritan thinkers, the Epicureans personified godlessness, consigning their school along with its emphasis on materialism to the dustbin of history.

....

In the mid-eighteenth century, a trove of Epicurean works was discovered in the ruins of a library in Herculaneum, buried since the eruption of Vesuvius in 79 CE. Thirty-seven papyrus rolls by Epicurus, a series of lectures, were recovered in damaged condition. The result is that, of all the ancient Greek philosophers, Epicurus became the one whose thinking we know best through an approximation of his own words, as opposed to accounts composed by later historians such as Diogenes Laërtius, which come to us sometimes centuries removed from the original. The timing was good, and in the aftermath of Puritanism, Epicureanism came to be widely reconsidered in intellectual if not ecclesiastical circles. Epicurean tenets such as the eternal existence of atoms, experience as the basis of knowledge, and physics being the science of probabilities sat well with eighteenth-century thinkers such as Jeremy Bentham, David Hume, Isaac Newton, and Jean-Jacques Rousseau. Society was not fixed and preordained, but continually evolving and changing. Challenges required practical solutions that worked with the natural order of things. There was no "divine right." If something needs fixing, it is not enough to pray to God, gods, or beg the favor of a divinely appointed leader. You have to get in there and set things straight on your own. Although the Roman poet Horace popularized the phrase "carpe diem" more than two centuries after Epicurus, it neatly summarized a core aspect of the philosophy, and appealed to the emerging social strata of the Enlightenment.

....

With the advent of Protestantism, the concept of *askēsis* received a boost and an unexpected transformation. According to early twentieth-century German sociologist Max Weber, a Protestant striving for wealth was in effect a form of extended worship. Religious life could no longer provide a refuge from the world. Under capitalism, the Puritans discovered a way to at once keep themselves from temptation and to fulfill God's will that they prosper: the sanctification of life became contractual—an extended business enterprise. Weber portrayed asceticism as forming a miserable framework for the capitalist environment. It was pessimistic and anti-humanist at its core, with one precept above all others: evil is inherent to this world. Overconsumption and corruption, the scale of which we have only an inkling, pervades life on Earth. For the Protestant, Weber argued, the sole path to God is through labor. The heavy, never-ending task of redemption requires vigilance, discipline, and sweat, with the inevitable consequence, as historian Eliezer Diamond has pointed out, that

> *any form of idleness, including any activity that was not seen as adding to God's glory, was not tolerated. This included overeating, oversleeping, ostentatious dress, "frivolous" engagement in the fine arts—in short, anything other than work, worship, and the carrying out of one's familial and social duties.*

Self-control is not only a matter of repression. It bridges a gap between classical and modern lifestyles. The asceticism recurrent throughout classical religions and ancient cultures, as manifested by fasting, allows us to function in contemporary society, while at the same time acknowledging our debts to the distant past. Can an ascetic tradition thrive on a purely humanist basis? While asceticism provides the spiritual framework for fasting, asceticism is for many a reminder of things more essential, more lasting, and therefore more "real" than what most of us value. It helps remind us, in the words of behavioral psychologist B. F. Skinner, that "a small part of the universe is *private*," because we quite literally contain a portion of the universe within our skin. And if you contain a cosmic fraction within yourself, it is rewarding to occasionally contemplate its existence.

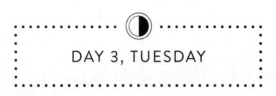
The Marvelous Machine:
What Happens to Our Body When We Fast

Not very far into the journey, but already I think I miss the conviviality of eating more than the eating itself: even while eating alone, you read the news or text friends. Life at present is calmer, but duller. There are fewer distractions from work and from doing what should be done—answering emails, doing the laundry, cleaning up the mess of my desk. C. and I strolled down to Washington Square and back, having what seemed to us a coherent conversation all the while. Feeling otherworldly, but otherwise no symptoms. Eating anchors us to this world: a meal fills us; it literally and figuratively weighs us down. Not eating casts us off, and up we drift. Floated a couple hundred yards to Home Depot, picked up heavyish box of household goods, floated back. Also not sure that unworldly feeling isn't just because I'm so unusually focused on every twinge in my body. Slight headache toward end of the day. I wonder if my senses are ramping up: A. was slicing a cucumber and I smelled it from across the loft, a good twenty feet away. An unmistakably fresh, distinctly springlike smell. Not sure I could do that pre-fast, or perhaps it's just that I never noticed. Had animated chat with D. in the afternoon. Told him about the fast, boasting a bit. He laughed, then said he was amazed C. and I hadn't killed one another. I said we would have, but we no longer had the strength. In actuality, I don't feel particularly weak, anxious, or irritated; I feel more like a lotus-eater than a berserker. It's interesting how even the *thought* of not eating becomes a threat to normalcy. It undermines stability, which we associate with a steady, plentiful supply of food. Even more than shelter, which offers us protection from emergencies, regular access to food (and drink) is our social glue. What's tough about this is making the commitment; it's getting over the pervasive, mind-consuming anxiety of not eating. When did we start eating three meals a day and why?

For the most part we willfully ignore what goes on beneath the membrane of the skin. When we do consider that hidden realm, it is with disgust. For at least four thousand years, our guts have been labeled the corrupt baggage we lug around on life's journey. In ancient Egypt, only souls whose corpses had been rid of impurities by having their insides scooped out could submit themselves to the judgment of the gods. Once a person died, Anubis, the jackal-headed lord of the dead, weighed the soul against a feather. Then Thoth, the bird-god of intelligence, thinking, and the creator of language, decided whether the petitioner might enter the afterlife.

In Europe, the notion of the tricky, unknowable body gathered momentum with the teachings of the *Hippocratic Corpus*, a collection of writings from the late fifth to the early fourth century BCE. As people came to identify the human body as the locus for undermining forces, anxiety increased about the lurking chaos within. Silent diseases festered in our mysterious interiors, only to spring out unbidden, afflicting the innocent and the guilty alike.

For the dozens of texts that make up what we think of today as the writings of Hippocrates—although we have no idea what he actually wrote—preventing a disease was more important than curing it, and the unseen body was a place that sheltered the demonic and could only occasionally be relied upon. Centuries later, emptiness was equated with cleansing and health by Aelius Aristides, who in extensive writings about his own ailments linked self-erasure with growth. Fasting, dieting, and purgatives of all sorts became his prescription for contending with what classics scholar Brooke Holmes elegantly terms the "Odyssean slipperiness of the body." With absence came regeneration. Our rejection of our "dirty" interior selves and our focus on clean exteriors continues in the twenty-first century. No horror film is complete without a generous expenditure of blood and guts; the revelation of things more customarily concealed, particularly where waste and genitalia are concerned, shocks most of us.

....

Day after day, we charge ahead, shoveling calories in one end and expelling waste from the other. If the process comes to a halt, the remarkable, intricate machine that is our body swings into action. The organism reacts first by sending out alarms that rapidly increase in intensity. At the most elemental level, our stomach growls. You can't control borborygmi, as Hippocrates called stomach growling, unless you eat something. Borborygmi occur as a consequence of the migrating myoelectric complex, or MMC, which in turn is triggered by an empty stomach. MMC stimulates wavelike contractions in gastrointestinal muscles known as peristalsis—and if there is nothing in the stomach, the borborygmi result. Peristaltic contractions move fluid and gas through the gastrointestinal tract. The stomach acts as an amplifier, and as we all know, the results can be disconcertingly loud.

For millennia, the stomach was seen as the source of courage and animal appetite. Hence the phrase "I can't stomach . . . ," meaning "I can't put up with . . ." Rumblings from that direction indicated a gathering chaos. It seemed as though the organ was distinct from the rest of the body, particularly the human spirit, which most ancient philosophers located in the chest, although Aristotle connected the warmth of the stomach with the warmth of the ensouled—the essence of the organism, without which a body is no longer human. For most, the stomach was the source of our animalistic instincts: Odysseus condemns his "shameless belly." No matter his troubles, his stomach always demands precedence. King Lear's loyal courtier Edgar, on the run and forced to disguise himself as Poor Tom, speaks to the growling devil in his own stomach when he says, "Hopdance cries in Tom's belly for two white herring. Croak not, black angel; I have no food for thee."

....

While we may think we depend on sensory outposts that deliver information on sight, smell, hearing, taste, and touch—that is all surface stuff. The gut is by far the largest sensory organ. In many ways, the stomach really does behave as an independent creature, no matter what our conscious desires might be. The question of which part of us is rebel-in-residence and which conformist overlord shifts on a regular basis: the gastrointestinal tract has one of the largest surface areas in the human body, and hosts a complex microbiotic ecosystem composed of tens of trillions of bacteria, protozoa, viruses, and even fungi that comprise hundreds or thousands of species—no one knows how many for sure. This miniature wilderness has shaped humans for longer than we can fathom. Certain of the tiny animals have been linked to simple, multicellular creatures known as placozoans that have been around for 600 million years.

That the gut plays a role in our sleeping and waking cycles was identified in the postwar period by a microbiologist working at the Argonne National Laboratory in Illinois. In the 1960s, as long-distance jet travel became widespread, humanity encountered a new opponent: jet lag. Gut science played its part through the persona of Dr. Charles F. Ehret. Ehret's initial area of scholarly focus was the mating habits of paramecia, leading a colleague to christen him "the Kinsey of the protozoa." At Argonne, Ehret shifted to chronobiology, or the science of circadian rhythms, and in 1982 he released the "Argonne Anti-Jet-Lag Diet," suggesting an optimum fast-feast eating schedule for jet-set travelers. It was quickly adopted by everyone from the Canadian national swim team to the U.S.

Secret Service. A U.S. military study conducted in 2002 that involved 238 soldiers confirmed the diet's effectiveness as an anti–jet lag tool.

While the Argonne diet is still widely recommended, more recently the simple act of fasting before a flight has proven to be just as useful, and easier to implement. A 2008 study conducted by doctors at Harvard Medical School and the Beth Israel Deaconess Medical Center in Boston found that the rhythm of eating can override the body's internal sleep monitor, normally ruled by the presence or absence of light. "We discovered that a single cycle of starvation followed by refeeding turns on the clock," Dr. Clifford Saper, a Harvard Medical School professor, said at the time. The fast-feast jolt "hijacks all of the circadian rhythms onto a new time zone that corresponds with food availability," according to Saper.

....

A human has about 16 billion cortical neurons, and in the tip of a woman's clitoris alone are 8,000 neurons—a man's penis has a pitiable 4,000. More than 100 million neurons (nerve cells) are in our stomach, and more than 500 million pack the enteric nervous system, which is sometimes called the "brain in the gut." This number is slightly fewer than the neurons in a dog's cerebral cortex. The stomach's cells and nerves translate what we eat or don't eat into neural signals that become the sensations that help define our existence. If the cries of the digestive network go unanswered, an amazing internal concatenation of biochemical machinery activates.

At the start of a fast, the stomach commands production of certain hormones, or signaling molecules. Among these are ghrelin, which stimulates hunger and lowers the level of the hormone leptin, which produces a feeling of fullness. Leptin is secreted by fat tissue in proportion to its mass, so the more fat, the more leptin. These hormones trundle along, taking up to ten minutes before their impact is felt. Ghrelin activates nerve cells within the hypothalamus—a part of the forebrain—and produces two proteins that cause hunger, neuropeptide Y and agouti-related peptide (engagingly associated with a large South American rodent, the agouti, because of the role that the peptide's molecular cousin—agouti-signaling protein—plays in coloring the bristles of the beast). These peptides are complemented by a recently discovered lightning-fast signaling node in the digestive system, a neural circuit that sends messages to the brain within milliseconds. The node operates via synaptic transmission: certain cells lining the stomach emit glutamate, a neurotransmitter that affects the vagus nerve, a neural highway between the brain, gut, hearts, and lungs. The body uses the same neurotransmitter in neuronal synapses from cells of the inner ear and retina. Researchers think the electrical signals provide the brain with "precise spatial and temporal information about gut contents."

Hormonal manipulations and electrical signaling engender more hunger pangs and growling, clear signals that all is not right with the world, just in case our consciousness has not already registered the fact that we are not plying ourselves with the usual amount of food. The primal self urges us to reach for a "friendly bite," a gentle reassurance that we're in familiar territory—safe, warm, and with a food supply readily at hand. At this point in the fast, to suppress such natural inclinations requires conscious redirection. For the mind to betray instinct is a rebellion of the most basic sort. The body is firmly on the side of instinct. The spirit is leading an insurrection, and the body responds by calling for a return to unthinking habit. This self-induced (mild) torture lasts anywhere from forty-eight to seventy-two hours, at which point the call for outside assistance diminishes, the body gives up the fight, and resorts to internal resources.

Certain foods provide carbohydrates (fibers, starches, and sugars), which are broken down via the digestive process into glucose, which provides most of the body's energy. As the fast proceeds, the body recalibrates, in effect going into lockdown mode. Our corporal machine continues along an alternate pathway, working toward a transformed self via gluconeogenesis (the process by which glucose forms) and adaptive thermogenesis (the process by which the body heats itself). It does so first by using up most of the excess glucose stored in the muscles and liver as glycogen, which can easily be processed into energy. There is a lowish reserve of glycogen to begin with, typically only enough to provide energy for a hard-driving athlete to perform for an hour or so. (A fasting person at rest has about sixteen hours' worth of glycogen to draw on.) As blood sugar levels drop, that underappreciated organ (at least for those of us without diabetes), the pancreas, joins the fray by producing glucagon, a hormone that acts on the liver, stimulating the production of glycogen and reducing consumption of glucose by the liver, all so the bloodstream can maintain a steady level of glucose. The priority is to keep the brain constantly supplied with calories in the form of glucose.

About three or four days into a fast, when glycogen reserves run very low, the body turns to fatty acids (adipose tissue triglyceride) derived from fat (adipose tissue) stored throughout the body. The brain can only use highly refined fatty acids, so low levels of insulin signal the liver to switch its production focus to metabolizing ketone bodies from fatty acids. Ketones are an emergency fuel that allow the body to go relatively long periods without food.

A reliable indicator of ketosis—highly elevated levels of ketone bodies—is the smell of acetone on a faster's breath and a distinct taste that has been variously described as lemon drops or walnuts: as the liver metabolizes fatty acids, it produces three types of ketones, one of which is acetone, the same stuff found in nail polish remover. Thanks to acetone's high vapor pressure (meaning that it is volatile, and evaporates more quickly), it can cross the membrane barrier into the lungs. The result is breath that smells of fruit or alcohol. Breath acetone concentration has been shown to be an effective way to measure fat loss; the more acetone, the higher the rate of fat loss.

As its beneficial effects have become known, an avalanche of studies and popular books extolling the virtues of induced ketosis has resulted. Since the 1920s, nutritional ketosis (where caloric intake equals energy expenditure) has been used as a treatment for epilepsy because ketones provide elevated energy to the brain, which causes a reduction in seizures. In 2008, the largely anecdotal evidence for the effectiveness of fasting as a treatment for epilepsy was backed up by a five-year study involving 145 children aged two to sixteen in England. All the children chosen for the study were suffering from a minimum of seven epileptic attacks a week. After going on a ketogenic diet for three months, 38 percent showed a decrease in seizures, while in the control group (those receiving medications as usual), 37 percent showed an increase in seizures. Seven percent of those on the ketogenic diet reported a drop in seizures of 90 percent or more, versus zero percent in the control group.

While the chorus is far from unanimous—some studies show that ketone bodies, because they are more potent than glucose, may adversely affect blood flow, leading to vascular damage and/or high cholesterol (hypercholesterolemia)—arguments for the health benefits of fasting accumulate on practically a daily basis, reinforcing the idea that it can be a powerful refresher for the body and help heal ailing cells. "Ketone bodies are not just fuel used during periods of fasting," wrote Rafael de Cabo, chief of the Translational Gerontology Branch at the U.S. government's National Institute on Aging, and Mark Mattson, professor of neuroscience at Johns Hopkins and former chief of the neurosciences laboratory at the National Institute on Aging, in the *New England Journal of Medicine*. "They are potent signaling molecules with major effects on cell and organ functions." Thanks in large part to these high-energy miracle compounds, metabolic switching induced by fasting prompts repair and renewal down to the molecular level. As part of a study of fasting's effects on aging, de Cabo and Mattson found fasting benefits for those suffering from obesity and diabetes mellitus, cancer, cardiovascular disease, neurodegenerative disorders, postoperative recovery, and even (on the basis of animal models) for people preparing to undergo surgery: "Intermittent-fasting regimens reduce tissue damage and improve functional outcomes of traumatic and ischemic tissue injury [resulting from poor blood circulation]. . . . Preoperative fasting reduces tissue damage and inflammation and improves the outcomes of surgical procedures."

In the course of their consideration of fasting, de Cabo and Mattson pointed to the Okinawa Centenarian Study, a Japanese Ministry of

Health–funded program to determine why such a remarkable number of Ryukyu Islanders live very long lives (Okinawa is the largest of the islands). Okinawans living a traditional lifestyle incorporated what is essentially a permanent fasting regime—a low-calorie diet from energy-poor but nutrient-rich sources (lots of green leafy and yellow root vegetables, small amounts of fish and meat). They had a mortality rate that was strikingly skewed compared to the rest of Japan. The three gerontologists who headed the research noted that "death rates from heart disease, cancer and cerebral vascular disease were found to be only 60 to 70% of that of the Japan average and the all-cause mortality rate for 60- to 64-year-olds was only half that of other Japanese. . . . Thus, life expectancy at older ages is extremely long in Okinawa. For the septuagenarian cohort, life expectancy from age 65 is the longest in Japan, and possibly the world, at 24.1 years for females and 18.5 years for males." There are four to five times the number of centenarians in Okinawa as in most industrialized countries. The trick is calorie restriction, even to the degree of eating on an energy *deficit*— Okinawan septuagenarians in the study ate "approximately 11% fewer calories (approximately 1,785 kcal per day) than would normally be recommended for maintenance of body weight." If growing old is the goal, long-term calorie restriction, which results in delayed aging in studied populations, seems a necessary component of the plan. As the population ages rapidly in industrialized countries—a fifth of the American population is expected to be over the age of sixty-five by the year 2040, more than double that in 2000; it was barely 4 percent in 1900—fasting in the form of caloric restriction is certain to become a topic of greater relevance.

....

After the first seventy-two hours or so of self-starvation, fasters often report feeling serene, even mildly euphoric. Such accounts may perplex non-fasters, who associate fasting with self-punishment. But there are a number of reasons this sensation is grounded in biological fact. In the 1950s, it was discovered that peristalsis (involuntary contractions in the digestive system) induced by fasting causes the body to release large amounts of the neurotransmitter serotonin, a signaling molecule that works to inhibit the secretion of gastric acid. Serotonin, present in high amounts alongside rich and diverse gut microbiota, is sometimes called the "happy hormone." Low levels have been associated with mental illness, depression, memory issues, and in general poor social functioning, as well as Parkinson's, irritable bowel syndrome (IBS), balance issues, delayed healing, and more.

Higher levels of endocannabinoids have also been measured in people who fast. As their name suggests, the molecular structure of these neurotransmitters is closely related to their plant-based cannabis cousins, and their function in the body is homeostasis—an organism's ongoing effort to keep everything in balance. The endocannabinoid system was discovered a little over thirty years ago, and its role in contributing to "the faster's high" is unclear. In daily life, however, it helps us adjust to changes, affecting mood, memory, sleep, and sensitivity to pain.

There is more to the ketone cocktail. The blissful sensation is compounded by the onset of ketosis, and is specifically due to the ketone body beta-hydroxybutyrate (BHB). BHB is a molecule that shares many properties with the synthetic drug gamma hydroxybutyrate, or GHB, also known as the "date-rape drug." The chemical formulas of BHB and GHB are the same, and contain the same number of atoms. The two differ only in the placement of one hydrogen and one oxygen atom, and bind to the same anxiety-reducing receptors in the brain. This means that fasting is not all about physical deprivation (fasters as hedonists!), and that it can introduce us to new forms of contentment and possibly enlightenment. The vision quests of many Native American cultures, including the Cree, Siksika (Blackfoot), Nez Percé, Anishinabe, and Inuit, all involve fasting from both sleep and food for several days, allowing ketosis to have its characteristic euphoric effect.

Recently, ketones fueling the brain have been shown to cause an increase in the gene containing instructions for making BDNF, brain-derived neurotropic factor, a protein molecule found in the brain and spinal cord that is crucial for all nerve connections. BDNF is important to cell regeneration and is "associated with the promotion of mitochondrial biogenesis [which maintains mitochondria, the so-called 'powerhouses of the cell'], synaptic plasticity [the ability of neurons to communicate], and cellular stress resistance." It also appears to act as an antidepressant. As BDNF increases, so does NGF (nerve growth factor), which has led some scientists to conclude that fasting may supercharge the brain, a finding corroborated by the legions of fasters convinced that refraining from eating sharpens their senses. Weirdly, low levels of BDNF have been associated with anorexia—a counterintuitive finding that at present remains unexplained. Low BDNF has also been connected to neurogenerative diseases such as Alzheimer's and Parkinson's, but the jury is still out on whether low levels play a factor in causing disease.

Yet another biochemical cause of fasting's association with well-being and sharpened senses seems to be heightened levels of the neuropeptide known as orexin-A. Caffeine, exercise, and fasting all increase the presence of orexin-A, which zaps the system, making us feel awake and alert. Low levels are associated with dullness, depression and, in extreme cases, narcolepsy (a disorder that causes people to fall into an immediate deep sleep). Blocking orexin-A is used as a way to fight insomnia. In one small study presided over by the Japanese National Institute of Public Health, ten women fasted between seven and ten days, and all saw their orexin-A levels jump on the third day and remain high throughout the fast. In other research that took place in Saudi Arabia, orexin-A levels in eight men increased during their daily Ramadan fasts. The conclusion was that the "finding supports findings from animal studies that fasting increases alertness." The most prominent animal study involving orexin-A suggested that the peptide improves cognition in sleep-deprived primates. Rhesus monkeys were prevented from sleeping for thirty to thirty-six hours and their puzzle-solving abilities unsurprisingly declined; upon taking orexin-A, they performed normally on short-term memory tasks and brain scans showed that they appeared to be fully awake.

Cesar Chavez, the cofounder of the United Farm Workers union, was an inveterate long-term faster. In a conversation with the novelist Peter Matthiessen, he described the onset of ketosis as giving access to a kind of enlightened, superhuman ecstasy: "About the third or fourth day—and this has happened to me every time I've fasted—it's like all of a sudden when you're up at a high altitude, and you clear your ears; in the same way, my mind clears, it is open to everything. After a long conversation, for example, I could repeat word for word what had been said. That's one of the sensations of the fast: it's beautiful." Sad to report, in my case, my memory never improved, but by about day three I did feel quite serene.

....

As the body runs out of carbohydrates to burn and ketosis ensues, fatty tissue—where many toxins are stored—diminishes, along with the AGEs (advanced glycation end products) that cells accumulate from elevated blood sugar. AGEs are waste molecules that arise in all living organisms from the reaction of glucose with proteins and lipids (the molecular group of fats and fatty acids). An imbalance of AGEs causes oxidative stress and damages cell lipids and proteins, resulting in cell death, inflammation, and various corporal dysfunctions. AGEs have been associated with aging and degenerative diseases such as heart disease, some types of cancer, and diabetes.

If the fast continues, with available reserves shunted to sustaining essential organs, other routine functions are neglected. The body's thermic regulation is first to go: you get cold. Metabolizing food heats the body, and less digestive activity means a lowered metabolism, meaning less energy expended throughout the body. Even limited calorie restriction has been shown to lower body temperature. That same lowered digestive activity prompts the release of somatostatin, a hormone that inhibits *other* hormones such as gastrin from doing their work and causes the stomach's acid levels to drop. It really is like a Fischli-Weiss sequence or

Rube Goldberg apparatus in there. It is a domino effect, but one simultaneously involving dozens of pathways and hundreds of different elements.

With still more fasting, the body's metabolism drops off a cliff. As thyroid hormones and iron levels drop, the result is cold hands and feet, as well as confusion, general weakness, and fatigue. Heartbeats may become irregular. Because of low blood sugar, blood pressure is likely to drop. The respiratory rate drops. Serotonin also plummets (after initially having increased), because the brain derives new serotonin only from tryptophan, an amino acid found in foods such as nuts, seeds, dairy products, oats, chocolate, and certain meats.

If the fast is prolonged and absolute in its regimen, after a few weeks, when the energy deficit is too great and fat reserves are depleted, the entire organism starts to break down any available protein, in a process called catabolism. As part of the unceasing effort to produce glucose, both liver and kidneys turn to deriving it from amino acids, the building blocks of protein. As the blood becomes more acidic, kidney and liver damage can occur, and acidosis, the evil twin of ketosis, rears its ugly head. Acidosis occurs when excessive amounts of metabolic toxins such as urea and ammonia accumulate in the body as catabolic by-products. Its outward symptoms are the opposite of ketosis: irritability, fatigue, weakness, and depression. As BHB, together with another ketone body, acetoacetic acid, builds up in the body as a result of extensive fasting, ketoacidosis, a "potentially life-threatening metabolic disorder," can result. Symptoms of ketoacidosis include abdominal pain, rapid and shallow breathing, vomiting, and dehydration.

Severely malnourished patients near death often exhibit a phenomenon known as the king penguin syndrome, named after king penguin chicks, which during winter months can endure five months or more without eating—a record-length fast—while waiting for their parents to return. They can experience a 70 percent drop in body mass. At the point people are diagnosed with king penguin syndrome, the body is dying from what is technically known as cachexia—general wasting syndrome caused by starvation—but paradoxically exhibits a surge in what is known as "resting energy expenditure," the number of calories a body burns while at rest. The protein has to come from somewhere, and without supply from fat reserves or an outside source, what food critic Ligaya Mishan has called "the crime beyond all crimes" occurs: the body in effect cannibalizes itself, feeding on the protein in its own muscles, including the heart, and wasting away. Everything must be sacrificed to keep the brain functioning. Eventually death results, often from cardiac arrest.

....

Much of what we know about the effects of long-term, unalleviated starvation on humans comes from a remarkable document that was smuggled out of the Warsaw ghetto in 1942, compiled by a heroic team of twenty-eight Jewish doctors working under unimaginable conditions. Translated into English as *Hunger Disease*, it documents the effects of starvation with precision and a certain literary license: in breaking starvation down into three stages, for example, it catalogues stage one, when surplus fat disappears, as being "reminiscent of the time before the war when people went to Marienbad, Karlsbad, or Vichy for a reducing cure and came back looking younger and feeling better." With time and no break in malnutrition, starvation enters stage two: "Gradually youth was drained and young people changed into withered old people. . . ." Finally, "like a melting wax candle," the patients slip into the terminal stage, stage three. What is the maximum amount of time a human can go without nourishment? It of course depends on the person, but without food or water, most people collapse within a few days. With support and monitoring, some can hold on considerably longer: the longest recorded hunger strike, supplemented by sugared water, was ninety-four days by Irish republicans held in Cork County Gaol in 1920, who ended the strike at the behest of their leadership after several of their group had died. In 2020, the Turkish lawyer Ebru Timtik, on a hunger strike to demand a fair trial, survived 238 days on water and vitamins before she expired.

....

For those of us who maintain moderate fasts over time (such as calorie restriction) and who stop fasting well before organ collapse, the initiation of gluconeogenesis—the process described earlier, in which non-carbohydrate-based glucose is formed in the body by combined efforts of the pancreas and liver—can aid in detoxification and more. Apart from good spirits, many people who clamp down on food intake while avoiding malnutrition report heightened energy and an increase in strength and endurance. The changes initiated by calorie restriction (CR) have their own highly complex series of pathways. At the molecular level, a jumble of nucleotides, fuel-sensing enzymes (proteins that enable the biochemical reactions in our bodies that produce energy, otherwise known as metabolic processes), and coenzymes are involved in the process, and they are commonly known in the medical community by a veritable alphabet soup of acronyms: among them ADP, AMP, ATP, NAD, and NMN.

To receive near-immediate benefit from CR on a physical level it doesn't even appear to be necessary to prolong the effort. A study headed by de Cabo, of the National Institute on Aging, notes adaptive cellular response can occur with just "a few hours of fasting." Beneficial adaptations can be measured in the changing ratio of certain organic compounds in the body, alongside other changes that trigger repair and block anabolic processes. An endless parade of influencers now tout the health benefits of CR. It occurs in myriad forms, such as alternate-day fasting, time-restricted feeding, and calorie restriction itself, each of which has its own set of proponents.

An important stage of any fast is its end. The longer the fast, the more carefully the emergence from the experience must be managed. Coming out of a long fast can be dangerous, and if done carelessly can result in a potentially fatal condition known as "refeeding syndrome." After a period of malnourishment, an abrupt resumption of a normal intake of calories, or—even worse—an abrupt intake combined with an excessive one to compensate for the fast, can cause an imbalance of fluids and electrolytes. Electrolytes are the micronutrient minerals such as sodium, potassium, chloride, calcium, and magnesium, which are crucial for normal body functions. During a fast, metabolic processes can drop by as much as 25 percent, and the body's requirement for these electrolytes declines along with their availability. Blood measurements may remain normal, because some nutrients remain inside blood cells. As refeeding begins and the metabolism revs up to normal levels, insulin pours into the system. Insulin, which helps process fat and protein, requires certain of these nutrients and stimulates absorption of others, and the result is that the supply of these essential electrolytes is further depleted. The consequences can be catastrophic.

Refeeding syndrome's symptoms are not universally agreed upon, but components of the malady can include double vision, nausea, trouble breathing, abnormally low blood pressure, seizures, and more. Yet it is not difficult to avoid. Recommendations on best practices for a safe entry back into the non-fasting world vary and depend on the faster and the length of the fast, but most researchers advocate a gradual transition back to a pre-fast diet, sometimes taking as long as a week or more, and starting with easy-to-digest foods that are light in fiber, sugar, and fat, such as dried fruit, fermented food (such as yogurt), and light soups.

Intermittent fasting—several days off, several days on—or partial fasting over prolonged periods, such as occurs during the month of Ramadan or the forty days of Lent, has rarely been associated with negative effects. Numerous studies have shown what effects there are (diminished body weight, fatigue) are not enduring. During Ramadan, the ninth month of the Islamic calendar, observant Muslims abstain from all meat and drink from dawn until nightfall. Depending on where a fasting Muslim is located and what time of year Ramadan occurs, the daily fasting period can be as long as eighteen hours (Ramadan moves ahead about eleven days each year and can occur in any season). Research shows that the performance of professional athletes on such strict diets has been affected minimally, if at all; for example, a study of Muslim soccer players in the Russian Premier League concluded that fasting during

Ramadan "had no negative influence on the running performance of elite Muslim professional adult soccer players during daytime matches." Other studies suggest that Ramadan fasting has minimal negative impact, and no lasting negative impact, even on growing children: one 2014 paper detailed the experiences of eighteen Tunisian boys participating in their first-ever Ramadan. The researchers found that while the adolescents' endurance declined during the fast, "short-term explosive physical activity" remained unchanged. These and other extant studies on human fasting are limited, and people considering a long-term fast should bear in mind that the above cases involved professional athletes on the one hand and the malleable bodies of adolescents on the other.

Such on-again, off-again fasting seems to have many benefits. Strangely, weight loss may not be among them, principally because of the body's natural pull back to a static weight level. A food cutback certainly results in weight loss—fewer calories in means the body turns to its own reserves—but if monitored over time, not only does half the loss occur in the first month (and "one fourth to one third thereafter is from muscle tissue"), it doesn't stick. At least two relatively recent, major studies corroborate this likelihood. A three-month-long University of California study in 2019, while not definitive, showed no statistical difference in weight loss between intermittent fasters and participants who maintained their usual diet. The results of a year-long study in 2022, published in the *New England Journal of Medicine*, involving 139 patients in Guangzhou, China, came to similar conclusions. Participants randomly assigned to an intermittent-fasting plan showed insignificant weight changes ("no weight-loss benefit") versus participants simply dieting as usual. A follow-up one year later confirmed the initial results. The Chinese scientists also found that the intermittent fasters enjoyed no advantages in terms of other risk factors such as blood pressure, sensitivity to insulin, and blood glucose levels. Dedicated intermittent fasters may in fact be more likely than most of us to be suffering from eating disorders. In one recent U.S. study of forty-four women and twenty men, "[m]en and women engaging in [intermittent fasting] scored significantly higher than community norms on all subscales of the Eating Disorder Examination Questionnaire" (a questionnaire developed by the Medical Sciences Division at the University of Oxford), with almost a third of the participants "at or above the clinical EDE-Q cut-off." The truth is that most people using intermittent fasting as a weight-loss tool gain back their weight within five years.

Obesity rates have escalated sharply since 2000 and have continued to climb, according to the health policy advocacy group Trust for America's Health. But an increasing number of anti-dieting movements such as "intuitive eating" argue that the bloated diet industry—estimated by the *Wall Street Journal* as generating $76 billion in yearly revenues—should be condemned as both racist and sexist. Dr. Sabrina Strings, a sociology professor at the University of California, Irvine, eloquently makes this case in her book *Fearing the Black Body* (2019).

As it happens, most types of dieting are ineffective. They can simply make people become more food-obsessed, and can lead to an unhappy binge-starvation cycle, with dieters putting themselves through a grueling and unhealthy roller coaster of gain and loss. This up-and-down sequence has been shown to put all kinds of debilitating stresses on the body, in particular the liver because of the extra work fasting entails. The heart can also be at risk: an American Heart Association study in 2019 of 485 women showed that those with a history of weight fluctuation were far more likely to suffer from heart disease. The more episodes of "yo-yo weight loss," the more risk factors accumulated. The lead author of the study, Dr. Brooke Aggarwal, a professor of medical sciences at Columbia University, said: "Achieving a healthy weight is generally recommended as heart healthy, but maintaining weight loss is difficult and fluctuations in weight may make it harder to achieve ideal cardiovascular health." And an imbalance in serotonin, the neurotransmitter that helps regulate mood and is involved in satiety and sleep, has also been documented in long-term fasters: "If you were to come to me and say, 'Well, Doctor, tell me how I can mess up my serotonin system,' I would say, go on an intense diet, go fast for a long time," Dr. Howard Steiger—director of the Eating Disorders Program at the Douglas Mental Health University Institute and a professor of psychiatry at McGill University—told me. "There's a very clear connection between calorie restriction and lowering of brain serotonin activity."

Fasting to lose weight is a bad idea, and fasting to improve your health is not a sure thing. Genetic differences determine, along with height and much of our behavior, somewhere between 40 and 80 percent of our body mass index. Intuition, directed by neural regulatory circuits responding to our environment and genetics, causes us to eat more or less—and generally pushes us to overconsumption. If that's the case, one might ask, why has the obesity rate risen over the years? One reason might be the sheer availability of snacking. Neurobiologist Stephan Guyenet cites the Food Marketing Institute in stating there were on average 15,000 items in stores in 1980 and 44,000 a decade later. The number is presumably much higher now. The inverse of what behavioralists call "sensory specific satiety," which describes how our attraction to a food declines as we gain access to more of it, comes into play: we feel full after eating a certain food and then we experience the desire to eat more when presented with something new. The same principle explains both why we overload our plates at buffets and have such difficulties in curtailing our online purchasing. It's the tyranny of choice. When we're faced with a wide selection, we want it all. Substitution rarely works, either. Kima Cargill, one of the most astute analysts of consumption, chronicles in *The Psychology of Overeating* how it does us no good to switch from, say, regular Coke to Diet Coke. Studies show that switching to diet drinks can lead to overcompensation in other areas of one's diet, "a deal with the devil," as she writes. Research suggests that artificial "sweeteners may actually increase caloric intake from other sources."

....

While permanent weight loss may not be a benefit, occasional fasting has been described as a workout for the cells, forcing them to adapt to changing circumstances. Vast amounts of research associate fasting with improving overall fitness and cognitive skills. While claims touting fasting as a cure-all are irresponsible and have no basis in fact, for someone in good health, fasting does seem to enhance many aspects of the body's system, helping protect against cancer, neurodegeneration, diabetes, and more. We may live longer by eating less—obesity is regularly associated with health risks such as diabetes, hypertension, cancer, and various cardiovascular issues (the number one cause of death worldwide)—but not necessarily better. A 2014 study by the USC Longevity Institute in Davis, California, found that prolonged fasting serves both to reinvigorate the immune system and to protect it against damage. It was therefore suggested that cancer patients, who frequently suffer immune system damage as a side result of chemotherapy, might benefit from fasting instead of the traditional advice to "bulk up." The study found that because the number of white blood cells drops during an extended fast, certain stem cells switch on from a dormant state and begin regenerating immune system cells. It is as though a portion of the entire immune system undergoes a reboot.

A number of subsequent studies have focused on the effect on cancer cells of fasting in combination with chemotherapy: essentially the effectiveness of curing cancer by starving it to death. Italian researchers, for example, have confirmed that short-term starvation protects normal cells, but weakens a variety of cancer cell types, opening up treatment possibilities. This induced vulnerability of cancer cells is due to the drop in adenosine triphosphate (ATP), a molecule present in all living cells. Most cancer cells depend on ATP for sustenance. ATP derives energy from food, passing power along to other cellular processes. While most of the fuel for normal cells—the synthesis of ATP from glucose—involves oxygen consumption, most cancer cells rely on oxygen-free processing to create ATP, a phenomenon known as the "Warburg effect."

Otto Warburg was a quirky physiologist who won the Nobel Prize in 1931 for his discovery of the cellular respiratory enzyme. That same year he was named director of the Kaiser Wilhelm Institute for Cell Physiology in Berlin, not long before the Nazis rose to power. Warburg hypothesized that damage to cells' mitochondria results in insufficient cellular respiration, fostering the growth of cancerous tumors. The complicated, intricate process was decoded by Warburg, who himself was complicated: brilliant, gay, born to one of Germany's long-established Jewish families, and who remarkably managed to continue his work (and his lifestyle) under the Nazi regime.

One of Hitler's many obsessions was cancer, and Warburg's conviction that cancer had dietary rather than genetic roots trumped both his Jewishness and his sexual preferences: Hitler's beloved mother, Klara, had died from breast cancer at the age of forty-seven, and for obvious reasons he embraced the idea that cancer was not the result of degenerate ancestry. Cancer was then thought of as a disease that was somehow "dirty," on par with an STD. It was something shameful to have contracted, as Barbara Ehrenreich wrote in *Harper's Magazine*. In the case of breast cancer, it was "a dread secret, endured in silence and euphemized in obituaries as a 'long illness.'" Despite being scrutinized by the Gestapo, Warburg remained in charge of his institute for the duration of World War II. He diligently focused on his work even as his relatives, professional associates, and friends were exiled or annihilated.

A characteristic of carcinomas is uncontrolled cellular growth, so a drop in ATP deprives cancer cells of fuel and sensitizes them to treatment. This state, in which normal cells are protected but cancer cells are debilitated through short-term starvation, has become known as the "anti-Warburg effect." In the case of certain particularly virulent brain tumors, for example, the anti-Warburg effect has been shown to aid in "differentiation therapy," which forces lethal cancer cells to transform into other, harmless cells. Fasting further suppresses the growth of new cancer cells by repairing mitochondria, increasing oxygen consumption, and restoring the metabolism. It has also been suggested that fasting's consequences may have beneficial effects "not only in cancer but also in other diseased cells."

....

As a fast proceeds and metabolism slows, the production of free radicals—molecular by-products of the normal mitochondrial process that draws energy from nutrients and produces ATP—also declines. Free radicals are molecules with an unpaired electron. This "free" electron makes the molecules highly reactive, causing them to function much as rust does on iron: as they grab an electron from other compounds with which they come into contact, they cause large chain chemical reactions and turn into agents of corrosion, or oxidation. Like low-level radiation and lead, free radicals accumulate in the body over time, leading to issues such as fatty formations in arteries (atherogenesis). For years, free radicals have appeared to be the primary driver of aging because of their relentless assault on mitochondria and other cellular components such as lipids, proteins, and DNA. In experiments on animals whose food intake was limited, a promising triumvirate seemed to reveal itself: as metabolism slowed, the production of free radicals declined, and life span was extended.

....

Genes are a sequence of organic molecules (nucleotides) that form segments of the body's coding, and in humans they number roughly twenty-three thousand. Thanks to what is often called the "genome within the metagenome" supplied by the microbiome, we are able to draw on a library of up to three and a half million genes. We contain interior galaxies and are outnumbered from the start, or perhaps it is that we are augmented more than we can imagine, at least genetically. We are just starting to learn about their interactions and the consequences for the larger organism. The molecular balance inside the body is like a seesaw: as fasting causes ATP levels to drop, the activity of sirtuins—the genes that play a central role in regulating the body's cellular health—increases. Sirtuins, a family of seven signaling proteins, were first discovered in the 1970s as "transcription repressors"—blocking the processes by which cells copy genetic information—in yeast. They have since been shown to appear in bacteria and other animals, including humans. They are present in the mitochondria, nucleus, and cytoplasm of many living cells, and work by changing the way other proteins bind to DNA. In the early 1990s, the first sirtuin discovered—SIR2—was found to extend the life span of yeast cells. Without SIR2, yeast cells died more quickly. With more SIR2, yeast cells lived significantly longer.

Since then, many thousands of research papers have been written about these notorious proteins, and there has been much publicity about their potential role in extending human life spans. While the evidence is tantalizing, the human connection remains to be parsed. What works in a single-cell fungus like yeast may not work the same in humans. Of course, health companies were quick to promote the virtues of anti-aging supplements that increase sirtuin levels in your body. As of this writing, you can buy a "year's supply" (no one is sure what that is) for only $480. At that price, immortality is cheap. All that has been documented for certain is that sirtuins are associated with a healthy lifestyle in humans: they help reduce inflammation, increase regeneration, and basically battle all the familiar aspects of physical decline, from Alzheimer's to losing our balance. And they increase with fasting.

....

In the first half of the twentieth century, the two world wars intensified scientific interest in the consequences of an optimal diet—and in the consequences of a lack of adequate nutrition. What did soldiers need to eat so they could fight most effectively? How little could they consume before their reaction time declined? Two American scientists were pioneers in this field, but they are almost never cited in the same context because, while they studied closely related phenomena, they had disparate goals. Clive M. McCay, a professor of animal husbandry at Cornell University in the 1930s, and Ancel B. Keys, a physiologist ensconced at the University of Minnesota during World War II, were both concerned with prolonged fasting. But Keys focused on extreme dieting, or semi-starvation, while

McCay was interested in a far milder iteration, what he called "very slow growth," and which came to be known as "calorie restriction."

Clive McCay's experiments on rats jump-started the field of gerontology when, after years of research, the nutritionist concluded that rats fed on a calorie-restricted diet, albeit one rich in vitamins and minerals, lived longer, in some cases up to 60 percent longer. Previous research had ignored the crucial element of nutrient deficiency. Seventy-five years after McCay's findings were released to the scientific community in a 1935 paper titled "The Effect of Retarded Growth upon the Length of Life Span and upon the Ultimate Body Size," researchers observed that "the importance of this publication to research in nutrition and aging cannot be overstated. . . . Calorie restriction (CR), also referred to as dietary restriction, remains the only nongenetic method that extends lifespan in every species studied."

McCay's great insight was that the body burns itself out on large quantities of food, and that a diet that provides minimal calories—accompanied by plenty of plant-derived nutrients—can extend life spans significantly. Both the average life span and the maximum life span (the longest-surviving members of the group) of his test subjects consistently increased. As Dr. Richard Weindruch, a professor of medicine at the University of Wisconsin, wrote in *Scientific American*:

> *This last outcome means that calorie restriction tinkers with some basic aging process. Anything that forestalls premature death, such as is caused by a preventable or treatable disease or by an accident, will increase the average life span of a population. But one must truly slow the rate of aging in order for the hardiest individuals to surpass the existing maximum.*

This ability to delay aging under certain circumstances—the ability of the metabolism to put itself on near-hold until better times return—amounts to scaled-back hibernation. It makes sense from an evolutionary perspective: with the reappearance of plentiful food, the reproductive process can resume along with "normal" eating. McCay also addressed the impact of undernutrition on growth. To the chagrin of millions of sailors during World War II, his principles were later put to work in the Department of the Navy, where he directed research on food and nutrition.

....

Ancel Keys was a world-roving adventurer, but his fame rests largely on his having devised combat rations (known as "K rations," probably in his honor) for the U.S. Army and subsequently directing the Minnesota Starvation Experiment of 1944 to 1945. He was more extreme in his interests than McCay, experimenting directly on humans instead of McCay's hapless rats. For six months, bracketed by a three-month lead time and a three-month recuperative time, Keys experimented on three dozen volunteers, all conscientious objectors to the war.

Keys's research was overseen and partially funded by the Department of the Army. He recruited his subjects by calling on their patriotism and arguing that the experiment would be to the benefit of Europe's starving millions, though precisely how was never made clear. The army was, of course, keenly interested in what transpired: it was essential to know how little (or how much) nutrition a fighting man needed to be an effective soldier. The men started with 3,500 calories a day, eating things like roast beef, mashed potatoes, and ice cream, and then dropped to an average of 1,570 calories a day, a semi-starvation diet. (The USDA's *Dietary Guidelines for Americans* today recommends 2,400 calories a day for men in the nineteen-to-thirty-year age range.) In this phase, the volunteers were fed meals designed to mimic European wartime conditions: cabbage and potatoes.

Keys's subjects battled with their intensifying, prolonged desire for a bit more food: some stole food on the sly, others were reduced to licking their plates, and several dropped out because of overpowering hunger. The men became obsessed with food: thinking about it and dreaming about it. They could talk of little else among themselves and to researchers. On average, their weight dropped by 25 percent (which was the study's goal), and as the weeks passed, most of the volunteers became demoralized, disoriented, and anxious—many of them became clinically depressed. They developed obsessive gum-chewing and cigarette-smoking habits. Their pulse rates, body temperatures, and reflexes dropped. So did their mental stability, if not their cognition. One man used an axe to chop off three of his fingers in an effort to be excused from the experiment. On his hospital bed, ashamed of his actions, he begged Keys to be let back in to the program. Keys magnanimously agreed. But while the men's morale dropped precipitously, their powers of logical deduction, memory, and analysis seemed to be unaffected. "No objective loss in intellectual ability and no faults in memory or logic were observed," and some of the study's participants maintained a full academic load during the experiment.

As someone who's undertaken more absolute but far shorter and thus far milder fasts, to me the regimen sounds like mutually agreed-upon torture, an example of a single-minded researcher exploiting the naivete of volunteers. Many of these volunteers had been accused of cowardice for refusing to take up arms and were undoubtedly anxious to prove their manhood. With a traditional fast, there is a steep learning curve. For most people, the first few days are challenging, but once past the three-day mark, ketones start to kick in and some notion of serenity emerges. And the importance of agency cannot be overemphasized. A fast is an opportunity to affirm control over one's body. Keys made his subjects sign away their own decision-making powers: while, of course, they could have dropped out of the program—and several did—they would have done so knowing that they had failed a test of endurance they'd agreed to undertake for the sake of the destitute masses. Although Keys worked with volunteers, he leaned on guilt to turn fasting into a test of manhood and an opportunity for alternative patriotic martyrdom.

Keys's experiment downplays the beneficial effects of controlled fasting noted by McCay and countless other practitioners and researchers. In the first half of the experiment, the most noticeable results of the drop in calories were weakness, fatigue, and confusion. Indications of increased tranquility, energy, and so on are nowhere to be found in the accounts, undoubtedly because they'd been subsumed by the weight of weeks of starvation. Depression increased along with the experiment's duration, and was only alleviated in the rehabilitation phase, when test scores for mood improvement correlated with calories received. Much of the explanation for this result may lie in the Minnesota project's having functioned almost as surrogate punishment for the conscientious objectors—punishment World War II America felt they merited and perhaps punishment that the subjects themselves felt they deserved. During any war, and particularly during a worldwide conflagration in the aftermath of an attack on the United States, COs are commonly regarded as despicable and therefore expendable in a laboratory context. A mere 42,000 Americans were COs in the Second World War, as opposed to the 16 million who joined the fight:

> As the war continued, these conscientious objectors grew increasingly restive. In an oral history compiled later, one man complained, "My God, you're talking about planting trees and the world's on fire!" Another remembered, "This is what finally got under my skin more than anything else: the sense of not sharing the fate of one's generation, but of sort of coasting alongside all of that; you couldn't feel you were part of anything terribly significant in what you were doing."

The Minnesota subjects saw themselves as sacrificing, as being deprived of normal routines. Suffering was synonymous with being helpful. Under the guise of science, fasting became once again mortification of the flesh. Almost sixty years after Keys's project ended, researchers tracked down nineteen of the thirty-six original participants. While many of the 2018 report's conclusions may be attributable to the characteristics of conscientious objectors and not to the consequences of long-term fasting, it found the nineteen to be uniformly well-educated and to have fully recovered from their ordeal. The researchers concluded that "voluntary severe food restriction for six months was not associated with life-long physical, cognitive or emotional adverse effects, despite significant individual suffering during the experiment. . . . All participants ultimately led interesting and productive lives, perhaps not unexpected in view of their voluntary participation as conscientious objectors and the original selection criteria for physically and psychologically healthy subjects."

....

One of the first researchers on caloric restriction remains one of the best known. Dr. Roy Walford was a longtime advocate of eating with more purpose. It was just after World War II when he began to consider the health benefits of fasting, feeling it was bound up inextricably with progressive activism. I met Walford when I published two books by him. Although his previous books had been released by the largest publisher in the country, by the time he approached my small independent publishing firm, he was seen as an extremist and a renegade. I'm sure he only came to us because he'd been turned down by the major houses. Not unlike Timothy Leary—another highly pedigreed researcher who explored the alternative and personally committed to his research by experimenting on himself—Walford both embraced his rejection by more conventional scientists and was pained by it.

Walford got his start by building on Clive McCay's research. A graduate of the University of Chicago's medical school and a professor of pathology at UCLA's School of Medicine, Walford was a lean and genial man with a perpetual air of serenity about him. With his bald pate, his low voice, and his gentle, steady admonitions to consume more thoughtfully, he had the stereotypical attributes of a Buddhist monk. That low-key presence belied a free spirit that sometimes ran counter to his public statements: after he graduated from medical school, together with his friend the mathematician Albert Hibbs (later the coauthor, with Richard Feynman, of the textbook *Quantum Mechanics and Path Integrals*), he analyzed the patterns of roulette wheels in Reno, Nevada, and made enough money to buy himself a yacht. After a December 1949 *Life* magazine feature on

Walford and Hibbs, casinos banned them—and also changed the way roulette wheels worked. Walford then went on solo treks across Africa and India, which intensified his interest in non-Western, alternative approaches to spirituality. When he had become a respected scientist, he was once appointed the master of ceremonies for a medical convention, which culminated with his standing silently onstage for ten minutes in front of hundreds of perplexed pathologists as if in homage to John Cage.

Walford encountered McCay's work early in his career and began writing about caloric restriction in the 1950s. His theories on the benefits of eating less were put into practice in Biosphere 2 some forty years later. Biosphere 2 was the massive experiment in Arizona that operated more or less as a self-contained environment over two years. Ill-fated from the start, beginning with its coy appellation—the planet was supposed to be "Biosphere 1"—the project was plagued by an aura of pseudoscience and hucksterism, but nevertheless produced some valuable data for students of CR. While it failed to generate sufficient oxygen and food for its eight participants and thus to operate as a truly independent mini-world, an unintentional food shortage resulted in its becoming a closely monitored laboratory of the effects of severe long-term calorie restriction on eight healthy men and women. Those results have never been refuted, and decades later are still being cited by researchers.

At sixty-seven, Walford was the oldest member of the team. He documented the unplanned fast, which soon restricted the Biospherians to roughly 1,750 calories a day, three-quarters of what had originally been planned for them. The body mass index of both men and women on the Biosphere team dropped to 20 (considered the knife-edge of normal; less than 18.5 is underweight, according to the Centers for Disease Control). "Their blood pressure, blood sugar, cholesterol and triglyceride levels all fell by at least 20% to extremely healthy levels. The team members also exhibited an increased capacity to fight off illnesses, such as colds and flu." In 2004, at the age of seventy-nine, Walford died of amyotrophic lateral sclerosis (ALS), which he contended stemmed from environmental conditions (specifically, not enough oxygen) in Biosphere 2.

Walford drew on research that extended into both the worlds of science and spirituality to conclude that an anti-consumerist outlook was restorative for both our bodies and minds. In many ways Walford was a throwback to the eccentric iconoclasts of ancient Greece in his willingness to live according to his principles, in his compulsion to challenge convention, and in his pursuit of what the Greeks called *arete*, personal excellence in one's behavior, more commonly translated simply as "virtue."

....

There have been only a few, limited studies involving humans and calorie restriction. CALERIE (Comprehensive Assessment of the Long-Term Effects of Reducing Intake of Energy) was a study jointly conducted by researchers at Washington University in St. Louis, Tufts in Boston, and the Pennington Biomedical Research Center in Baton Rouge from 2007 to 2009. The first randomized controlled effort to test the metabolic effects of CR, CALERIE involved 220 people on calorie-restricted diets. The goal was to determine what happens to people who reduce their daily calories by 25 percent over an extended period. (Twenty-five percent was settled upon because laboratory animals begin to die when their calorie intake is cut by half. But up to that point, with more intense calorie restriction, life span continues to increase until the 50 percent threshold is reached—studies have shown that animals under an extreme CR regimen live up to 60 percent longer than what is expected. The lower range was determined because it was both feasible and still likely to have measurable effects on aging.)

The results pointed back to McCay's thesis. "Aging and chronic diseases are often viewed as inextricably linked. We now know that this is not true, because in mammals it is possible to prevent the development of chronic diseases," wrote Luigi Fontana, the doctor in charge of the Washington University trial. "Although it is currently not known if long-term calorie restriction with adequate nutrition extends maximal lifespan in humans, we do know that long-term calorie restriction without malnutrition results in some of the same metabolic and hormonal adaptations related to longevity in calorie restriction rodents." A follow-up study ten years later called CALERIE Phase 2 involved fifty-three people and provided "new evidence of persistent metabolic slowing accompanied by reduced oxidative stress." Based on studies on animals, it appears that the determining factor is not simply "leanness": while exercise alone also burns calories and is good for you, only calorie restriction can "slow down aging and increase maximal life span."

More recent research suggests that, while free radicals are significant players in the process, it is our genes that determine our rate of senescence. Instead of aging being the result of damage over time, we are genetically programmed to age by the same processes that control our growth. As much as we depend on these developmental sequences, their unceasing efforts lead to decrepitude and with the passage of time become pathological. The result is that humans join cars, cell phones, and many household appliances in being subject to obsolescence, except that in our case it's a dynamic process caused by unending growth.

Traditionally, aging has been seen as a period of loss. Sarcopenia—age-related diminishment of muscle mass and power—is a recognized medical condition. Even without the medical diagnosis, all of us experience a decline in strength, agility, and cognition as we grow old. Inevitably, however, the process is also one of accumulation—of adding clutter to an unsullied original: the weak bones, the stuttering heart, the clogged veins, the failing memory, and so on. And because it does increasingly appear that it is the pace and extent of development that wears us out—that it is not so much that cells are damaged over time, but that they function inappropriately—the ways that fasting may assist us become more apparent.

In one study, in 2022, mice treated with growth suppressants had significantly extended life spans, a result that correlates with familiar observations about organisms such as slow-growing trees and tortoises. It is as though we drink from a life-giving faucet that can't be shut off, and we end by gagging on its output, choking on too much life. The result is apoptosis, or programmed cell death, which comes not from injury or infection but from the combination of the passage of time and relentless energy input. This developmental hypothesis of senescence may also explain why fasting delays aging. By slowing growth, fasting tamps down the continuation of processes that sabotage the healthy body and lead to the organism's decline. "I think aging is a program. It is not random wear-and-tear," says molecular biologist Wolf Reik, a Cambridge professor of epigenetics (the science of studying heritable traits). If that conclusion is correct, the possibility presents itself that "dying of old age" may some day become as rare (or as restricted to the impoverished) as dying from smallpox.

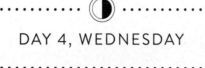

Ascetic Roots 2:
The Abrahamic Traditions

Strange dreams, all about conflict, reflecting what I suppose is something of a daily struggle. Did morning exercises, but skipped push-ups. Felt more fragile this morning. Still seem to be fairly coherent, or at least no less coherent than usual. Lots and lots of miso soup and tea. Adding some chopped parsley to the soup felt like a major decision. I am knowingly betraying the purity of the project, which is a relief. We spend so much time measuring, and to a real degree our lives are constrained by this awful, pervasive habit. We measure our age, our weight, our sleep, our calories, our steps. . . . Too easily we get diverted by the triviality of these measurements and miss the meaning. Walked a quarter mile (measuring!) to the post office and back, didn't feel winded or muscle fatigue, but it definitely was an effort. Looked up "fasting" on Google. It would seem that by now ketones must be kicking in. The cleansing process must be well underway. In the evening we sat down with A., who was eating a salad. I found myself mesmerized by its color: a dark green, a stormy sea green. I could get lost in that salad. I could dive in, cover myself with a blanket of leaves. I feel I'm less of a person than I was, and not just in terms of body weight. . . . No dark circles under eyes or other outward manifestation of our heroism. Hand trembles, but hasn't it for some time now? By end of the day WE ARE ON THE HOMEWARD TREK.

Wondering if it isn't getting a bit hard to focus. Watched *Godzilla vs. Kong* and couldn't decide which one to cheer for. Don't find myself obsessing about food, not bothered at all by the thought, until I sit down to ask myself what foods I am missing. A large, cool bowl of plain yogurt would hit the spot, but I'm okay.

> *"Hast thou found honey? Eat so much as is sufficient for thee, lest thou be filled therewith, and vomit it."*
>
> —Proverbs 25:16

When we leave our starting point, the self, and give the world greater importance, we recognize the power of the extracorporeal. The Epicureans showed that materialism can lead to social change as easily as it can to decadence. Recognition of the self's tenuous place in the world is essential to fomenting change. Materialism is as useful to advocates of reform as it is to landlords, said Sartre. Those who want to change their reality "know themselves from the outset on the basis of the world that crushes them, and they want to change this world that is crushing them." What unites Roman moralists such as Cato and radical philosophers such as Sartre is not anti-consumption, but a criticism of *how* things are consumed. For Romans, profligacy threatened the social order because it diminished inherited wealth, which was a key component of *virtus*, a civic value derived from ancestry, wealth, and personal merit. For Sartre, wanton consumption was only possible as a result of indifference to the plight of the many.

For the past several thousand years, virtuous self-deprivation has played a central role in Judaism. While fasting was not unknown to the Greeks and Romans, a ritual abstinence from meat and drink—along with circumcision and the keeping of the Sabbath—were the signal traits of Jews. In the Torah, fasting is regularly associated with mourning, self-punishment, and supplication, and this tradition helped shape

Christian and Islamic attitudes toward the discipline. Judaism is not generally associated with ascetic impulses; its students and practitioners are consistently concerned with matters of the physical world and life-affirming traditions. Communal activity and procreation ("Be fruitful, and multiply") are divine commandments. An ascetic lifestyle, if carried to extremes, could therefore be seen as a prideful turning away from the divine creation. Appropriate to both the deliberative, fluid nature of ancient Judaism and the contradictions of fasting, some scholars warned of fasting's moral dangers: "'Too many fasts trouble the community unduly'; 'Whosoever fasts [for the sake of self-affliction] is termed a sinner'; 'How could then a man be called holy seeing he humiliates God (who dwells within him) through fasting.'" At the same time, the rabbinic dictum for "the way of the Torah" sounds like the very definition of extreme ascetic living: "You shall eat bread with salt, drink water by measure, sleep on the ground, and live a life of discomfort while you toil in the Torah." But as I try to suggest in these pages, aspects of asceticism and its most visible analogue—fasting—can help us focus on issues of importance to the here and now.

Recent work by scholars such as Daniel Boyarin and Eliezer Diamond have complicated the idea that asceticism resides outside the Jewish tradition. The Jewish God pervades the world, and therefore a near-absolute withdrawal from the world, as opposed to a more measured renunciation, amounts to a rejection of the divine. Yet these scholars convincingly make the case that asceticism is inseparable from Judaism: commonly accepted elements of ascetic practices (among them self-betterment in terms of both morals and knowledge, fasting, renunciation of luxuries, and veneration of spiritual values) are familiar to Jews. Excessive celebration of the physical is a sin. For instance, during Passover—one of the most important Jewish holidays—Jews read from a prayer book known as the Haggadah, which contains a ritual question-and-answer exchange involving the "good son," the "wicked son," the "simple son," and the "son who doesn't know to ask." "In general," writes Boyarin, "medieval and early modern Haggadahs feature the wicked son as some form of martial figure, almost always, in fact, a knight in shining armor." The wise son comes to his beliefs through contemplation, analysis, and piety; the wicked son is obsessed with the material. The Jewish ideal is withdrawal from immediate physicality as a way to get to the deeper meaning of things. As in the *Zhuangzi*—the Chinese text from the third century BCE—it is only possible to attain true understanding by using the intellect to "reach across" a space. The son who immerses himself in the hard tangibility of the present will never transcend the obvious.

The Jewish forerunner of liberal humanism, the Enlightenment philosopher Baruch Spinoza (1632–1677), rejected Cartesian dualism and saw the inability to manage one's desires as itself a form of imprisonment, a crushing burden that could only be relieved by the imposition of a modicum of discipline. While Spinoza is rarely associated with asceticism, his admonitions to moral behavior often sound like those of any Desert Father or Mother. In one of the best-known passages in part 4 of his *Ethics*, he wrote: "Man's lack of power to moderate and restrain the affects I call bondage. For the man who is subject to affects is under the control, not of himself, but of fortune, in whose power he so greatly is that often, though he sees the better for himself, he is still forced to follow the worse." Unusually for someone in the Jewish community, Spinoza was excommunicated—and by his own congregation at that. He was also stabbed by a fellow Jew, although biographers differ on whether this was because of his heretical beliefs or because he was owed money by the person who attacked him.

....

Fasting peppers both the Old and New Testaments. In the Bible, at least three Judaic leaders (Moses, Elijah, and Daniel) prove their spiritual worth and God's special favor by showcasing an ability to survive prolonged fasting on a mythic scale. Before receiving the Ten Commandments, Moses fasted for forty days in the Sinai. Jesus also fasted, echoing the supposed forty-day fast of Pythagoras. Why forty? Judaism regards the number as particularly powerful. In the Bible, it signifies testing. Citations of the number in both the Old and New Testaments include the Flood (when it rained for forty days and nights), Exodus (where it is the number of years that the Israelites wandered through the desert), and Acts (where it is the number of days between Jesus's resurrection and ascension). Forty was once the approximate number of years of a generation. In the Talmud, at the age of forty a person proceeds to a higher level of wisdom. The word "quarantine" (from Latin for "forty"), where people are set apart from the crowd—just as they are set apart during fasting—owes its existence to the belief in the mystical properties of the number. After forty days of quarantine, people's impurities were supposed to have been removed.

According to tradition, Moses's descent from Mount Sinai with the Ten Commandments under his arm coincides with the one fast day clearly specified by the Torah, the Day of Atonement, otherwise known as Yom Kippur, which is the holiest day of the Jewish year. Yom Kippur marks both a period of expressing sorrow for past sins and a time of cleansing. The day also asks consideration of the potential for change, brought about by the delivery of divine directives in the form of the stone tablets. (The great anarchist Emma Goldman, who identified as a Jew culturally if not religiously, regularly observed Yom Kippur by partying: she once came dressed as a nun and "cleared the dance floor for her rendition of 'the anarchist slide.'" For Goldman, religious fasting was a symbol of conformity and self-righteousness.)

Similarly, Elijah, having busied himself slaughtering 450 "false prophets," is visited by an angel, who delivers a meal that enables him to endure forty days and nights without sustenance. The obvious conclusion is that the most devout and favored followers of the one true God have no need of earthly fare. Fasting is associated directly with the divine. Daniel, best known for his adventures in the lions' den, fasts twice. First, he rejects the meat and wine offered to him by his Babylonian captors (the first hunger strike on record?) and eats only vegetables and drinks only water. Fasting does not have to be absolute to be effective, and like Achilles,

Daniel's explicit refusal to accept what is offered to him sets him apart. Later, Daniel undertakes three weeks of mourning, manifested by a similarly partial fast ("no pleasant bread, neither came flesh nor wine in my mouth"), at the end of which time he is rewarded with a holy vision. Daniel's waking dream is one of the more spectacular in a section of the Bible that is rife with them, and all are brought about by fasting, perhaps with a bit of help from the ketone body beta-hydroxybutyrate:

> *A certain man clothed in linen, whose loins were girded with fine gold of Uphaz: His body also was like the beryl, and his face as the appearance of lightning, and his eyes as lamps of fire, and his arms and his feet like in color to polished brass, and the voice of his words like the voice of a multitude.*

As recounted in the Gospels, Jesus is tempted by Satan three times during his forty-day fast in the desert. He is challenged to turn stones into bread, to prove his authenticity by leaping off the temple's pinnacle, and finally he is offered all the kingdoms of the Earth if he consents to worship the devil. Jesus responds by paraphrasing Deuteronomy 8:3 ("It is written, 'Man shall not live by bread alone, but by every word of God'"). He refuses to prove himself or forsake his beliefs. From a nonreligious standpoint, what is interesting here are the dual acknowledgments that a voluntary fast makes even the best of us hungry—because if Jesus were not hungry, the devil's offer would not be tempting—and that a fast can be fortifying, as the philosophers Lerat and Charbonnier remind us:

> *When we fast, we have the chance . . . to discover that other kinds of nourishment exist: it nourishes us to empathize with others, it nourishes us to contemplate nature, to breathe, to touch. There is other sustenance, and there are other hungers. When we eat, it is often with the delusional—and partly unconscious—intention of appeasing another hunger.*

This forty-day fast was demonstrative for Jesus, serving to legitimize his claim to the mantle of Moses. But for many Christians, it was the embrace of the fast's end that helped distinguish the new teachings from Judaism. The Catholic scholar John Dominic Crossan liked to say, citing Luke 7:33–35, that John the Baptist came to fasting and Jesus to feasting. It was the reemergence into the physical world that was emphasized, as opposed to the purity of the fast. Crossan held that "you fast in preparation for what's coming"—also a departure from Jewish tradition.

Jewish lore holds that there are as many ways to interpret the Torah as there were Jews who followed Moses out of Egypt, the implication being that there are hundreds of thousands of ways to interpret holy law. For people from a Jewish heritage (such as myself), a disparate tribe that generally celebrates debate, fasting has been a point of unity. It signals penitence and sadness. "The relevant biblical passage says you should 'afflict the soul,' which the rabbis interpret as going without food, water, and even shoes," the Jewish scholar and rabbi Michael Strassfeld explained to me. Rabbi Strassfeld is particularly known in Jewish circles, together with Sharon Strassfeld, for having organized and written *The Jewish Catalog*, modeled on the *Whole Earth Catalog*.

Fasting's primary role in Judaism is as an indication of mourning, but also as an apology to the Supreme Being. It is associated with the days marking the apostasy of the Israelites who turned away from Judaism to worship the golden calf; with the destruction of the First Temple in 586 BCE, and then the Second Temple in 70 CE. It is a sacrifice to a God that forbade sacrifices (see Abraham and Isaac), an act of mourning and penitence: it is paying God his due.

"You don't rend garments on fast days and you don't fast when a loved one dies, but they share that aspect of marking tragedy," Strassfeld explains. "For example, there's a custom that mourners would sit on the floor or a low chair. For the fast that commemorates the destruction of the Second Temple by the Romans, there is a tradition that when the book of Lamentations, which describes the destruction of Jerusalem by the Babylonians, is chanted in the synagogue, you sit on the floor or on a low chair. So there is some overlap with mourning customs. And similarly on that day the tradition is that you don't wear leather shoes, which are supposed to be comfortable. There's kind of a constellation of customs around mourning, some of which get applied to the national and some to the personal."

Students of the Talmud—the collections of ancient rabbinic writings that seek to unravel hidden meanings in the Bible and in the world—might see the destruction of the Second Temple as a manifestation of *tzimtzum*, the withdrawal or emptiness that makes creation possible. While the temple stood, Jewish scholarship was based on oral tradition. Only the Bible was written down. The Second Temple's elimination made room for the development of rabbinic Judaism and the Talmud itself. So, too, a fast might be seen as a "little destruction," a fleeting imposition of emptiness that allows for something else to flourish. This is similar to the process known in Christian traditions as kenosis, which is derived from the Greek for "emptying," as laid out in Philippians 2:7, wherein Jesus is said to have emptied himself to become humanity's servant.

Some have argued that in her recurring references to "decreation"—or the Supreme Being's abdication—Simone Weil also borrowed from the concept of *tzimtzum*. But Weil inverted the principle, as well as John the Baptist's "He must increase, but I must decrease," by connecting existence to imperfection and emptiness to divinity: "I am God's abdication. The more I exist, the more God abdicates. So if I take God's side rather than my own I ought to regard my existence as a diminution, a decrease." Self-nullification, while unattainable if we remain in the land of the living, is a return to what is holy. Weil wrote that the divine lay in the *lack* of creation. This is close to what philosopher Arthur Schopenhauer meant in *The World as Will and Idea* when he referred to "the unrestricted existence and assertion of the body" in opposition to "the complication of circumstances." Weil pursued this intriguing idea with increasing intensity. It may have contributed to her death at the age of thirty-four from tuberculosis exacerbated by severe undernourishment.

Decreation was however not an argument for inaction: Weil both believed and demonstrated that a moral person could not be an accomplice to corrupt behavior. She protested on behalf of workers' rights, took up arms for the anarchist Durruti Column during the Spanish Civil War, and volunteered for the Resistance in France and the Free French in England during the Second World War. She quit in disgust after the exiles refused to let her put into motion her absurd plan to organize a parachute drop of a brigade of nurses into occupied France with her spindly, nearsighted self at the head. That episode led Charles de Gaulle to quip that Weil was *folle*. In a way, she was; but the "patron saint of twentieth-century anorexics," as Francine du Plessix Gray has called her, reasoned quite logically that physical actions have moral implications, and she was frustrated at the prospect of sitting idly by while the world was burning. Weil's two driving moral impulses were in perpetual conflict. On the one hand, the decreative imperative to "stand down," to retire from the world, and so allow for divine presence; and on the other, the moral obligation to stand up and fight injustice. It is tempting to see in Weil's conflict the archetype for fasting: an action that at once signals determination and an embrace of vulnerability, a withdrawal and an engagement with something different. As we have seen, a faster steps off the path of the ordinary. To fast, she must refuse conventional codes of conduct, which in the normal course of things serve to protect us from reality. Habit is a shield against unpredictability. Someone who never considers challenging "this continuous process of consuming and being consumed," in W. G. Sebald's words, is not thinking about the process. That is not to say s/he is callous. Almost all of us participate in the process of avoidance. New media theorist Douglas Rushkoff has built on this concept with his idea of "degrowth," which is not regression, but moving forward with less. It is fasting on a society-wide scale.

....

For believers of all stripes, fasting is also a way of getting God's attention. In the book of Esther, Queen Esther fasts for three days before appealing to the king for mercy on behalf of the Jewish community that he was planning to slaughter. Jehoshaphat also called for a fast throughout Judea when he was faced with a seemingly insurmountable army of Ammonites and Moabites. In both those cases the Jews were saved, but the Old Testament God was fickle: fasting didn't help King David when his son was struck down by disease. The boy died. In the eyes of devout Jews, the difference in God's response may lie in David's appeal for personal, as opposed to community, benefit.

"The Bible doesn't tell us why it says you should 'afflict,' but I think it is to get you to focus on your soul, on your spirit, on the task at hand, which is to repent," Strassfeld tells me. "In a way, it's a technique of concentrating, paying attention to what is supposed to be central. To engage in this process of *teshuva*, or repentance, is challenging. It's about cultivating a technique of focusing and not being distracted by things which are irrelevant." *Teshuva* literally means "return," and repentance becomes a return to the path outlined for us by the prophets, the path that we habitually lose sight of in the fog of our daily affairs. As Strassfeld points out, "If you didn't commit the sin, you wouldn't need the purification." And it would seem that none of us, religious leader or not, is exempt from sinning. For Jews, fasting became another way to confirm their Jewishness: congregants saw themselves as suffering together, as mourning together.

From absence comes creation: in the wake of the destruction of the Second Temple in 70 CE, when Jewish leaders feared oral traditions would be lost in the wake of the pervasive destruction wrought by Roman legions, the Talmudic laws, which include extensive commentary on fasting, began to be gathered. The Talmud refers to two immensely layered collections of observations and analyses by generations of scholars on Jewish religious practices, one compiled in Palestine in about 200 CE, and the other two centuries or so later in Babylon, which came to supersede the first. By the time of the Babylonian Talmud, the intellectual aspect of "sacrifice" had been elevated over the blood-soaked ritual of slaughtering a fellow creature, the scapegoat. The sacrifice had moved away from being foisted on a third party and had become a matter of personal, individual responsibility in the form of a fast.

In twelfth-century Egypt, the philosopher and physician Maimonides combined the two Talmuds together with his own considerable scholarship and wrote his version of the Mishneh Torah, an intricate fourteen-volume code of religious law. It is still regarded among Orthodox Jews as an authoritative arbiter of law and custom. Within the Mishneh Torah, an important section is devoted primarily to fasting (with diversions along the way on things such as when it is appropriate to request rain from God). While Yom Kippur is the one fast demanded by the Torah, the Maimonides Code specifies seven additional fast days (six public and one private or individual, the latter to be observed only by the first-born son). A *ta'anit* (Hebrew for "fast") can be absolute: from food, water, sex, laundry, self-adornment and, nowadays, even deodorant. On Tish'ah b'Av, the fast devoted to commemorating the destruction of the First and Second Temples, "it is forbidden to wash in either hot or cold water; it is even forbidden to place one's finger in water."

Maimonides wrote that a fast is a response to tragedy. It is done to begin the process of *teshuva*, reminding us of our ancestors' sins as well as our own. This humiliation leads to openness and a desire for improvement and, it is hoped, actual betterment—resulting in fewer calamities visited upon us from on high. An impending sense of doom hovers over this kind of fasting, providing an explicit link to the nature of fasting as a doorway to death. During fasts, "all the people go out to the cemetery after praying and weep and offer supplications, as if to say, 'Unless you return from your [sinful] ways, you are like these deceased people.'" According to Talmudic commentary, this passage emphasizes the just nature of the world: we suffer because we are being punished for being unvirtuous—and furthermore, that the living need the dead to intercede on their behalf. The alleviation of present unhappiness depends on connections to the past, and these connections are opened through fasting. Trouble in the world creates the need for contemplative fasting, according to the Talmud. "When there is peace in the world and the

Temple is standing, these days will be times of joy and gladness; when there is persecution and troubles for the Jewish people, they are days of fasting; and when there is no persecution but still no peace, neither particular troubles nor consolation for Israel, the *halakha* is as follows: If people wish, they fast, and if they wish, they do not fast."

Jewish fasting was not, however, a way to earn divine mercy, as it often was for the Puritans. Fasting came after the calamity and was an investment in the future. It was a holy act, but not a magical one. A quote from Talmudic literature, cited by classicist and food historian Veronika E. Grimm, underscores that Jewish fasting needed to occur in a time of tranquility:

> *Fasting was forbidden to the inhabitants of a city under siege or one endangered by floods, to those on board a ship, "for a person pursued by Gentiles or by brigands or by a demon, for all these it is not right to afflict themselves by fasting, otherwise they would not conserve their strength." The concern with saving life and health generally overrode the wish for fasting.*

....

For several centuries until the destruction of the Second Temple, a mystic Jewish sect of communitarians known as the Essenes flourished in the Dead Sea area. While there is considerable debate over who the Essenes were and what they believed, according to accounts by contemporaries such as Pliny the Elder and Josephus, all possessions, including clothing, were held in common in these ascetic centers. Any income derived by sect members was turned over to a purser, whose responsibility it was to purchase food and anything else the group could not make for itself. Like the Shakers of eighteenth-century New England, they lived simply, valued prayer and fasting, and did not engage in sexual relations.

The Essenes disappeared after the destruction of Jerusalem by the

Roman general Titus. Most likely they were victims of a push toward a strictly cohesive orthodoxy by the surviving Jewish spiritual leaders, the Pharisees, who in the aftermath of the chaos resulting from the destruction of the Second Temple insisted on a unified religion. The Pharisees became the rabbinate, a loose confederation. The desert dwellers, once revered for their devotion to the spiritual, were characterized as renegades and were eventually even physically attacked. Their communities were disbanded. Now everyone hated and feared these anarchists: early Christians shared an anti-Essene bias with the Jewish rabbis, but for different reasons. The Jewish sect seemed uncomfortably close to the early Church, which shared its beliefs, ideals, and rites. While some scholars say that John the Baptist was a member of the Essene community, primarily due to his austerity and his association with fasting, for many Christians the suggestion that Christianity was the outgrowth of a ragged bunch of Jewish outcasts, rather than a new and revolutionary way of worship, is the worst sort of blasphemy. The Essenes, like the Epicureans, disappeared as both a living community and an obvious spiritual influence.

In 1947, in the desert around Qumran in what is now occupied Palestine, the Bedouin shepherd Muhammad ed-Dib was looking for a lost sheep when he discovered a cave containing a number of ancient Hebrew scrolls. Another cave containing scrolls was discovered in 1952, again by Bedouin shepherds, and then many more caves were discovered in the following years. Most historians—with the notable exception of certain rabbinic scholars, who to this day seem to nurse an anti-Essene bias—felt the scrolls were the remnants of the Essene community mentioned by Pliny the Elder and others. The result has been a postwar explosion of interest in the Essenes and their pre-Pharisaic Judaism.

Although the Essenes have become a byword among many New Age followers for a certain kind of ascetic, desert-centered lifestyle, the so-called "Essene diet" is based on the notorious forgery of an early-twentieth-century Hungarian psychologist. Nonetheless, the Essenes do appear to have followed an ascetic philosophy that focused on fasting in its various forms in their religious life. By turning away from worldly goods, they exemplified an enduring strand of fasting philosophy, one that heavily influenced the early Church.

The early Christians saw mind and body as one. Just as the body influences the mind through pain or ecstasy, mind and spirit influence the body. Ecstatic self-mortification was a way to come closer to God: additionally, gluttony led to out-of-control sexuality. Tertullian, a second-century Christian theologian who declared fasting central to his faith (and who praised the Epicureans for their reliance on the power of the senses), went so far as to declare that "food destroys or damages all discipline." The ideal was represented by Moses or Jesus, who each persisted without food for forty days, and who were then rewarded with a one-to-one relationship with God. And besides, fasting had a practical purpose, argued Tertullian: "An emaciated body will more readily pass the narrow gate [of paradise], a light body will resurrect more rapidly, and in the grave a wasted body will be preserved best." This near-literal interpretation of Jesus's camel/needle's eye quote ("It is easier for a camel to go through the eye of a needle, than for a rich man to enter into the Kingdom of God") was a common view. Emaciation was next to godliness, corpulence was indicative of depravity. This viewpoint was often carried to extremes, bolstered by the reasoning of Galen of Pergamum, active in the second century CE.

"The character of the soul," opined Galen, "is corrupted by bad habits in food, drink, exercise, sights, sounds, and music." Galen codified and developed medical principles based on what he understood of Hippocrates. Thanks largely to attentive self-promotion—he wrote at least two books about his own books, in translation titled *On My Own Books* and *On the Order of My Own Books*—his writings became popular and remained in the medical canon for the better part of 1,400 years. Galen saw the body as a sort of miniature weather system, prone to imbalance, one that required extreme vigilance to maintain. Imperfection was a constant. The self was therefore in continuous need of recalibration. When the four "humors"—blood, yellow bile, black bile, and phlegm—were out of balance, trouble manifested itself in the form of disease, depression, anxiety, licentiousness, and so on. Each humor was associated with two of four characteristics: heat, cold, moisture, and dryness. To restore equilibrium, patients often had to undergo bloodletting and fasting. A lustful person, for example, might have an excess of blood, and therefore an excess of heat and moisture. He would need to follow a dietary regimen of the strictest abstinence. His body would cool and dry as he ate less and avoided flesh, and the likelihood of sinning would diminish as good health returned.

Galen's theories were embraced by the early Church (as they were by later Arab scholars, who helped preserve and spread his teachings) and still influence us today: every time you eat a bowl of cornflakes—introduced in 1898 as a way to tamp down the sexual impulses of hot-blooded Americans—or munch on a graham cracker, you're unwittingly adhering to Galenic dictates.

It is no accident that in Galen's short list of "bad habits" that corrupted the soul, food was number one. From its outset, Christianity has had a tortured relation with food and eating. As the first sin, gluttony is at the origin of all other cardinal sins, notes food historian Ken Albala:

> *Avarice, or failure to practice charity with surplus food; pride, in showing off one's bounty; sloth, in the consequent torpor that derives from overeating; envy, from the desire to obtain luxuries enjoyed by others; and, most importantly, wrath and lust, which were considered the physiological by-products of gourmandism.*

It seems appropriate that the second-century inventor of the asterisk, Origen, was a prolific faster and a champion of the practice. What is occasional fasting but a series of prolonged asterisks appended to the text of life? And food has always been associated with temptation. Apart from the consumption of a luscious apple causing the expulsion from the Garden of Eden, it was during dinner, Origen wrote, that the devil corrupted Judas Iscariot. In his writings Origen often expounded—over the course of much verbiage; he reportedly wrote more than six thousand works, of which plenty have survived—on the power of faith as a means to stave off hunger and thirst on both a spiritual and physical level. "Who could ever thirst if he had a spring inside himself?" he asked. The Egyptian theologian was a pacifist with a tolerance for new ideas unusual for the era. He believed that the Bible was full of allegories not meant to be taken literally, and that the accumulation of wisdom—his own included—was an organic process, one that developed over time. Except where he professes his absolute belief in the power of the Church, Origen often admits to not being sure that he has reached the perfect solution to a problem under consideration. His hesitancy is what makes him a continuing subject of fascination. Long after his death, Origen's belief that knowledge evolved and therefore that change was often positive led to his being condemned by Christian theologians and the Byzantine emperor Justinian I, who burned Origen's books for the philosophical threat that they represented to the concept of empire and eternal, unchanging order.

The fasting ascetics of the first half of the first millennium included the proudly illiterate St. Anthony, otherwise known as Anthony the Great or Anthony of the Desert, the "Father of Monks." The illiteracy was not a by-product of his asceticism, but integral to it. Anthony, the quintessential desert recluse, is described as *choosing* not to learn how to read (and as a child, choosing to avoid friendships) in the *Life of Anthony*, attributed to a follower of Origen. These decisions should not be mistaken for a rejection of the need for additional learning, or, in the case of Anthony's self-estrangement, mere unfriendliness. It was fasting from earthly knowledge. By committing himself early on to a life of total fasting—rejecting not only conventional amounts of food and comfort, but conventional knowledge and relationships—Anthony sought to become the empty vessel of Philippians 2, opening himself up to an emptiness that allowed space for divine enlightenment. It also enabled him to participate in an oral tradition that eliminated any intermediary between him and holiness. In one anecdote in *Life*, when Greek visitors remarked on his apparent ignorance, Anthony asked them which came first, the mind or letters—and did the mind cause letters, or letters cause the mind? The answer that the mind came first led to Anthony's questionable conclusion that, with a sound mind, literacy is unnecessary. The Greeks left, "astonished" at Anthony's rhetorical brilliance. Writing is at the mercy of its author, Anthony has reminded them, and it is corrupted by its passage through the flawed filter of human understanding.

The distrust of written knowledge is also at the heart of another kind of fasting, the fasting from speech reflected in the vows of silence undertaken by many of the hermits and later monastic orders such as the Trappists. If writing is a step removed from understanding, so is speech itself. The very act of speaking, the physical breathiness of uttering a word, transforms and debases it. And yet, for the early Christian ascetics, ascetic discipline was "a science of imitation," with the best students the closest to God. The new religion attracted unusual devotees such as Simeon the Stylite, revered for sitting atop his column for thirty-seven years (and then for impassively observing his gangrenous leg as it rotted). Control of the self was paramount, but so was intensity of devotion. The asceticism of the desert cultists became almost a contest: when Macarius of Alexandria heard of other hermits who ate less than he, he restricted himself to eating "only a few cabbage leaves on Sundays." Admittedly, the image of desiccated old men trying to outdo one another in extremes of self-deprivation is not the most enticing argument for fasting.

....

Extreme fasting, and fasting from society, was not exclusively the domain of men, or even primarily of men. In the early fifth century, an official at the court of Byzantine emperor Theodosius II commissioned a report on the desert ascetics now known as *The Lausiac History*. Its author, Palladius, estimated that the number of women living the ascetic life outnumbered men by two to one. Yet until recently, the formative role of women in early Christian asceticism has been at best glossed over and more often completely ignored. Church historians' focus on the Desert Fathers made it seem as though women were irrelevant to the movement.

In fact, their contributions may have been methodically eradicated. The *Asketikon* or *Rule* of St. Basil of Caesarea, who was active in the fourth century CE, has long been credited with setting the standard for asceticism in a communitarian setting. The historian Susanna Elm convincingly makes the case that Basil had codified the example laid out by his mother, Emmelia, and his sister, Macrina, several years previously. The women, who came from the wealthiest stratus of Cappadocian society, had subdivided their possessions, freed their slaves, and abolished any class distinctions in their extended circle, planning an egalitarian model for a monastic community on the southern coast of the Black Sea. Such an act, while not unprecedented in the ancient world (recall Epicurus's willingness to treat slaves as equals) was unusual. These Desert Mothers had shattered a social barrier and transformed "an ascetic household into an ascetic institution."

While a few women in this period openly rejected the standard maternal route and lived the physically and spiritually demanding life mandated by desert asceticism, others did so undercover. The Greek Orthodox Church records ten holy women who dressed as men and lived in male-only monasteries, and others must have passed unremarked. Of the acknowledged women monastics, one of the most celebrated was Amma Theodora of Alexandria, who in the fifth century CE dressed as a man and spent two years in a monastery. Reviled by her fellow monks for her extreme piety, she was expelled on trumped-up charges for fornicating with a woman in a nearby village, "even being presented with a child as evidence of her sin." Her deception was only discovered upon her death. Persistent if brief references to other female ascetics establish that Theodora, Emmelia, and Macrina, while not typical ascetics, were not outliers. These independent-minded women participated in all ascetic practices, including extreme fasting:

> Once some travelers heard in the desert the groan of a sick person.
> They discovered a cave, where a "certain holy virgin" lay on the ground.
> She said: "Behold, I have passed eight and thirty years in this cave

and I have satisfied my wants with grass, for I labor with Christ." ...
Having said that, she died on the spot.

As Susanna Elm observes, for "the perfect ascetic the question of male or female no longer exists, because he or she has risen above the limits determined by the body; asceticism means annihilation of sexual distinction. The desert 'mothers' present the opportunity to introduce yet another nuance into the development of this concept."

But ascetic purity withered in the face of intractable misogyny. One of the leading ascetics was the fourth-century priest and historian Jerome of Stridon, later known as St. Jerome. Although Jerome was aware of Buddha—Jerome refers to him as having been born from a virgin—he apparently did not absorb Buddha's message of the middle way. He was a fanatical proponent of fasting, which he took as a marker of the Christian hero:

I saw monks: one lived as a recluse for thirty years on coarse barley bread and muddy water; another subsisted on five dried figs a day. . . . These things will seem unbelievable to those who do not believe that all things are possible for those who believe.

The saint, whose work became a cornerstone for early Christian thinking, devoted much of his study to documenting the sexual depravity of women, and generously offered his advice to his wealthy female devotees. His exhortations are couched in loathing and what has been characterized as "extreme hostility" toward women, who in his eyes tended to overeat and overheat in every sense. In his many letters, he urges women to avoid dining for pleasure, to hold themselves apart, and "to fast for the sole purpose of cooling their 'hot little bodies.'" By this point, thanks to Emperor Constantine, Christianity had become the official religion of the Roman Empire. Jerome's reactionary outlook correlated with imperial needs. It also tied fasting to physical self-hatred and extremism, associations that still color many people's view of the practice.

Jerome was both fascinated and repulsed by women, as he was by his antecedent Origen, whose work he annotated and condemned. In Origen's extensive analysis of the raciest parts of the Holy Bible—the Song of Solomon ("Let him kiss me with the kisses of his mouth: for thy love is better than wine. . . . A bundle of myrrh is my well-beloved unto me; he shall lie all night betwixt my breasts")—he had made the case that agape (spiritual love) and eros (physical love) were one and the same. In Jerome's eyes, this argument flirted with outright blasphemy.

From Jerome's own writing, it is clear that he found serenity elusive at best. His constant battle was against longing. No gesture or mode of living was innocent. His acolyte, Paula, fasted from cleanliness, maintaining that a dirty mind revealed itself in a clean dress: too much attention to worldly values, including cleanliness, meant vanity. A carelessness in presentation of the physical self, or so the reasoning went, revealed sacrifice of the ego and therefore personal virtue. This logic is hardly surprising given the female menace outlined by male theologians of the period. Women were more than sexual mates, but less than intellectual partners, and always a threat. They represented the ties of home and society, of body and family, of all things the holy men wanted to leave behind. They were a pull to the physical. Women who wanted to join the ascetic community therefore had particular obligations placed on them. They knew to suppress the awareness of their bodies to avoid outside attention. Their burden was particularly heavy, as their most remote ancestor (Eve) had brought about the Fall—they were forever tainted.

For Jerome, the unquenchable hunger for purity substituted itself for the unquenchable hunger for food. Fasting became Jerome's scourge of the sin of fornication. Food was the source of body heat, and heat generated in the belly was related to heat generated below the belly, what Daniel Boyarin has aptly called the "antics of the lower body." Appetite should be suppressed in all things—particularly women's appetite. Jerome's view was not unique for the era, but he pursued the idea of women's innate frailty and wickedness with a singular intensity. His devotions to the necessity of female asceticism likely led to the death by starvation of at least one of his followers, Blaesilla. Jerome had convinced Blaesilla—the aforementioned Paula's eldest daughter—to remain a widow after the death of her husband. She would be married only to Jesus, cooling any latent passions by severely restricting her intake of food. When she starved to death in her early twenties, Jerome proclaimed her "the victor in the struggle against Satan." The wisdom of her choices was later affirmed when the Church named Blaesilla a saint.

In the aftermath of Blaesilla's death, many Romans were outraged and blamed Jerome, and he was forced to flee the city together with some of his followers. Years later, another of his cult, one Laeta, sister-in-law of the unfortunate Blaesilla, petitioned Jerome for advice on the upbringing of her daughter, also named Paula. In a wide-ranging response in 403 CE, Jerome condemned "long and immoderate fasts" on the one hand and on the other hand acknowledged the heroic quality of the perpetual faster (see his "Letter to Laeta"). For "the virgin and the monk," indefatigable Christian warriors, there could be no intermission from fasting. He wrote admiringly of the "cold chastity [of a Christian virgin who] seeks to put out the flame of lust and to quench the hot desires of youth." For many Christians of this period, the importance of devout ascetics' fasting seemed to have less to do with echoing the martyrdom of Jesus than with purification and smothering the lustful, avaricious enemy that lurked within.

Unlike Jewish scholars, who saw fasting as a means of making spiritual atonement real, for Jerome fasting was a weapon with which to mortify the flesh and to preserve chastity. His fear of the body and his obsession with sex became important guidelines for the Church. His teachings were leavened somewhat by the gentler words of his North African contemporary Augustine of Hippo, a faster for whom food was medicine, as he wrote in his *Confessions*. In contrast to Jerome, Augustine, the most humane of saints (he reprised his youthful self's prayer to God in book VIII of the *Confessions*: "Give me chastity and continence, only not yet!") urges moderation as the ideal where food was concerned (sex was another matter).

Gluttony was abhorrent, but so were all forms of excess. In a return to the classic Judaic interpretation, fasting was a means to an end. Augustine was a convert to Christianity from Manichaeanism, a religion that came out of Persia in the third century CE and to which fasting is integral. For Manichaeans, the devil Ahriman was committed to an ages-long war in which he drained divine light from the supreme deity Zurvan, trapping portions of the light in physical matter. Permanent fasting for the religion's spiritual leaders during daylight hours helped slow the transfer of divine light to corporeality.

Augustine imagines the body as the "servant" of the soul, its master, just as the soul is a servant to God. While the soul holds in check the body's desires, these longings cannot be permanently extinguished, and an attempt to do so would be disastrous. Fasting is not about giving up food altogether; it is about abstaining from food that particularly gives pleasure. Augustine applies the principle of self-denial to fasting itself: overindulgence is bad in any form.

....

The sayings of the desert sages, which began to circulate widely in the fourth and fifth centuries CE, have a certain Zen-like, ultra-Stoic quality. "Think on the loss, and feel the pain." "Wherever you stay, be in no hurry to move." The man who "controls and forces himself to be content with necessities and nothing more, that man is a monk." "Go and sit in your cell, and your cell will teach you everything." The fifth-century philosopher John Cassian, sometimes known as John the Ascetic, was actually a cosmopolitan by any century's standards. Although his origins are unclear, he spent time in Bethlehem, Constantinople, and Rome, studied under various Egyptian hermits in the Nile delta, and founded a monastery in Marseille. His writings helped spread Greek theories of ascetic spirituality and became central to monastic life throughout Europe. Although a proponent of fasting, Cassian also advocated for regular mealtimes and a balanced diet. He taught that the hermit, for him the exemplar of a Christian way of life, was as directed and driven as any merchant: the immediate goal (*skopos*) was purity of heart, and the ultimate goal (*telos*) was the kingdom of heaven. Here he quotes one of the Egyptian sages on hermetic life: "For this [ultimate goal] he endures every kind of labor tirelessly, even gratefully. For this he grows not weary of fasting, enjoys the fatigue of watching in the night, is not tired by the continual reading of the Scriptures and meditation upon them, bears even the naked and grinding poverty and loneliness of life in this desert."

The attraction of self-mortification is clear: the further an adherent can push herself, the closer she can come to God and to the body's "natural" Edenic state, self-sufficient and needing minimal sustenance. Eccentricity and extremism became occupational hazards for devotees of the young religion, and fasting was fundamental to the process, valued primarily for its role in attacking the flesh. Ascetics were not so much in pursuit of spiritualism as they were lusting for extreme discomfort and pain:

> *Reading the lives of fourteenth- and fifteenth-century women saints greatly expands one's knowledge of Latin synonyms for whip, thong, flail, chain, etc. Ascetic practices commonly reported in these* vitae *include wearing hair shirts, binding the flesh tightly with twisted ropes, rubbing lice into self-inflicted wounds, denying oneself sleep, adulterating food and water with ashes or salt, performing thousands of genuflections, thrusting nettles into one's breasts, and praying barefoot in winter. Among the more bizarre female behaviors were rolling in broken glass, jumping into ovens, hanging from a gibbet, and praying upside down.*

The medieval concern with gluttony can scarcely be overemphasized. Sumptuary laws were enacted on a regular basis to restrict commoners from wearing certain types of jewelry and clothing, and even from using beeswax candles. These laws were adopted largely on the principle of tamping down excessive consumption, which was thought to be "un-Christian." The laws also served to reinforce class barriers and to associate earthly authority with divinity. Some laws specifically referenced "Christian morals" and were seen as "a way to curb the sins of pride, vanity, gluttony, and even lust." Even something as seemingly innocent as breakfast was a step on the road that led straight to hell. In his *Summa Theologica*, the medieval philosopher Thomas Aquinas concludes that eating "hastily" (or too soon) is symptomatic of one of the deadly sins—gluttony.

Aquinas felt that to wake up, leap to the table, and gobble down breakfast forestalled a considered and controlled ingestion of food. For early Christian ascetics, a lack of appetite was not necessarily as symptomatic of depression as it is today; the desire for breakfast was an indication of runaway appetites that didn't stop at the stomach. The suppression of such appetites was a sign of devotion to a higher power. In the fifth century, the *Rule* of Benedict of Nursia, later known as Saint Benedict, specified that the monastic community was generally to partake of two meals, with exceptions being made for fast days and Lent, when eating was postponed to the afternoon.

What was called *inedia*—fasting to the point of death—was valued by the Church and was one of the criteria for canonization. By simultaneously urging moderation and venerating people who starved to death, it is no wonder that the religion fostered self-starvation in its most devout followers. Ordinary people, whose commitment was less than absolute, could not withstand the rigors of genuine devotion.

It was several generations before fasting's role as a signifier of spirituality, rather than a weapon against the sins of the flesh, was reaffirmed. For Meister Eckhart, *Gelassenheit*, or "letting-go," and *Abgeschiedenheit*, or "detachment," were essential for an understanding of the divine. Throughout his work, he returned again and again to the idea that it is only through emptying oneself that one may approach spiritual "fullness": "What is inferior is always empty, what is perfect is never so." And again, "No cask can hold two different kinds of drink," he wrote, echoing St. Augustine. "If it is to contain wine, then they must of necessity pour the water out; the cask must become empty and free. . . . To be empty transforms nature; emptiness makes water flow uphill and other marvels of which we need not now speak." Eckhart's concern with fullness was both literal and symbolic. He abjures us to leave what would later be called ego behind, to observe ourselves and to leave ourselves.

Fasting and Christian asceticism were seen as implicitly "feminine" exercises. Fasters and ascetics rejected the physical and sought to be impregnated with spiritual insight. Claims that Origen had castrated himself (which he denied) reinforced the impression. Christian ascetics of both sexes referred to themselves as "brides of Christ," wanting nothing more than to be filled solely with Christ's Word: Hildegard of Bingen had a vision of "Woman," dressed as Eve, collecting Christ's blood and hearing a voice telling her to eat and drink it in order both to annul Eve's sin and to receive enlightenment. And Eckhart explicitly wrote that "For a man to conceive God in himself is good, and in his conceiving he is a maiden." Eckhart cited as an inspiration the eleventh-century sage Solomon Ibn Gabirol, a Jewish poet who lived in Al-Andalus (Muslim Spain). Given his open reliance on a Jewish sage, it is unsurprising that Eckhart was tried as a heretic by the Inquisition; he died at the age of sixty-eight before a verdict was reached. According to the pope, Eckhart supposedly recanted his beliefs on his deathbed.

....

Some scholars of religion argue that the traditional male/female division was further eroded by the image of Jesus himself, who embraced fasting, self-denial, and embodied reversal; a slight and suffering lord, even one who himself became female: "a lactating and birthing mother, nurturer of others." Similarly, argues Caroline Walker Bynum, so did the female fasting ascetics often reject traditional roles as nurturers and become bold spiritual recipients of holy wisdom. "In union with the dying Christ, women became a fully fleshly and feeding self—at one with the generative suffering of God. Women's eating, fasting and feeding others were synonymous acts, because in all three the woman, by suffering, fused with a cosmic suffering that really redeemed the world."

From medieval times through to the first part of the twentieth century, extreme adherence to fasting signaled not only virtue but access to the spiritual plane. Such fasters were therefore seen as emissaries possessed of special knowledge. Often but not exclusively, women who renounced marital life in favor of taking God as their husband, the saints who battled their bodies without mercy, were treated as sages who not only had a divine connection but had undertaken the task for the sake of all humanity. As documented by scholar Rudolph M. Bell in his study of Italian women whose fasting feats were detailed in the Catholic Church's *Bibliotheca Sanctorum*, these women were consulted by popes and kings, elevated by their conspicuous self-sacrifice to a prominence that they were unlikely to have otherwise achieved.

Catherine of Siena, one of the best-known of all holy fasters, was a confidante of Pope Gregory XI, whom she addressed as *dolcissimo Babbo* ("sweetest Daddy"). Many other examples abound: the fifteenth-century Swiss ascetic saint, Nicholas of Flüe, who was supposed to have fasted for nineteen years, living solely on water and communion wafers, is often cited as the Ur-father of modern Switzerland for his supernatural ability to bring about peace between the warring rural and urban cantons. But medieval fasters who rejected daily routine and opened themselves up to the supernatural realm were not always assumed to be in contact with the divine. Often they were suspected of being possessed or influenced by the devil, which was a dangerous accusation during the Inquisition. Even Catherine of Siena was accused of being fed by devils at night. Jerome's constant inveighing against women contributed to the belief in the pervasiveness of witches, who were almost exclusively women. This public panic gathered momentum in the fifteenth century with the publication of the ominously titled *Malleus Maleficarum* (*The Hammer of Witches*), a 1486 witch-hunting manual written by two inquisitors for the Catholic Church. While formerly belief in witches had been deemed to be heretical, now *failure* to believe in their existence was heretical. Witches were held to be part of "an international Satanic movement aiming at blasphemy and the undermining of the Roman Catholic Church."

They were known to have little flesh on their bones; their lack of a fleshy anchor proved their connection to the devil. Witches could fly because the good earth rejected their unholy tread.

The fact lay at the root of a peculiar method to prove bewitchment: the "weighing test." The design of this test was of staggering simplicity. If a woman's weight on the scale turned out to be less than what might be reasonably expected considering her stature, this was evidence of bewitchment.

Whether diabolically or divinely inspired, extreme fasting was proof of connection to the supernatural. Even if it was seen as not outright devil's work, it presented a problem. Since suicide or self-harm was a mortal sin, Christian leaders regularly associated excessive fasting with the sin of pride, and reminded monks and nuns to moderate their fasts. God had provided food for humanity to enjoy, and some theologians felt that extreme fasting demonstrated a childlike rejection of this divine gift. Moderation itself, whether in fasting or in eating, is an ancient virtue; in the original Aramaic, Abaddon ("doom," also the "angel of the bottomless pit," the angel that knows no satiety) is paired with Sheol, the place of the dead, in Proverbs 27:20: "Sheol and Abaddon are insatiable." An unending appetite for abstinence was no more a sign of spiritual understanding than an unending appetite for luxuries. In the King James Version, this passage is translated as "Hell and destruction are never full; so the eyes of man are never satisfied." This modification of the original strengthens the association of constant dissatisfaction, the ceaseless quest for more, with destruction and the place of the dead. But there were other, more practical reasons to oppose extreme fasting, particularly in religious communities: it deprived monasteries and convents of much-needed labor, as long-term fasters were too weak to help their brethren and furthermore required the ministrations of others to help them survive. They became a burden.

....

During Ramadan, the only fasting period specified in the Quran, observant Muslims regard daily fasting as fulfilling the promise of the fourth of the

Five Pillars of the religion. (The other pillars are the profession of faith, prayer, charity, and the hajj, or pilgrimage to Mecca.) The monthlong fast requires complete dawn-to-sunset abstinence from food, all forms of liquid, smoking, and sex. Ramadan holds out the offer of forgiveness for the sins of the previous year. Distinct from Islam's ancestor religions, this period of fasting is imbued with the promise of celebration and excitement. For Jews and Christians, fasting carried the threat of divine menace. In Leviticus chapter sixteen of the Torah (a holy book in Islam as well, known as the Tawrat), God imposes the Day of Atonement on his followers shortly after having incinerated Aaron's sons Nadab and Abihu for the sin of offering "unauthorized fire" at the holy altar. The gravity of the day is reiterated in Leviticus chapter twenty-three, wherein the Lord decrees that non-fasters will be shunned ("cut off from among his people") and that more obdurate non-fasters—those who continued working as usual—would be killed ("the same soul will I destroy"). In contrast, the fasting of Ramadan comes as a gentler, soothing request. In the Quran, the holy period is presented almost as an offer, a vacation from daily cares:

> So any one of you who sees in that month should fast, and anyone who is ill or on a journey should make up for the lost days by fasting on other days later. God wants ease for you, not hardship. He wants you to complete the prescribed period and to glorify Him for having guided you, so that you may be thankful.

The Quran states that even believers for whom fasting is simply too daunting can be exempted. In that case, non-fasting Muslims are expected "to feed a needy person."

For devout Muslims, fasting is not a door to something else, as it is for Christians during Lent, the long gateway before the resurrection of Easter. The fasting of Muslims is an end in itself. And it is not a burden to be endured as proof of religious devotion or sincerity of repentance, as Yom Kippur (the Day of Atonement) is for most Jews. The close of

Ramadan is capped by Eid al-Fitr, the "feast of the breaking of the fast," when people give gifts, visit their families, and bestow blessings. A typical Eid blessing is "May Allah accept all your prayers and forgive all your faults." Another is simply "*Eid Mubarak*": "Blessed feast." In Ramadan, the emphasis is not on fear and trembling; it is on joy, thankfulness, and quiet contemplation. Its festive character sets it apart from the heavy themes of regret and guilt that mark both Christian and Jewish fasting. Ramadan is also not associated with a particular period of the year, as Lent is with winter's end and Yom Kippur is with the autumn. Muslims follow the lunar year, which is shorter than the solar year by eleven days. Within a thirty-three-year cycle, Ramadan moves through all the seasons.

Shaykh Suhaib Webb, a scholar in residence at New York University's Islamic Center, tells me that he sees the unity brought on by Ramadan's fasting as a way to counter "the hyper-individualism of Western spirituality, which is rooted in untethering yourself to find meaning." For most Muslims, God is found through "the legal conformity of Islam." "Through that adherence to the law, you are now engaging the knower of all, the transcendent God, who is going to give you *kesh*, the capacity to lift the veils," he says. Webb cites the nineteenth-century Moroccan scholar and mystic Ahmad Ibn Ajibba, who wrote that the highest spiritual state is freedom, but a distinct type of freedom brought about through submission to the divine. Essential steps on this path involve turning away from narcissism and hubris, "living vicariously through faith instead of letting faith live vicariously through us—and within that very clearly is included fasting." Webb tells me that "in Arabic, the passive is meant to inspire awe—the crux of it is, by minimalizing your intake to that of sustainability instead of opulence, you are freed from being overly and unhealthily attached to the material, so that now you can have a relationship with something that transcends the material, and that's really the goal of fasting." The material world in Islam is not necessarily evil, but it is transient. In Arabic, the word *dunya* is used to describe the earthly realm: a stopping place for souls on their way elsewhere.

In recent years, the Ramadan fast has become a focus of the Chinese government's determination to stamp out independent streaks in the Uyghur and Turkic Muslim communities. In the Xinjiang Uyghur Autonomous Region of western China, a vast area of about 26 million people, officials have severely restricted the number of those permitted to fast in an attempt to "Sinicize" Islam and to avoid "negative effects on children's minds," according to one village administrator. Only a limited number of the elderly and people without children are allowed to fast. Violators can be sent to one of the many internment camps scattered throughout the region, where approximately 1.8 million people have been undergoing involuntary reeducation since 2017. Authorities have told those living in the region that they must provide names of anyone fasting, which has been labeled a terrorist-adjacent activity promulgated and practiced only by extremists. Some Uyghurs understandably feel that the best course of action is to assert that no one is fasting during Ramadan. "Oh, no— there's no such thing now," said one local when asked if he intended to fast during Ramadan. But Islamic traditions, and consequently fasting, stubbornly persist. "Fasting in the eyes of the Chinese [government] is not about eating less and peacefully staying at home," Shohret Hoshur, an expatriate Uyghur journalist, wrote me. "[It is] about gathering together with religious fervor, sharing grievances with one another, getting angry after grievances, and then making plans to act against the Chinese. So fasting worries and scares the Chinese authorities." Hoshur cited two episodes in recent history as evidence: the 2013 Aykol incident, where several people were killed, and the Elishku massacre, where by some accounts two thousand Uyghurs were killed. "Both happened on the last day of Ramadan," Hoshur pointed out. Even within a traditional religious framework, fasting disrupts daily routine. If you fast, you reconsider. Such an action is necessarily inimical to dictatorship.

....

With the Christian Reformation, extreme fasting in the West, at least as a doctrine of everyday religion, underwent a decline until the dawn of the Industrial Age. Increasingly, the Catholic hierarchy frowned on the practice: apart from the dangers of committing the sin of pride and imposing a burden on the religious community, a growing understanding of how the body works, the exposure of fasting frauds, and the threat of unsanctioned interpreters of the divine made a strong argument for clerical opposition to the holy fasters. At the same time, while the philosophers of the Reformation—Martin Luther, John Calvin, and Ulrich Zwingli—all rejected fasting as essential to salvation, they incorporated many of its tenets into the ascetic core of the movement. For these reformers, limited fasting on specific occasions was seen as a means for affirming a shared history, generating communal empathy, and responding to adversity. Fasting under Protestantism became both symbolic and spiritual preparation for receiving the divine Word. It was not a path to salvation, as it had been for Catholics: Catholics fasted to purify their bodies in preparation for receiving the physical body of Christ.

For Protestant factions such as the Puritans, fasting was a method of self-improvement. The Cambridge academic Thomas Cartwright (1535–1603), the preeminent leader of the Puritans in the era of Elizabeth I, placed rigorous fasting at the center of worship. A fasting Puritan abstained from food, but also sex, "fancy clothing," and even sleep. Likely influenced by Cartwright, the English parliament at the time regularly called for civil fasts in response to all variety of crises. Cartwright is presumed to be the author (as indicated by the initials "T.C.") of the 1580 treatise *The Holie Exercise of a True Fast, Described out of God's Word*, which at its start observes:

> that like children newe come into the worlde, we know not when to eate, and when to forbeare eating, no further then we have our declaration of God's Word. But it is yet more marvell, that in so small a matter, scarse the hundred person, of those which professe the name of Christ, know either how to enter into this way, or howe to turne them in it when they are entered, to any glory of God, or profite to themselves.

Cartwright spends much of the book inveighing against the "Popish" and their fasting habits, which he deemed insufficiently rigorous. During fasts, Catholics and members of the Church of England concocted elaborate meat substitutes that molded sugar, spice, eggs, nuts, and fruits into the shapes of birds and beef, making the fast a period of celebration instead of mourning, a practice of which Cartwright strongly disapproved.

In 1604, Englishman Nicholas Bownde wrote *The Holy Exercise of Fasting*, laying out the principles of fasting for Puritans. A fast was done on two levels, the "outward" and the "inward":

> *The outward appertaineth to the body, and is called a Bodily exercise,*
> *as to abstaine from meat, drinke, sleepe, and such like; . . . the other*
> *is belonging to the soule, and consisteth in the inward vertues and*
> *graces of the minde holpen [helped] forward by this bodily exercise.*

The fasting tradition quickly took root in the Puritans' overseas colonies. Once established, it persisted for several centuries, particularly in the New England area. In emergencies, it provided a way to appeal directly for divine intervention. Just three years after they had established themselves at Plymouth, in the spring of 1623, the Puritans found their settlement on the edge of collapse. "Half-naked" and "full of sadness," they were slowly starving to death—and then they were hit by a two-month drought. The leaders called for a day of fasting and humiliation. Historian Martha L. Finch dramatically depicts the scene:

> *Throughout the "parched" day, hour after desperate hour, they sat in*
> *the close, still air of the meetinghouse in fervent supplication, while*
> *outside "it was clear weather, and very hot, and not a cloud nor any*
> *sign of rain to be seen." Yet, in the evening, as they returned to their*
> *homes, "it began to be overcast, and shortly after to rain, with such*
> *sweet and gentle showers" that "the earth was thoroughly wet and*
> *soaked therewith, which did so apparently revive and quicken the*
> *decayed corn and other fruits, as was wonderful."*

Subsequently, the English colonists called for hundreds of days of fasting in response to disaster and hardship (and, alternately, a thanksgiving in response to bountiful harvests). These were constant reminders of their tenuous hold on physical existence in tandem with their unshakable dependence on divine providence—providence that was granted or withheld only in accordance with their piety. Fasting, too, was an implicit rebuke to selfishness: "The Fatter the Soil, the Ranker the Weeds" went a Puritan saying. The Reverend Cotton Mather, the second-generation Puritan preacher, who together with his father, Increase Mather, was an advocate of witch-hunting (and defended the results of the Salem witch trials in his *The Wonders of the Invisible World* [1693]), was a firm believer in the powers of fasting (accompanied by prayer) as a cure for all ills, but also warned of its dark side: he cautioned that extreme or "long fasting is not only tolerable but strangely agreeable for such as have something more to do with the Invisible World," meaning witches.

While the New Englanders were the most fervent of the colonizers in their application of fasting, Dutch Reformed congregations in New York and numerous groups from South Carolina to New Hampshire were also committed to the practice. Fasting was later adopted by rebels throughout the colonies. "A day of fasting, humiliation, and prayer" was the immediate answer Thomas Jefferson and other members of the Virginia House of Burgesses in 1774 put forth to protest the Intolerable Acts imposed by George III. While as president Jefferson held that prayer should be a private choice and not a national mandate, he saw the fast day as a means to rouse "our people from the lethargy into which they had fallen." This tripartite form of self-denial ("fasting, humiliation, and prayer") became a sort of American Protestant mantra. The Continental Congress regularly declared national days of fasting and prayer "to frustrate the cruel purposes of our unnatural enemies," as John Hancock wrote in 1776. All understood fasting to be a *natural* exercise, one that comes from our untutored nature and is unsullied by artifice. It takes us back to our origins.

National fast days in the young nation were special, but not extraordinary occurrences. Continuing the long tradition of fasting in response to crisis, President James Madison decreed a fasting day not three months after the destruction of Washington, D.C., by the British in 1814 and just before peace talks with the English were scheduled to begin. When "Old Tippecanoe"—President William Henry Harrison—died in 1841, just one month after his inauguration, a national fast was declared. President Zachary Taylor made "a recommendation" that August 1, 1849, be observed as a national day of "Fasting, Humiliation, and Prayer" because of "a fearful pestilence, which is spreading itself throughout the land." And Abraham Lincoln declared at least three national fast days during his presidency. In March 1863, a few days after a Union attempt to take Vicksburg failed, Lincoln decreed in his Proclamation 97 "a day of humiliation, fasting, and prayer," saying that Americans had become "intoxicated with unbroken success" and "too self-sufficient to feel the necessity of redeeming and preserving grace, too proud to pray to the God that made us!" For Lincoln, humility came first.

While fasting had regularly been a means for mobilizing the faithful through churches and was a stern reminder of patriotic obligations by national and local governments, it wasn't until the suffragists that it was used as a tool for mass protest. In 1899, the newly formed Afro-American Council declared June 4 a day of fasting to protest the surge in lynching throughout the South, but this was unusual: fasting had, to that point, only been employed as a sort of nationwide "note to self," a self-admonishment that would, it was hoped, bring divine favor.

Richard J. Foster, a popular Christian theologian and fasting proponent, feels that together with prayer and meditation, fasting leads to a more profound understanding of religion. He writes that fasting became a casualty of modernity's aversion to medieval fanaticism, a result of "the decline of the inward reality of the Christian faith." Extreme fasting, self-flagellation, and other physical trials were once seen as proof of godliness, and "modern culture reacts strongly to these excesses and tends to confuse fasting with self-mortification." He blames the ongoing avalanche of propaganda urging us to consume for our squeamishness with fasting: we're constantly being pressured to stuff ourselves, as though nothing were worse than being less than full. Fasting seems unnatural to a consumer society. As soon as we are placed upon the planet, we are required to ingest.

Fasting once had a competitive element that Americans found relatable. Professional fasters were on a par with champion weight lifters at the height of the Victorian period. Fasting become an odd proof of manliness, whereas among women fasting was known as the "wasting disease," or anorexia, evidence of either nervousness or some other anomaly (and in the eyes of most mainstream doctors, malingering or fraud). But these women, or "fasting girls," such as Mollie Fancher and Sarah Jacob, similarly attracted throngs to witness their extreme vulnerability, which represented a kind of womanly ideal. Fasting's popularity as a spectator sport overlapped neatly with the era's obsession with moral degeneracy, temptation, and self-restraint in personal and public behavior as manifested in endless treatises on proper decorum delivered both from the pulpit and on the printed page.

In modern Protestantism, fasting, once out of favor, seems to be coming back into vogue. But some things remain constant: achieving a fasting milestone is not for outward display, as Dr. Michael Bos, minister at New York's Marble Collegiate Church, explained to me. And even as a path to inner change, Bos said that "fasting has more of a place in churches that stress personal transformation." Bos explained that "Matthew tells us to do the best as you move forward, so that what you're doing is between you and God."

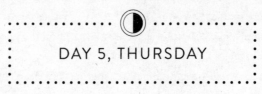

The River of Kings:
Fasting as Protest

Feel clearheaded, quite comfortable today. Decent night. Stretching seems easier. In hiking, it often seems the homeward stretch is the one where you have an accident. We shall see; things don't seem so threatening just now. What would I like to eat? The thought seems increasingly irrelevant. I think of Kafka's "A Hunger Artist," a strange story that I haven't read for half a century. I just now reread it and was happily enjoying submersion in the world of humiliation and grotesquerie, but then was jolted by the apex of the story: the Hunger Artist lies dying. The Supervisor approaches and asks him why he has undertaken such a long fast. And the Hunger Artist whispers that he hadn't been able to find a food to his liking. A macabre joke on the arbitrariness, the meaninglessness of everything—there is no meaning in eating, there is no meaning in not eating. There is a connection here to Bartleby's inability to commit (I hope not symptomatic of my own decision to fast), but Kafka's protagonist seems more self-aware. Even at this stage of his near-disappearance, the Hunger Artist recognizes he is shackled to desire, to wanting to desire. Through creating a state of want (in the sense of not having), what "healthy" fasting can point us to is a place where we want less. Today I heard a lecture by Carlo Rovelli, who was talking about the basics of quantum physics. "Properties are relational," he said. He cited the Middle Way of Nagarjuna, and said: "Entities by themselves don't exist: all the way down is relations," perhaps a reference to the joke at the beginning of Hawking's book *A Brief History of Time*: the world isn't floating in space, it rests on a giant turtle, which rests on another, and so on. It's turtles all the way down. "To be conscious is to be affected by the external world," says Rovelli. Maybe he has it wrong: to be conscious is to be affected by the internal world. The external is mechanics; he's presumably not saying ants, plants, and rocks are conscious. Or maybe he is? Rovelli also mentioned Alexander Bogdanov, a Russian pioneer of systems theory among other things, who placed emphasis on relations, in opposition to Lenin, who called him an anti-materialist, which, Rovelli says, was a misunderstanding of the position. This evening, I went to a movie theater, first time in over a year. Went out to see the film *Minari*— feasted on images of delicious Korean food. I overstate: it looked good, but I remained detached, calm. C. and I each had a "turmeric tonic" and our companion, A., had a glass of wine and a lemon square. I had no desire to have a bite, and that felt freeing.

"*Power depended upon public obedience, a will to submit.*"

— Vladimir Bukovsky, *To Build a Castle* (1978)

"*He has chosen death:*
Refusing to eat or drink, that he may bring
Disgrace upon me; for there is a custom,
An old and foolish custom; that if a man
Be wronged, or think that he is wronged,
And starve upon another's threshold till he die,
The Common People, for all time to come,
Will raise a heavy cry against that threshold,
Even though it be the King's."

—W. B. Yeats, *The King's Threshold* (1903)

How to dissent in the face of overwhelming power, and to do so effectively and peacefully, is a recurring dilemma. As the American sociologist and anti–Vietnam War activist William Gamson argued, when the authorities fail to respect the rules of the game, the most effective means of dissent are not the ones provided by institutions. For those looking for an alternative to what Gamson promoted as the "tactics of the street" (although he was careful to specify "feistiness" over violence), fasting can yet again offer a solution—but it is a solution that also carries the potential of disastrous consequences for its practitioners.

....

The River of Kings, or *Rājataraṅgiṇī*, is a twelfth-century saga of the kings of Kashmir. Throughout the saga's eight books (known as waves, or *tarangas*), the praiseworthy concept of *prāya*, fasting to the point of death, appears. In classical Sanskrit, *prāya* carries with it the connotation of a warrior's action, of sallying forth to battle. While the act of fasting might seem at an opposite extreme to the behavior of a warrior, there is a recurring cultural link between the two: the yamabushi in Japan—famed for defeating samurai in single combat—and the sannyasi in India—Hindu ascetics who developed martial arts—both valued extreme fasting. In the sixteenth century the sannyasi fought the Mughals, and in the late eighteenth century, during the Sannyasi Rebellion, they again rose up in opposition to the British East India Company. (They lost.) The routines of the Knights Templar, medieval Christian warriors, involved fasting on a regular basis. In biblical times, Jews fasted before going out to do battle with their enemies, which is today still commemorated by some during the Fast of Esther. For ancient warriors, fasting provided not only spiritual strength but martial vigor.

Prāya is normally cited in epic narratives as a means of coercing wrongdoers into correcting the error of their ways. That errant behavior could include something as ordinary as refusing to acknowledge lingering debt, or a more serious crime against oneself, or a person in one's own household. Self-harm or suicide from despair is a sin in Buddhism and Hinduism, disdained as a destructive act and "self-abandonment." But as in Christian traditions, exceptions are made for holy men and women, ascetics and martyrs.

When other means had failed, the elite Brahmans (priests), or royalty, employed *prāya*. It made a private dispute part of public discourse: the wronged person would go to the reprobate's house and there lie on his side, fasting in the doorstep until the complaint was satisfied. Onlookers would have made an immediate connection to the reclining Buddha. According to dogma, Buddha lay on his right side during his final illness, before leaving the karmic cycle and entering before attaining *paranirvana*—which in Hinduism, Jainism, Sikhism, and Buddhism has a different connotation from the loose English cognate of "paradise." In its original religious sense, nirvana is a place of absence where *sunyata*, or emptiness, has been attained. For a Christian community, the equivalent to *prāya* would have been someone blocking a doorway with arms outstretched, silently evoking the Crucifixion. But *prāya* was not merely a moral weapon. It was a very real threat with potentially drastic results. A fast-unto-death opened a door onto a mystical realm. Those who ignored fasting supplicants and allowed them to starve would themselves spend eternity in hell.

The tradition appears in the most revered writings of the period, such as the *Mahābhārata*, the *Rāmayana*, and the Laws of Manu, and has been traced back to 600 to 300 BCE. In terms of fasting, as Sanskrit scholar John Nemec has detailed, what is intriguing about *The River of Kings* is that it contains several instances of priests and nobles fasting for the benefit of others, and therefore of fasters putting themselves at risk for the sake of a community. The fasting Brahmans chronicled in the epic do so in order to change the way the regime operated in Kashmir, "often for the good of Kashmiri subjects in general and not simply for the limited ends of selected individuals." In one episode in the saga, Brahmans enter *prāya* while debating whom to select as the next Kashmiri king—in effect fasting with *themselves* as the target, since they would starve if they could not speedily agree on whom to consecrate. *Prāya* in these instances is manifestly unselfish. It is what we would call a hunger strike.

....

I've tried to suggest that a fast is not a turning-away-from, but instead is an intensification of experience, a turning-toward. When familiar tools for dissent are stripped away, forbidden, or simply ineffective, only the body remains as an amplifier of disagreement. When it is used as a means of protest, fasting becomes a hunger strike. It is a two-pronged strike, both in terms of its refusal to participate and its assault on the sanctimoniousness of authority. This fasting subset not only proclaims a rejection of someone else's claim to dominion, it announces that other options exist. It is a way of forcing the discussion when those in authority have proclaimed the discussion over. As metaphor, a hunger strike is a powerful tool for pro-testers: by embracing hunger and often thirst, dissenters make the lack of justice palpable, translating an abstract notion ("You are being unjust") into the physical realm. Even today, when the mystical is often regarded with cynicism, the targets of a hunger strike are routinely referred to as being "besieged," as though committing to abstinence were a physical assault and the injured party were not the hunger striker (who is often incarcerated) but the authorities who are being challenged.

Like asceticism, the hunger strike has probably been present from the outset of organized human society. In imperial Rome, the strike was regularly used as a manipulative tool, or statement of righteousness, at the highest levels of society. To give a prominent example, the professional life of the emperor Tiberius was bracketed by fasting. As a middle-aged man, the future emperor undertook a hunger strike in 6 BCE. This decision came after years of a successful career as a general commanding legions in Germania, Armenia, and elsewhere, during which Tiberius expanded Rome's borders to the Elbe River. Tiberius had then retired to the island of Rhodes, in defiance of the wishes of his stepfather, Emperor Augustus Caesar, and his mother, Livia Drusilla, both of whom had great plans for their hero son. According to the Roman historian Suetonius, when his parents increased pressure on Tiberius to return to Rome, he started a fast in protest, refusing all food. This is a miniaturized echo of Buddha's great fast, which he also undertook just before he was supposed to take the throne. However, apart from his glancing commitment to fasting, Tiberius shared few of Buddha's attributes—including his commitment to fasting. After a mere four days, the imperial couple relented, as those in authority often do in the face of such clear determination.

The general's victory was only temporary. Tiberius eventually left Rhodes and, despite his earlier reluctance, became Rome's second emperor in 14 CE after his stepfather's death, just as his parents had schemed. Ironically, one of the first recorded deaths from a hunger strike occurred during his reign. The Roman historian Aulus Cremutius Cordus starved himself to death in 25 CE in apparent moral outrage after being accused of committing a crime against the emperor, and of thus violating the *lex maiestas*. The intensity of his beliefs that led him to offer his life as evidence of his sincerity argue eloquently for his innocence, as they were intended to do. Wrote the historian Tacitus of the death of Cordus: "And so one is all the more inclined to laugh at the stupidity of men who suppose that the despotism of the present can actually efface the remembrances of the next generation. On the contrary, the persecution of genius fosters its influence; foreign tyrants, and all who have imitated their oppression, have merely procured infamy for themselves and glory for their victims."

Similarly, Marcus Cocceius Nerva, "a man always at the emperor's side, a master of law both divine and human, whose position was secure and health sound," again according to Tacitus, also went on a hunger strike in this period. Nerva, grandfather of the eponymous emperor, determined to starve to death to protest "the miseries of the State": the corruption and violence he saw around him, particularly that perpetrated by the Praetorian Guard. Tiberius reportedly rushed to his bedside, begging Nerva to desist from his protest on the grounds that his death would damage the imperial reputation, but to no avail, and the jurist starved to death in 33 CE, four years before the end of Tiberius's reign.

Historians generally agree that despite Tiberius's proven skills as a general and his promising start as an emperor, his rule ended in chaos. When Tiberius was murdered at the age of seventy-eight, smothered by one of his retainers, the masses celebrated in the streets. The poor man should have stayed on Rhodes.

In Ireland, the history of fasting in protest long predates the arrival of Christianity on the island and is a powerful practice known as a *troscead* or *cealachan* that once had its own codified set of rules. Lawbreakers, and in particular debtors, were "fasted against" and would suffer the ignominy and supernatural peril of a hunger strike at their door. Crucially, fasting was only applied against a person in power, and involved a public shaming. As with the Indian institution of *prāya*, if the dispute continued, a kind of "stomach duel," or "fasting duel," then ensued. If the debtor, whether chieftain or wealthy farmer, denied the claim, he was obligated also to take up a fast until he either offered food to his creditor and pledged to settle the debt or submitted to a third party's ruling on the matter. According to the *Senchus Mór*, or the Great Book of Irish Law, which was composed in the fifth century CE from oral traditions, fasting was seen as evidence of moral rectitude. It followed that a failure to fast was not only antisocial; it revealed moral depravity. Resolute non-fasters forfeited their legal rights: "He who does not give a pledge to fasting is an evader of all; he who disregards all things shall not be paid by God or man." As with *prāya*, someone who spurned a faster on his doorstep was a thorough renegade, a person who had no regard for moral values or the rule of law. Fasting was so highly regarded and revered as a kind of mystic weapon that "fasting illegally" merited a fine.

When Christianity swept the island in the first part of the fifth century, obliterating almost every trace of druidic rites, the *troscead* remained and was elevated in status. As we've seen, fasting was essential to early Christianity as evidence of ascetic commitment to the religion's principles, and fasting's preexisting centrality in Irish culture undoubtedly facilitated the conversion of the Celts. Fasting—and in particular fasting as a tool for change—was closely associated with no less an authority than St.

Patrick himself. At the age of twenty-three, kidnapped from Wales by Irish pirates even before he had begun to proselytize, the saint claimed to have heard a voice praising him for his fasting. Tírechán, an Irish bishop writing in the seventh century, reported that the saint fasted for forty days, while "being assaulted by large birds" on the summit of what is now Croagh Patrick. He didn't specify why Patrick did so; Tírechán presumably wished to associate his forebear with the distinguished line of forty-day fasters in the Bible, particularly Moses, who undertook his fast after ascending Mount Sinai.

Subsequent mythologizing as chronicled in the ninth-century collection known as the Book of Armagh held that Patrick, in fury at the obstinance of the pagan Irish, undertook this epic fast directly against God. According to legend, Patrick demanded the right to judge the Irish at the Last Judgment and only resumed meals when he was assured of God's capitulation. The twelfth-century *Lebor na gCeart*, or *Book of Rights*, attributed the "fall of Tara"—the ancient seat of the high kings of Ireland—to Patrick's fasting. And in the early medieval *The Tripartite Life of Saint Patrick*, Patrick is described as fasting against kings and heretics to variously convince them of his sincerity and the twin necessities of compassion and conversion. He fasted against King Trían of Ulster to compel him to treat his slaves mercifully and fasted against Irish followers of the Pelagian heresy (Pelagius was a fourth-century ascetic who argued that we are not tainted by original sin, and that perfection is possible through divine grace).

The pagan Irish and the Christian missionaries found common ground in fasting, which was used as a legal lever in Irish traditions and as proof of devotion to Christ and penitence before God in Christian ones. For centuries after Patrick, the *troscead* retained its fearsome power, continuing its work for Christian priests as it had for the druids. Máel Ruain, a bishop and saint who died in 792 CE, was said to have fasted three times against one of the high kings of Ireland: "After the first fasting, the king's leg, it is recorded, broke in two; after the second, the fire fell and burned him from top to toe; after the third, the king died."

Beginning in 1875 with Sir Henry Maine —a civil servant who had been stationed in India in the 1860s—a succession of cultural observers made the connection to the same traditions applied continents and centuries away. In India, *prāya* had morphed into dharna over the centuries, a similar but less absolute tool to achieve justice that is derived from a Sanskrit word meaning variously "pious" and "dutiful." Even today, people "sit in dharna," or wrongdoers are "put in dharna." Dharna does not necessarily involve fasting from food. It is a sit-in obstructing the normal course of business, and makes a powerful public statement. Like more common forms of fasting—withdrawal-in-order-to-engage—dharna must be done in the open, and may take place in the doorway of an individual or institution, or even in the middle of a road. Significantly, dharna was suppressed by the British from the earliest days of their occupation of India, beginning in the eighteenth century. The colonial authorities failed to eradicate the practice, and throughout contemporary India, activists of all stripes regularly "stage dharna" or "join dharna," protesting everything from poor road conditions to corruption and worse.

India's best-known hunger striker since Gandhi is the "Iron Lady," Irom Sharmila. In November 2000, days after an Indian army massacre of ten civilians in Manipur, in the northeast of India, the slight twenty-eight-year-old intern at a human rights organization sat in dharna at the site of the shooting. Her goal was to repeal the Armed Forces Special Powers Act (AFSPA) of 1958, which allowed the army to use extreme measures—including shooting people on sight—to crush anti-government insurgencies. Under the law's protection, soldiers had executed, tortured, and raped Manipuri citizens for decades, free from any consequences. A crowd quickly gathered. After six days of sitting in dharna, Sharmila was arrested and charged with attempted suicide. She maintained the hunger strike, and after sixteen days she was force-fed. Though prison policy stated that she had to be force-fed through a tube inserted down her throat, she convinced authorities to put the tube through a nasal passage. "If she was force-fed through her nose," wrote one observer, "she reasoned she was holding to her promise not to eat until AFSPA was repealed." When she ripped the tube out of her nose, she was put on an IV glucose drip.

Sharmila was held in isolation and force-fed three times a day over a period of sixteen years. The police copied the English strategy of catch and release that had been applied to the hunger strikers of the suffrage movement in the early part of the century: once a year they freed her, then rearrested her on the same charges in order to comply with the letter of the law that limited a prisoner's detention to a year without trial. Always alone, she "rose in the middle of the night to walk in circles in the corridors. She held yoga positions for hours. She fought the maddening dryness of her mouth—having also eschewed water—by sucking cotton balls to keep saliva flowing."

As long as she was fasting, Sharmila's most fervent supporters came to see her as a saint or a divine incarnation, a holy woman sacrificing herself for the community. But she was frustrated both with them and the Indian government: Manipuris seemed content with her status as a remote deity rather than an example to emulate. They failed to rise up. The authorities simply continued to feed her, instead of engaging in dialogue on the issues. When in July 2016 the Indian Supreme Court finally demanded an investigation into the extrajudicial killings in Manipur, Sharmila saw an opportunity to end her fast with dignity. The next month, after 5,574 days of fasting, she terminated the strike. When Sharmila quit the fast, those who had worshipped her were outraged. She had returned to the mortal level. Instead of being hailed as a courageous leader, she was condemned as "a big joke" and "a prostitute" and had to leave Manipur.

Dharna persists. To take one of many examples, in southern India in the spring of 2022, Mamata Banerjee, a prominent political aspirant, sat in dharna to protest the refusal of the electoral authorities to allow her to campaign. An approving local journalist noted that her sitting in dharna "amplifies the sympathy factor," "highlights [her] street warrior credentials," and "underscores her image as Bengal's defender."

The Indo-Celtic connection is interwoven throughout the history of fasting, and fasting has served as an enduring cultural link between the two nations: Gandhi, Jawaharlal Nehru, and others consciously drew on the history of the Irish struggle, which became a model for how to resist a well-established force that to all appearances had an overwhelming advantage. The cultural and historical ties between the distant nations may at first appear startling, but the connection was reaffirmed via a shared history as a British colonial possession. Hard on the heels of his surrender to allied French and American forces at Yorktown in 1781, Lord Cornwallis was named governor-general of India. While there, as administrator of the East India Company, he enacted the "Permanent Settlement" based on the principles of the Anglo-Irish tenant farming system and its land agents. Cornwallis empowered an elite group of native Indian landowners known as zamindars to collect fees and taxes from tenant farmers, thereby creating both a revenue stream for the company and establishing a privileged intermediary between the English rulers and their subjects. It was a natural promotion for Cornwallis when he was named lord lieutenant of Ireland in 1798. As long as the colonial legacy persisted, the English conflated the two countries. "Those Englishmen who know something of India, are even now those who understand Ireland best," wrote the philosopher and economist John Stuart Mill in 1868. "Persons who know both countries have remarked many points of resemblance in both the Irish and Hindoo character. . . ."

In both India and Ireland, massive, prolonged famines under English colonial rule were attributable at least in part to the bureaucracy, which created pressure to grow cash crops (to pay off rent and other debts to the authorities). These policies disenfranchised small local farmer/tenants, making them little better than serfs beholden to absentee landlords. The widely reviled administrator for British relief in Ireland at the time of the Great Famine of the 1840s was Charles Trevelyan, who served the empire in India both before and after his time in Ireland. After a million Irish had starved to death and another million emigrated—causing a population drop of 20 percent—Trevelyan insisted on continuing grain exports. His actions inadvertently laid the foundation for a regime-shaking kind of fasting, a refusal to participate in the prevailing mechanism, a new development in fasting technology that came to be known as "the boycott."

Another Indo-Celtic form of nonviolent protest that was later taken up by Gandhi and many others, boycotting remains a variant of fasting in that it requires specific, physical actions of self-restraint. As traditional fasting does, it leverages the social and economic impact of people not in power, and it is nonviolent—and often hugely effective. A fast-from-contact, a boycott is obstructionist at its core, and neatly employs fasting's trickster element of reversal, highlighting both the strength of the entity being boycotted and the exploitation of those boycotting: the former depends on the latter for their support, which the latter withhold. The tactic was first given a name in the late nineteenth century when tenant farmers in County Mayo, inspired by the Irish patriot Charles Stewart Parnell and the Irish Land League, shunned English land agent Captain Charles Boycott in 1880. Boycott was known for being a particularly merciless rent collector on behalf of his absentee landlord employer, the Right Honorable John Crichton, the third Earl Erne. With the devastating Great Famine of 1847 to 1851 still a vivid memory—areas in Ireland's west, such as County Mayo, had been the hardest hit—the disenfranchised, poverty-stricken Irish enthusiastically embraced Parnell's suggestion, which fit neatly with ancient Celtic traditions, again echoing or paralleling those of the Indian subcontinent: "For a king of bad conduct there is no other medicine than shunning [him]."

Shops refused to serve Boycott and workers on the estate refused to perform their allotted tasks. "He was jeered on the roads, was hissed and hustled by hostile crowds in Ballinrobe, and required police protection." Boycott alerted the English press, complaining bitterly that he was being driven to financial ruin, with the result that thousands of pounds were raised to help the self-proclaimed "victim." Anglo-Irish volunteers, escorted by a thousand troops, arrived to help collect the harvest. But the action was a success in the eyes of the nationalists, in that the seemingly insatiable avarice of the English landholders was again exposed, as was the stubborn unwillingness of Irish farmers to submit to the rule of the colonizers.

....

Through the ages, a hunger strike has signaled purity of intent and action. But while it gives evidence of a oneness with principle, a hunger strike also suggests a breakdown in communication: if two sides fruitfully exchange ideas, there's no need for drastic action. And because a striker is putting her most basic commodity on the line—her body—the act suggests a moral importance to the disagreement that a mere exchange of words cannot convey. It is an attempt to redirect the parameters of an argument, to focus the discussion.

The precariousness of the hunger strike lies in its appeal to shared values, that we share a common humanity and deserve to be heard. If the opposing side simply doesn't care if the hunger striker lives or dies, the strike may permanently injure or kill the person who wields it. Typically, hunger strikers seek change: death is rarely the goal. But it can be. This kind of purposeful, lethal fasting occurred an unknown number of times during the Middle Passage, when kidnapped Africans made clear that they preferred death to slavery and refused to eat. That they did so on a regular basis is evidenced by the documented use of the *speculum oris*, an instrument originally used by physicians and adapted by slavers to keep Africans from starving themselves to death. One abolitionist account from 1836 described the device: "It opens . . . by a screw below with a knob at the end of it. This instrument was used by surgeons to wrench open the mouth in case of lock-jaw. It is used in slave-ships to compel the negroes to take food; because a loss to the owners would follow their persevering attempts to die." What one scholar has termed "subtle resistance" (as opposed to active rebellion, or "band resistance") became an effective means of protest at the unspeakable horrors that the prisoners were forced to endure.

The watershed year of 1989 saw one of history's most notoriously brutal responses to peaceful mass protest. After the death of Hu Yaobang, a party leader widely seen as friendly to democratization, many Chinese hoped that change would come as those in power assessed his legacy. A stream of activists from around the country converged on Tiananmen

Square in mid-April. The demonstrations had been underway for almost a month when 160 students there announced a hunger strike on May 13, explicitly declaring their allegiance to the Chinese government and their intention not to seek death but dialogue. While the gathering had, of course, been the focus of government concern, the hunger strikes upped the intensity of public sympathy and official alarm. "There's such a feeling in China about food because of the thousands of years of famines that they've had," explained Canadian journalist Jan Wong. "So when the students went on their hunger strike, it really moved people to tears." After six days, following failed negotiations with officials, the students called off their strike. But they had claimed the moral high ground. One day before authorities sent in tanks and soldiers to clear the square, resulting in the deaths of up to three thousand people, the poet Liu Xiaobo and several others called for a second hunger strike on June 2. "We appeal! We repent! We are on a hunger strike! We protest!" it began. "We are not in search of death; we are looking for real life."

> We must do this because hatred can produce only violence and dictatorship. We must adopt the spirit of tolerance. We must begin to build up Chinese democracy with a democratic spirit of tolerance and concept of cooperation. Democratic politics is politics based on mutual respect, mutual tolerance, and mutual compromise, through consultation, discussion, and the electoral process.

....

As the struggle for constitutional representation gathered momentum in imperial Russia, tales of hunger strikes by imprisoned activists protesting inhumane treatment by the czar's regime began to percolate out of the country. While the origins of Russian hunger striking are unclear, for anyone steeped in the culture, a hunger strike would have come naturally enough, as there are more than two hundred fast days in the Russian Orthodox Church. Godliness was bound up in fasting. For the devout Russian Orthodox, only boiled vegetarian dishes are permitted during the forty days of Lent, and everything else—meat, sweets, and dairy products—are forbidden. To any Russian onlooker, a hunger strike would have instantly conveyed a message of oneness with the highest moral authority. But that did not assure success.

Occasionally, the Russian strikers got their way. More often than not they were beaten by the guards, or worse. The prisoners called their self-starvation *golodovka*, a word that in prerevolutionary times meant "famine" or "want." In 1906, the American journalist George Kennan (cousin of the noted historian George F. Kennan, a generation after) wrote that "even the most 'brutally insensible' Russian wardens were alarmed by the 'pitiful weapon' of 'political hunger-strikers' because of its potential to unleash a firestorm of public outrage and violence." Kennan wrote that, despite the best efforts of the secret police and prison authorities to suppress news of the hunger strikes, word percolated out of prisons, with the result of public reactions in the form of "uprisings, prison sieges, and assassination threats aimed at prison officials and guards." And not only threats. In 1878, political prisoners in St. Petersburg from a notorious group known as the Group of 193—193 students who had been accused of treason and sentenced to hard labor and Siberian exile—went on a hunger strike to protest the conditions in which they were being held. After three days, the prisoners' families petitioned the czar's chief of secret police, General Nikolai Mezentsev, for mercy. Mezentsev reportedly said, "Let them die, I have already ordered coffins for them all." Later that same year, Mezentsev was stabbed to death in the streets of St. Petersburg by a revolutionary, Sergius Kravchinsky. Kravchinsky fled to London, where he started a journal called *Free Russia*, the first issue of which highlighted hunger strikes led by women prisoners in Siberia.

....

The publicity surrounding the Russian hunger strikers combined with memories of the ancient *troscead* traditions to inspire some of the most effective tactics of the Anglo-American suffrage movement. London had long been a haven for revolutionaries of all stripes. In 1849, Karl Marx was exiled to London and spent his days working on *Das Kapital* in the reading rooms of the British Museum. A decade or so later, the Russian anarchist Mikhail Bakunin collaborated with the socialist Alexander Herzen in London on a newspaper. After his 1902 escape from Siberia, Leon Trotsky (who had initiated a hunger strike among his fellow political prisoners while being held in Kherson prison in 1898) hobnobbed with Lenin in London. While in exile, these activists and dozens more publicized the plight—and tactics—of their Russian brethren. The Russian hunger strikers may have been doomed without the framework of a receptive government, but they called attention to a morally convincing alternative to street protests, bombings, and assassinations.

The "Russian method of the hunger strike," as one English voting rights activist described it, proved to be a transformative weapon in the fight for the right of women to vote. In England, the combination of a responsive public, determined hunger-striking activists, and a tradition of relatively free press created a juggernaut that helped reshape society. After witnessing a period of political awakening that coincided with the social and philosophical revolutions of the 1840s, English and American women campaigned with increasing intensity beginning in the 1860s. Decades of polite debate had gotten them no significant advances, and the movement was in decline. By the early 1900s, a new breed of suffragists appeared on the scene. (The first use of the word "suffragette" was in the UK tabloid the *Daily Mail*, which even in 1906 was stridently reactionary. The newspaper made the word diminutive, sneering, "It was not surprising that [the leader of the Conservative Party, former prime minister Arthur] Balfour should receive a deputation of the Suffragettes." Subsequently, English activists adopted the insult for their own, although in the U.S. the word "suffragist" retained its prominence.) These powerful women were impatient with what the great English suffragette Sylvia Pankhurst called the "incorrigibly leisurely" methods of their Victorian predecessors. They were physically committed to making substantive change happen within the immediate future: they overturned cars, smashed windows, burned the Great Yarmouth pier, horsewhipped then home secretary Winston Churchill on a railway station platform, and at least once attempted to assassinate the prime minister. They also, and with enduring effect, engaged in hunger strikes.

The first voting rights advocate to adopt the hunger strike was an aristocratic artist and writer, Marion Wallace-Dunlop, who had been born in a Scottish castle and was related to the legendary rebel William Wallace. A veteran suffragette, in 1909 she was arrested for the third time on behalf of the cause, on this occasion for having stenciled—in violet ink—a sentence from the 1689 English Bill of Rights on a wall of the House of Commons: "It is the right of the subject to petition the King, and all commitments and prosecutions for such petitioning are illegal." She was in the midst of stenciling the quote when she was arrested and released the same day. She returned to complete her stencil and was again arrested. (Wallace-Dunlop later said she had stenciled the words on the wall because there was "danger of their being forgotten by legislators.") On her second arraignment, she was required to pay a fine. She refused, and was sentenced to a month in prison, classified as a "second division," a criminal prisoner. Like generations of activists to follow, Wallace-Dunlop demanded to be categorized as a political prisoner. Her request was denied, and she went on a hunger strike. Wallace-Dunlop wrote the governor of Holloway Prison:

> I claim the right recognised by all civilised nations that a person im-
> prisoned for a political offence should have first-division treatment;
> and as a matter of principle, not only for my own sake but for the sake
> of others who may come after me, I am now refusing all food until this
> matter is settled to my satisfaction.

This was an experiment on her part, and it set a precedent for generations of activists to come. "I wondered what I could do to help the cause in prison and I decided to try a hunger strike," she later wrote. On the first day of her strike, she threw "fried fish, four slices of bread, three bananas and a cup of hot milk out of the window." Official threats of force-feeding only fortified her: "'You may feed me through the nostrils or the mouth,' I added; 'but suppose you get 108 women in here on Friday, all requiring to be fed through the nostrils?' At this the doctor's face was a delightful study."

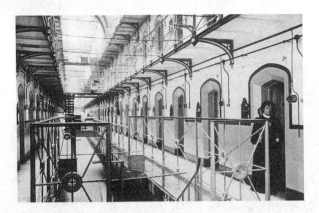

Holloway Prison, London, where Marion Wallace-Dunlop and many suffragettes were held.

Already a patient in the prison hospital due to her poor health, Wallace-Dunlop was released after a hunger strike that lasted only ninety-one hours. While her letters to government officials to be recognized as a political activist and not as a common criminal had been ignored, when she put her own body in the path of the prison machine it was obliged to respond. Women's rights activists immediately recognized the effectiveness of the strategy, and collectively decided to apply the tactic as often as possible: the day after Wallace-Dunlop's release, fourteen imprisoned women petitioners went on staggered intervals of hunger strikes, carefully coordinating their protest to maximize news coverage. A few weeks later, after a wave of attention in the press, the women were released.

Government authorities also quickly changed tactics. It was decided to subject the women to force-feeding. Ironically, force-feeding was an innovation of the Enlightenment in late-eighteenth-century France. Philippe Pinel, a pioneering precursor of modern psychology, was the first to advocate force-feeding for mentally disturbed patients, arguing they needed sufficient nutrients to get well. At the time, the prevailing view was that the insane could not feel hunger and required little food. Then, a century later, German physician Adolf Kussmaul, after experimenting on a professional sword swallower, introduced the mercilessly direct antidote of the stomach tube. Asylum doctors quickly embraced the method as a way to curtail fasting and to break the resolve of their patients.

For someone unfamiliar with the process, force-feeding does not sound like a terrible imposition. After all, it is only done to keep someone alive. It would appear to be for the hunger striker's own good. But force-feeding is physically and mentally devastating, employed to suppress the defiance, empowerment, and interiority that fasting engenders. To anyone who has observed the procedure, force-feeding is abuse, coercive punishment in the extreme.

Force-feeding satisfies the requirements of any reasonable definition of torture. It can involve full-body restraints and an apparatus of metal or heavy plastic to force open the relevant orifice. In force-feeding, tubes are inserted into the mouth, the nostrils, or the rectum to convey nutrients. If a tube is improperly inserted into the throat, food can enter the lungs, and suffocation or infection can result. Soft tissues can be damaged. Even if done voluntarily, getting food through a tube is a painful process: although liberated concentration camp inmates

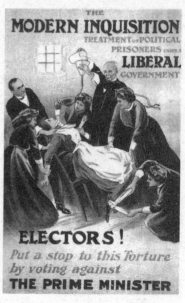

An anti-force-feeding poster.

at Bergen-Belsen had experienced some of the worst forms of torture imaginable, they considered the stomach feeding tubes implemented by well-meaning relief workers "a new form of torture." Whatever the method employed, force-feeding requires utter physical subjugation of a prisoner. And yet it can paradoxically reinforce the impact of a hunger strike: the brutality proves the striker's argument. As one doctor pointed out at the time, the authorities tacitly acknowledged the cruelty of the process by calling it "artificial feeding," which sounds much nicer, and a reasonable medical procedure.

In the winter of 1909, the American suffragist Alice Paul was sent to prison for a month in the aftermath of her attempt to disrupt the Lord Mayor's banquet. Following Wallace-Dunlop's precedent, she refused to wear prison clothes and went on a hunger strike for twenty-four days. On the second day, her food was forced upon her. She wrote:

> During this operation the largest wardress in Holloway sat astride my knees, holding my shoulders down to keep me from bending forward. Two other wardresses sat on either side and held my arms. Then a towel was placed around my throat, and one doctor from behind forced my head back, while another doctor put a tube in my nostril. When it reached my throat my head was pushed forward. Twice the tube came through my mouth and I got it between my teeth. My mouth was then pried open with an instrument. Sometimes they tied me to a chair with sheets. Once I managed to get my hands loose and snatched the tube, tearing it with my teeth. I also broke a jug, but I didn't give in.

In the span of just six months, between February 1913 and July 1914, the formidable Sylvia Pankhurst was arrested eight times and force-fed eight times.

An outcry arose as details of force-feeding were released to the English public. The government was in a quandary: order had to be maintained. Letting an Englishwoman, even a suffragette, starve to death was unacceptable. What was evidently the ongoing torture of prisoners had a bad look, not least because of the genteel background of many of the suffragists. The solution was the so-called Cat and Mouse Act, the Prisoners (Temporary Discharge for Ill Health) Act, of 1913, which allowed prisoners to be temporarily released when doctors determined their hunger strike had rendered them too weak to be kept safely. Once the prisoner had recovered, she had to return to finish her sentence, and the cycle began again.

The protesters earned a certain grudging respect in the media, and politicians on both sides of the Atlantic increasingly found it difficult to countenance the harsh methods of police and prison officials. In contrast, the working-class male activists of the Industrial Workers of the World (IWW), the "Wobblies," received little public sympathy when they engaged in hunger strikes. The same year that Alice Paul was sent to jail, hundreds of members of the IWW staged a fasting protest in Spokane, Washington, against the exploitation of itinerant laborers. Officials and media refused to accord them the dignity of fasters, instead labeling their action a "starvation strike." A hunger strike was recognized as an intellectual decision, something a morally upright person could undertake. But starvation and famine, as historian Nayan Shah has pointed out, are associated with poverty and social collapse. "Newspaper editors ridiculed Spokane's mass 'starvation strike' as pitiful, a desperate effort to neither work nor pay fines."

....

The first to use a hunger strike as a modern political tool in Ireland was the English activist Elizabeth "Lizzie" Barker in Dublin to disrupt the tumultuous 1912 visit of Prime Minister Herbert Asquith. During his visit, Asquith narrowly missed having his head split open by a hatchet thrown by suffragette Mary Leigh (the projectile instead lightly wounded Irish Parliamentary Party chief John Redmond). Barker was a veteran suffragette and signatory of the 1866 Women's Suffrage petition. She was freed within days after declaring her fast. From that point on, the hunger strike became an essential tool in the arsenal of Irish rebels, both women and men.

The suffragists were well aware of the rich history of fasting from both a religious and a political standpoint. Doris Stevens, an American leader of the movement, cited the Laws of Brehon and the rule of *troscead* in her 1920 memoir, *Jailed for Freedom*. In ancient Ireland, she wrote, "it became the duty of an injured person, when all else failed, to inflict punishment directly, for wrong done" and to use fasting "as compulsion to obtain a request." As in England, the Americans turned to hunger strikes in 1917 after being refused status as political prisoners, despite having committed their offense in the public interest and not for personal gain.

> *And so at first it aroused tremendous indignation. "Let them starve to death," said the thoughtless one, who did not perceive that that was the very thing a political administration could least afford to do. "Mad fanatics," said a kindlier critic. The general opinion was that the hunger strike was "foolish." Few people realize that this resort to the refusal of food is almost as old as civilization. It has always represented a passionate desire to achieve an end.*

It was in the context of the sacred that the suffragists invoked the fasting tradition in the United States. Many were careful to document the ordeals they underwent in order to emphasize the authorities' obsession with control and the threat they (correctly) saw in self-imposed fasts. If the prisoners became martyrs, so much the better.

....

The movement for Irish independence gathered intensity in the first years of the twentieth century, sparked by the bravery of the suffragists (and the intense media coverage of the women's struggles with prison authorities). The struggle was augmented by Ireland's own history of fasting. It was natural for Irish patriots to adopt the hunger strike, a tactic that demanded commitment but little else in terms of matériel and yet served to highlight the cruelty of those in authority. A number of prominent dissenters such as Charlotte Despard, Constance Markievicz (the only woman sentenced to a firing squad after her role as co-commander of the 1916 Easter Rising—spared only because of her gender), and Hanna Sheehy-Skeffington were active in both suffragist and independence movements, and the hunger strike was never far from the minds of the republicans. The first to revive the tradition of fasting-in-protest in the name of Irish independence were the Irish Volunteers, a paramilitary organization formed in 1913. The Volunteers fully expected to be arrested and sentenced. One of their principles was "to hold drill parades in public in the presence" of the Royal Irish Constabulary, and when sentenced "to go on hunger strike for political prisoner status." Between 1913 and 1923, approximately ten thousand Irish prisoners went on hunger strike. While the press outside Ireland was not widely sympathetic to the rebels, fasting took its toll on government staff: in 1916, a doctor at an intern-ment camp in Wales "threw himself into a quarry reportedly due to the mental stress of dealing with up to two hundred fasting Irish prisoners."

A grim turning point both for Irish independence and for the role of the hunger strike came the following year, when Thomas Ashe, a thirty-five-year-old Dublin school principal, was arrested along with thirty-nine members of the Volunteers. Ashe, a founding member of the Volunteers and a participant in the Easter Rebellion, was imprisoned for a speech he had made. Charged with "attempting to cause disaffection among the general population," he went on a hunger strike, demanding to be tried as a political prisoner or released. After a week of force-feeding, Ashe collapsed. He died within five hours of his hospitalization. His death in Dublin's Mountjoy Prison on September 25, 1917, was barely noted outside Ireland, but three thousand uniformed members of the Irish Volunteers turned out to accompany the funeral procession, and "tens of thousands" of mourners lined the streets. The revolutionary leader Michael Collins delivered the funeral oration, and Irish newspapers emphasized Ashe's "strength and brute masculinity" to highlight force-feeding's cruelty. The effect was to lead sympathizers to conclude that, since Ashe was neither suicidal nor particularly vulnerable, the system had murdered him. With Ashe's death, the prisoners arrested with him were released, and force-feeding was temporarily suspended. While hunger strikers didn't need to die to be effective, their deaths amplified their message: as Yeats wrote in *The King's Threshold*, "The man that dies has the chief part in the story."

After Ashe and until the death of ten members of the IRA in 1981, the most notorious self-sacrifice in Ireland was that of the Lord Mayor of Cork, Terence MacSwiney, who died in October 1920. MacSwiney's acceptance speech when he became mayor in April of the same year, shortly after the assassination of his predecessor, embodies the hunger striker ethos: "This contest of ours is not on our side a rivalry of vengeance but one of endurance—it is not they who can inflict the most but those who can endure the most who will conquer." Arrested at Cork's city hall while presiding over a court of arbitration, MacSwiney was charged with sedition and sentenced to two years in prison. He died on the seventy-fourth day of a hunger strike.

MacSwiney's death by self-starvation was the first to be widely reported on outside of Ireland, and inspired worldwide sympathy for the Irish cause, notably on the part of Gandhi. Also paying close attention to the news of MacSwiney was a certain Vietnamese immigrant to England—a dishwasher at the Carlton Hotel in London, who later changed his name to Ho Chi Minh. "A nation which has such citizens will never surrender," he is re-

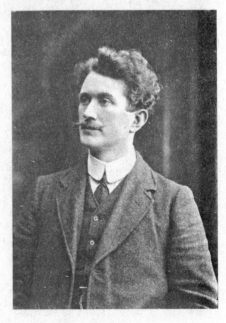

Thomas Ashe.

ported to have written upon hearing of MacSwiney's death. Other Irish hunger strikers died of starvation with much less fanfare: Liam Lynch and, on the same day that Lord Mayor died, another member of the Irish Volunteers, the American-born Joseph Murphy, who died on the seventy-sixth day of his fast in Cork Gaol. At the time, his death was overshadowed by MacSwiney's. But Murphy has not been forgotten; on the hundredth anniversary of his death, dignitaries and relatives hailed his commitment to the cause.

Were the Irish hunger strikers defying the Church in their pursuit of goals that were unlikely to be achieved, and therefore effectively committing suicide? Both supporters and opponents acknowledged that the dead hunger strikers became martyrs to the cause. The government position was best articulated by Bonar Law, Conservative leader of the House of Commons at the time (and later prime minister), who scoffed: "It would be perfectly futile if men are to be released because they choose to refuse food." The apparent disdain for hunger strikers persisted for decades among officials up to and through the 1980s (as Prime Minister Margaret Thatcher explicitly made clear). But from the start, Catholic clergy recognized a profoundly traditional, Celtic stance in the hunger strikers' behavior, and were reluctant to condemn the quest of the rebels as suicidal. Even the Catholic chaplain at Mountjoy Prison saw the strike as an "efficient political weapon." He wrote, in the *Irish Ecclesiastical Record* of 1918, that the hunger strikers' determination was "invincible": "This obstinacy did not arise altogether from attachment to the leaders to whom they had submitted, and who made no account of my representations; their strength of purpose was, in great part, derived from their conviction that they had in support of their action sufficient theological authority."

....

In the classic Hindu tradition, sannyasi (male) and sannyasini (female) have renounced material attractions. Beginning around the second century BCE, these "renunciants" performed their own funeral rites as a way of marking their rejection of worldly dharma, or duties. Although they came from the upper social strata, these Hindus were socially dead and owned nothing besides a begging bowl and old clothing. The Sanskrit word *sannyasa* literally means "renunciation of the world, profession of asceticism, abstinence from food." While Gandhi may be the best-known modern incarnation of a sannyasi—he identifies with the concept throughout his writings—such renunciants have occurred in many cultures and throughout history.

"For modern Hinduism, and for someone like Gandhi, fasting is part of a larger set of practices which are all negatively defined," Faisal Devji, professor of Indian studies at the University of Oxford, tells me. "Nonviolence is the larger term under which all of these practices fit. They include noncooperation, nonpossession, fasting, celibacy, and spinning—or manual labor. You might see that as a positive act, but Gandhi saw it as a way of pulling back *from*. Spinning was meant to transform you internally, to serve as an example, precisely because it was seen as an archaic and non-modern act." Gandhi's embrace of the spinning wheel made sense precisely because the mechanism was unable to provide cloth for India's people on an industrial scale. His was a call to reject industrialization and capitalist growth (and the reliance on imported British textiles at the expense of Indian manufacturers).

My thoughts turn to Melville's champion of diminishment, Bartleby the Scrivener, and his habitual "I would prefer not to," which so fascinated the philosopher Gilles Deleuze. The story's plot is itself magnificently minimal: it has the banal setting of a solicitor's offices on Wall Street. Its subject is, like its author, an unsuccessful writer—in Melville's case, because critical and commercial success eluded him until decades after his death, and in the case of Bartleby, because the pointlessness of any action overwhelms him.

Bartleby retreats into an unassailable fortress of neither/nor. At first he surprises, then frustrates, and then panics the story's narrator, who is a respectable attorney. The formula "stymies the speech acts that a boss uses to command, that a kind friend uses to ask questions or a man of faith to make promises," Deleuze wrote. "If Bartleby had refused, he could still be seen as a rebel or insurrectionary, and as such would still have a social role. . . . It makes Bartleby a pure outsider to whom no social position can be attributed." It is crucial to Bartleby's persona that, in contrast to others in the attorney's office, he never goes out to dinner and survives on handfuls of nuts—an unprocessed, elemental food. He doesn't consider himself a part of the office community, and this abstention destabilizes the entire office, eventually causing the attorney—in theory the man with all the power, social respectability, and money—to flee. And when Bartleby graduates to "I prefer not" from "I prefer not to," Melville means us to take him at his word. Bartleby actively prefers *not* to unthinkingly preferring *something*. He has achieved the *Zhuangzi*'s ideal of an absolute fast of the mind, absent the quality of what one scholar has called the "responsive awareness" of the Chinese text. His fasting has taken him beyond speech, beyond decision-making, into a Buddha-like state of otherness where nothing is what he prefers.

....

If an opponent refuses to recognize himself as your opponent or even relevant to your situation, it is very difficult to dislodge him. In the same way, a hunger strike, by deflecting the issue of opposition, can become an effective tool for dissenters. It is not an obviously aggressive act and can only extend its effects beyond the perpetrator's immediate circle if an outside force takes interest in the action. Although Gandhi held that it was not possible to go on an effective hunger strike against a tyrant, a fasting prisoner demands intervention, and forces either capitulation or violence—whether overt, in the form of force-feeding, or subtle, in the form of neglect. Instead of an orderly, obedient subject, the faster, ignited by a perceived wrong, becomes the source of chaos and disarray.

How to effect positive change without violence, assertion, or conquest was the driving question for Gandhi. While in his childhood he became familiar with fasting on Hindu fast days such as Ekadashi, he writes in his autobiography that he did so as a matter of rote, with no sense of its ultimate importance. "The idea," says Faisal Devji, "was to make change happen by withdrawal, by non-cooperating, and to allow your enemy to collapse of its own accord. Fasting can serve as a rejection of violence, which then might serve as a persuasive model for others, not because you are making them suffer, but because you are suffering yourself. So it's directed inwards, rather than outwards."

Although Gandhi held that one must not "play religion by employing fasting for spectacular purposes," he regularly employed it for leverage against the British. Gandhi saw both fasting and boycotting as manifestations of satyagraha, a portmanteau derived from the Sanskrit words for "truth" (*satya*) and "insistence" (*agraha*), which he defined as "firmness for truth." Satyagraha was active (as opposed to passive) resistance. Gandhi had revived the use of boycotts, a long-standing Indian practice, first in the early twentieth century in South Africa and then as part of his decidedly spectacular 1930 campaign against the salt tax imposed by British authorities. He sought to identify the practice as a kind of warfare, albeit one waged without weapons. The boycotting activists were courageous fighters in contrast to the "quaking," more obedient citizens:

> *The liquor and foreign cloth shops can be picketed. We can refuse to pay taxes if we have the requisite strength. The lawyers can give up practice. The public can boycott the law courts by refraining from litigation. Government servants can resign their posts. In the midst of the despair reigning all round people quake with fear of losing employment. Such men are unfit for* Swaraj [self-rule].

....

"I was familiar with the old tradition of fasting in Ireland," Pat Sheehan, a former member of the Irish Republican Army, told me. At the time of our interview, Sheehan was a Sinn Féin representative for Belfast West in the Irish parliament, but in 1980 he was imprisoned along with a number of Irish fighters, among them Bobby Sands. "You know, if someone committed an injustice against you, you would go on fast on their doorstep, to try and have them right whatever the wrong was and to bring moral pressure to bear on whoever had inflicted an injustice on you." Sheehan cited not only the deaths of MacSwiney and Murphy, but also the many republicans who died while on hunger strikes in the 1940s and 1970s. "There has always been a tradition that Irish republicans would assert the right to be treated as political prisoners, and hunger striking has always been seen as a weapon in the armory, not to be used willy-nilly, but you know, as a sort of last resort." Ten prisoners, including Sands, starved to death in what became one of the most consequential hunger strikes of the twentieth century.

As the unionists maintained their hold over Northern Ireland through voting restrictions and gerrymandering, and as police refused to protect peacefully protesting Catholics, tensions increased. By the early 1970s, close to a thousand prisoners were held without trial under the Special Powers Act at Long Kesh Detention Centre, a former air base outside Belfast better known as the Maze or H-Blocks. A turning point came when British soldiers attacked a nonviolent demonstration on January 30, 1972, resulting in a massacre of fourteen unarmed civilians that came to be known as "Bloody Sunday." A hunger strike later that year resulted in IRA prisoners gaining "special category" status, giving them the right to be treated as political prisoners in everything but name. They were permitted to wear their own clothes, to receive one visit a week, to receive food parcels, and were accorded other privileges distinct from criminal detainees. When special category status was withdrawn in 1976, an upsurge in hunger strikes occurred, culminating in the strikes of 1980 to 1981.

At the time, the British government was well aware of the dangers that hunger strikers posed to its standing with the public. When IRA detainees declared another strike on October 27, 1980, Conservative bureaucrats were alarmed. Humphrey Atkins, the British secretary of state for Northern Ireland, had earlier warned Prime Minister Margaret Thatcher that a hunger strike was "a ruthlessly determined act." The government needed to loudly proclaim its own determination, and so a few weeks later, in a slightly more refined version of General Mezentsev's statement, Thatcher told a radio interviewer that "if these people continue with their hunger strike, it will have no effect whatsoever. It will just take their own lives, for which I will be profoundly sorry, because I think it's a ridiculous thing to do." On December 18, the first strike "ended in failure," according to Sheehan, with the authorities conceding nothing.

Then twenty-seven-year-old Bobby Sands decided to put his life on the line. As "officer commanding" of the IRA members being held in the Maze, Sands declared a second hunger strike over the objections of other IRA prisoners. Sands was by then a legally recognized local official: he had won election to the district of Fermanagh (on the "Anti H-Block/Armagh Political Prisoner" ticket). "That made all the difference," Sheehan said to me. The hunger strike and the subsequent death of Sands on May 5, 1981, after sixty-six days of fasting, brought worldwide recognition to the prisoners' protests. Nine other strikers died around the same time, but it was the death of Sands that resonated. It became a kind of "post-mortem ventriloquism (literally: speaking out of their stomachs)," as one scholar put it. No less an authority than the BBC called Sands's death a pivotal point in the long and bloody Irish conflict. Were the prisoners suicidal? After all, a number of imprisoned Irish rebels had starved to death in relative obscurity (or achieved only local notoriety). Sheehan reacted emphatically to the suggestion. "We were healthy young men, with life ahead of us," he told me. "It was never our intention to die."

Without the public spectacle, hunger striking became far less effective for imprisoned activists. For that reason, in October 1988, the British government banned interviews on state-regulated media with not only the IRA but with its legal political wing, Sinn Féin. The government said it wanted to deny them the "oxygen of publicity." What authorities gained in terms of order, however, they lost in terms of credibility, as human rights organizations, free speech advocates, and opposition politicians—many of whom disagreed with the Irish republicans—objected to the heavy-handed measures.

....

America's best-known radical activist, Angela Davis, was arrested in New York City while on the run in 1970 from murder charges connected to a failed attempt to free "Soledad Brother" George Jackson. Sent to the Manhattan House of Detention, commonly known as the Tombs, she was placed in solitary confinement. Davis was told it was to prevent her from being attacked by other prisoners. It quickly became clear that other prisoners were just fine with her presence, and the goal was to prevent her from radicalizing other inmates. Davis decided to turn to fasting to "dramatize the situation by declaring myself on hunger strike for as long as I was kept in isolation." Other inmates joined her strike in solidarity. On the tenth day, when she had "persuaded [her]self that [she] could continue indefinitely without eating," the courts ruled that she was being penalized for her political beliefs and that she should be let back into the general prison population, and she ended the protest.

A mass, nonreligious fast that is not quite a hunger strike can still be a communal recognition of injustice, and that is what the annual fast known as Black August has become in the United States. Founded by a group of inmates at San Quentin in 1979 to commemorate George Jackson (shot to death by a tower guard at the prison in 1971), it is meant to serve as "a constant reminder of the conditions our people have faced and still confront. Fasting is uncomfortable at times, but it is helpful to remember all those who have come and gone before us." The concept has since been embraced by a number of Black activists, who each August fast between sunup and sundown "to honor and stand in solidarity with all Black political prisoners, those we've lost to racial violence, systematic racism, and extrajudicial murders."

Fasting and hunger strikes have been an essential part of the struggle for civil rights in the U.S. from the time of slaveholders to the present. In 1960, Eroseanna Robinson, a veteran activist and member of the Peace-makers, an American pacifist organization that worked with Dorothy Day's Catholic Worker Movement, refused to pay taxes to a government she saw as immoral—perpetuating racism and warmongering. Robinson, a champion athlete (she held the women's high jump record) had previously led the fight in the early 1950s to desegregate Cleveland's Skateland roller rink at great personal risk. She was repeatedly attacked by white skaters and thrown to the ground. She kept returning, insisting on her right to skate, and suffered "substantial injuries," including a broken arm. Arrested for nonpayment of taxes, she practiced total noncompliance, was carried into court by U.S. Marshals, and sentenced to a year in jail, where she refused to eat. During 115 days of fasting and noncooperation, she suffered painful and dangerous bouts of force-feeding before she was finally released. Her extraordinary self-discipline and skills as an athlete had given her an ability to endure an ordeal that would have caused most of us to capitulate.

At any one time, there are dozens, perhaps hundreds of people undertaking hunger strikes around the world. Many of these strikes go unremarked, but the fasts are a binding agent within the groups that undertake them. The line between fasting-as-protest and a hunger strike is largely one of semantics. A hunger strike draws on the language of labor movements to evoke a work stoppage, an action by community members. A fast suggests a moral goal. But in reality, there is little difference between the two. More than a protest against conditions or a call for attention, fasting in protest can express solidarity, and solidarity means trouble for even the most powerful adversary. Fasting in a group shows a fearsome amount of power. It eloquently states that the incarcerated and their allies are united in purpose.

Even when rights are stripped away, a hunger strike can serve to amplify voices of dissent. As issues around immigration have become more urgent, treatment of economic and environmental refugees has purposefully become more harsh. In 2014 at the Northwest Detention

Center in Tacoma, Washington, a U.S. Immigration and Customs Enforcement facility run by the GEO Group, detainees were subjected to inhumane and unsanitary conditions. They were told they were not prisoners, merely in "civic detention." Yet solitary confinement was regularly used as punishment, the food was thick with maggots, and guards controlled all aspects of the detainees' personal lives. A hunger strike that arose from discussions at a Bible study class included 1,200 of the 1,575 detainees, who came from all over the world—primarily Mexico, but also the Philippines, Canada, and just about every country on the planet. Operating in relays, the strikers continued their protest for fifty-six days, demanding decent food and better treatment by the guards. Wrote one of the detainees in a letter: "We have a profound respect for food, we honor it, we know that it is vital and necessary for many here and in the rest of the world but to make it known that we are here, we exist, it seems like the only alternative to say, 'we are here.'" Sandy Restrepo, an immigration attorney who represented several of the strikers, characterized the hunger strike as "a profound exercise: they put their bodies on the line, saying, 'We believe so strongly our rights are being violated and this is the only way we can protest, by refusing to eat.'" Restrepo said that two of her clients, who had each fasted more than forty days, were put into solitary and threatened with force-feeding. They were ultimately deported—Restrepo felt their activism "definitely prejudiced the judges"—but "a veil was lifted, and they were able to create a direct line of communication with the outside world. It really had a ripple effect on how detention is viewed here."

Many of the strikers were deported, but a number were released and reunited with their families. The week after the strike ended, President Barack Obama ordered a review of his administration's immigration policies, and he met with immigration activists. In the years since, immigrants held at the Tacoma facility have regularly gone on hunger strikes (most recently, 115 detainees in the spring of 2023), which continue to generate publicity for their plight.

The hunger strike's potential may lurk within us all, yet it is a strange weapon, because it can only be wielded by the more vulnerable of disagreeing parties. It works in one direction: up, toward authority. You can undertake a protest fast against government, against your parents, against corporations, and even against allies with whom you adamantly disagree (as was the case with Mahatma Gandhi and the union organizer Cesar Chavez), but it's difficult to imagine a hunger strike directed down, toward people utterly lacking in power. It is more than a symbol. A hunger strike becomes a part of the process of change, even if it is aborted. The results are uncertain, but in seemingly hopeless situations, forcing a reconsideration of the existing equation can result in positive recalibration.

Despite their drastic consequences, hunger strikes are often near-spontaneous reactions to overwhelming events and authority. They seem to be an innate part of the human psyche, done at all times by all ages, whether or not people are cognizant of the long history of hunger strikes that precede them. In the fall of 2021, a number of young activists from the environmental group Sunrise Movement went on an extended hunger strike against climate change in front of the White House. Interviewed in the immediate wake of his eleven-day fast, twenty-four-year-old Paul Campion, one of the older members of the group, said to me that the fast was undertaken with minimal preparation. The young activists felt stymied. "Biden was not at all fighting for his own agenda, and seeing corporate Democrats hack to bits the Green New Deal was really frustrating. . . . There was no fight, no public pushback. So a few of us were talking about what could we do, how could we shift the conversation away from budget details and backroom politics, and really clarify the stakes and demonstrate that the courage that we needed to see from Biden was more than he was demonstrating." The Sunrisers held a Zoom conference on a Thursday, traveled to Washington, D.C., the following Monday, and began the fast that Wednesday—less than a week after coming up with the idea. Campion said the protesters felt they had few options. "It really came together as this question: Would a hunger strike meet the moment?" They obviously felt that it did: "We knew we weren't the first people doing this," he told me. Campion said they had all "read some articles" about the history of hunger strikes, but that the legacy of hunger striking wasn't the main motivator. It was an effective, elegant tool to rally the media, public sympathy, and perhaps prominent politicians, to their side.

Sahar Francis, the director of the Addameer Prisoner Support and Human Rights Association in Israel, notes that Palestinians have a long history with hunger strikes, beginning in the 1960s. She told me that prisoners first used the strikes "to guarantee basic things for their daily needs, such as a mattress, a pencil, and paper." Francis, who has been involved with asserting prisoner rights for more than twenty years, said that the first important, politically directed Palestinian hunger strike was instituted against the Palestinian Authority itself, after the Oslo Accord was signed in 1993, when the issue of hundreds of prisoners held without charge under "administrative detention" in Israeli jails was excluded from the discussion.

Almost every Palestinian in Israeli prisons—at the time, some eight thousand in total—participated in an extended hunger strike in 2004 for improved conditions. Officials were sufficiently concerned by the action that they tried to break the strike by "grilling meat in the cellblocks and putting civilian Israeli prisoners, who are not on hunger strike, among the Palestinians" and secretly filmed one of the strikers eating in an attempt to discredit him. After eighteen days, the strike ended with Israeli officials denying that they had capitulated to the strikers' demands, but with Palestinians claiming most of the demands had been met. Whether the strike had been broken or not, the Palestinians had succeeded in redirecting the gaze of their jailers, and forcing them to engage in dialogue, however brief. The extent that officials went to in order to minimize the strike's impact suggests the importance that they attached to its failure.

Palestinians, whether longtime activists or civilians caught up under the sweeping powers accorded to the Israeli military, remain committed to the use of a hunger strike as a response to arbitrary detention. Khader Adnan, a baker from the West Bank affiliated with the political wing of the

Palestinian Islamic Jihad (PIJ) movement, had been arrested twelve times over a period of nineteen years by the government and never charged with acts of violence. On his thirteenth arrest, he began a water-only hunger strike, by some accounts his sixth strike. After almost three months on the hunger strike, he died on May 2, 2023, in Israel's maximum-security prison in Ramla. Adnan had spent eight years in detention, including nearly six years in administrative detention without trial. His death led to international condemnation of his treatment, with Palestinian fighters erupting in outrage and the European Union calling for "a transparent investigation" into his death.

....

In the 1970s in the Soviet Union, the dissident writer Vladimir Bukovsky was repeatedly imprisoned for public outrages such as unsanctioned poetry readings. Bukovsky's experience mirrored that of the suffragists mentioned previously: prison authorities were alternately infuriated and baffled by his actions—they knew they had to respond, but weren't sure how to do so. Several times Bukovsky protested unreasonable prison strictures with hunger strikes, which never failed to upset officials, who then resorted to more brutality. In his memoir, *To Build a Castle*, Bukovsky vividly describes force-feeding. "The authorities always turn savage when you back them into a corner," he wrote.

> But that is precisely the moment to break their backs.... They strait-jacketed me, tied me down to a bed, and sat on my legs so that I wouldn't jerk. The others held my shoulders and my head. My nose is bent a bit to one side—I used to be a boxer as a boy and damaged it. The feeding tube was thick—thicker than my nostril—and wouldn't go in for love or money. Blood came gushing out of my nose and tears down my cheeks.... But they kept pushing until the cartilages cracked and something burst—enough to make you howl like a wolf. But fat chance there was of howling when the tube was in your throat and you

could breathe neither in nor out. I wheezed like a drowning man—my lungs were ready to burst. The doctor watching me also seemed ready to burst into tears, but she kept shoving the tube farther and farther down. Then she poured some sort of slops through a funnel into the tube—you'd choke if it came back up. They held me down for another half hour so that the liquid was absorbed by the stomach and couldn't be vomited back, and then began to pull the tube out bit by bit. . . . On the evening of the twelfth day the authorities surrendered.

Eventually, Bukovsky's stubborn determination to undertake hunger strikes became known throughout the Russian penal system. "Prison governors had grown terrified of Bukovsky. His mere presence, they believed, would cause other inmates to mutiny." The Soviets resolved the problem by exiling Bukovsky, his mother, and his nephew to Switzerland.

....

In postwar America, few groups have suffered worse indignities than migrant workers, whose backbreaking labor brings fresh fruit and vegetables to American tables. In the wake of the Great Depression, new labor laws were implemented in the 1930s, but many of those protections did not apply to migrant farmworkers, who worked in dangerous conditions and did so for minimal pay. They had little money and less influence over local politicians, who were beholden to the farmers and businessmen who employed the workers, often illegally. Cesar Chavez, the cofounder of the United Farm Workers union and one of the twentieth century's great labor activists, repeatedly turned to fasting as a way to draw attention to the farmworkers and their struggle.

In 1968, Chavez undertook his first hunger strike in protest not against the bosses, but to convince his fellow farmworkers of the power of nonviolence. At the time, some strikers advocated violent responses to strikebreakers and their employers. Chavez was adamant about the necessity for self-control. As opposition to his approach grew, he undertook a liquid-only fast, which simultaneously extinguished talk of violence and attracted great attention to what became universally known as "the plight of the farmworkers."

Chavez began his fast privately, telling people only on the third day. He was then drinking only Diet-Rite Cola. He switched to water the next day, and vowed to continue even as family and friends told him that he was crazy and bent on self-destruction. Others were convinced the act was one of self-aggrandizement. As his fast continued, his supporters became more adamant in their demands that he resume eating. Debilitated as he was, Chavez stood firm. In Peter Matthiessen's profile of Chavez, *Sal Si Puedes (Escape If You Can)*, Chavez recounts an amusing anecdote that occurred several days into the fast. He had "never felt better"—his sinusitis, chronic headaches, and back pain had cleared up—but many farmworkers were concerned that he was damaging his health, perhaps killing himself. A nearby workers' committee in Merced, fifty miles away, delegated one man to save Chavez. The man had said that if the group paid for his transportation, he would force Chavez to eat. The farmworker showed up one evening, drunk, with a pail full of tacos "and all kinds of tempting things," Chavez told Matthiessen.

> *I tried to explain to him, but he opens this lunch pail and gets out a taco, still warm, a big one, and tries to force me. And I don't want to have my lips touch the food—I mean, at that point, food is no temptation, I just thought that if it touched my lips, I was breaking the fast, you see, and I was too weak to fight him off. . . . First he gave me a lecture and that didn't work, then he played it tough and that didn't work. Then he cried and it didn't work and then we prayed together, and that didn't work, either.*

During the entire episode, the drunk worker was sitting on the chest of a supine Chavez. He was finally pulled off the labor leader by Chavez's brother and some others, at which point Chavez again explained his reasoning to the man. When Chavez broke his fast after twenty-five days, six thousand people, among them U.S. senator and presidential aspirant Robert F. Kennedy, gathered to celebrate.

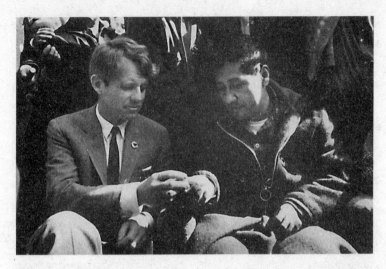

March 10, 1968: Sen. Robert F. Kennedy offers Cesar Chavez food during a special Mass in Delano, CA, attended by 6,000 people. Chavez ended a twenty-five-day fast that he had undertaken to rededicate the farmworkers' movement to nonviolence.

To call this fast a "punishment" on the part of Chavez for himself or for his followers, as some have done, seems a profound misunderstanding of the situation. It began as an internal, private decision, and evolved into a way to galvanize his fellow strikers: to convincingly demonstrate both the sincerity of his beliefs and his own toughness in the face of accusations that he was afraid of physical confrontation. Chavez wasn't condemning violence because he was afraid of its consequences. He was doing so because he felt that violent actions were worse than ineffective, that they undermined the movement. Both outside sympathizers and the workers themselves saw the fast as "a defining moment for the union," one where its leader affirmed the bedrock principles of nonviolence, self-determination, and dignity for all.

Chavez was consciously echoing Gandhi's 1924 hunger strike, which Gandhi had undertaken to appeal to striking mill workers inclined to violence. Chavez was a devoted reader of the Mahatma's writings. He knew that when people talk about committing violence, they mean it. Both leaders used nonviolence as a tool to reform an unjust system, and both were convinced that workers would undermine their own cause if they departed from the path of ahimsa (nonviolence), a concept at the core of classical Hinduism, Buddhism, and Jainism. In the case of Chavez, ahimsa fit neatly with his own Catholicism. Chavez also borrowed from Gandhi's example in his implementation of the most successful boycott in American history, the California grape boycott of 1968.

For Chavez, the grape boycott became not only a way for the farm-workers to directly pressure the growers but a means by which sympa-thizers around the nation could show their support for the effort, and feel good in doing so, thanks to their fast from grapes. The boycott, which started when growers refused to protect the workers from exposure to pesticides such as DDT—which was commonly sprayed over the vine-yards whether or not workers were present—gathered support from other unions, from celebrities, and from politicians. Across the country, not eating grapes became a mark of one's political affiliation. As the farmworkers accumulated allies, right-wing politicians such as Ronald Reagan—at the time the governor of California—expressed sympathy for the growers. Finally, after five long years of struggle, the farmworkers and growers together settled their case.

Fasting was an essential organizing tool for Chavez. It worked on several levels, as an aid to market the struggle, as a means of empower-ment, and as a practical tool to pressure employers and attract outside sympathizers. It clearly signaled that the system as it existed was unten-able, but that the farmworkers rejected doing violence to others. It was a shield and a sword. Chavez went on three significant public fasts, lasting longer than twenty days each. His final fast was in 1988, when he was sixty-one years old. He fasted for thirty-six days, again as a response to farmworkers pushing for violent demonstrations, this time against the wanton use of pesticides in fields. (As with the vineyards, farmers often sprayed their fields while unprotected workers were still working in them.) At the end of the fast, he said:

> A fast is first and foremost personal. It is a fast for the purification of
> my own body, mind, and soul. The fast is also a heartfelt prayer for

purification and strengthening for all those who work beside me in the
farmworker movement. The fast is also an act of penance for those in
positions of moral authority and for all men and women activists who
know what is right and just, who know that they could and should do
more. The fast is finally a declaration of non-cooperation. . . .

....

Hunger strikes by prisoners held without trial at Guantánamo Bay—
the notoriously brutal U.S. detention camp—began almost as soon
as it was opened in 2002 by the Bush administration. (Prisoners had
to refuse nine consecutive meals for the military to officially declare
a hunger strike was taking place.) Shortly thereafter, the military
implemented force-feeding as a matter of policy. It may seem strange
that a hunger strike often compels those in power to step in and try
to stop it; a hunger strike is meant precisely to attract attention. But
if prison authorities let a strike continue to its logical conclusion,
ridding themselves of an irritant, they cede control. To let a prisoner
decide their own fate deprives the state of its object lesson, and may
mark the prisoner's transition from a ward of the state to its arbiter.

At one point, 131 of the 500 prisoners in Guantánamo were being
force-fed, making it the largest mass force-feeding in history. The method
preferred by the U.S. military authorities there was to insert tubes through
a prisoner's nostrils. Bioethicist Jacob M. Appel, himself a doctor, wrote
of the procedure: "Forcible feeding through a naso-gastric tube ranks
alongside the most unpleasant and downright horrific experiences that one
human being can inflict upon another." Alternatively, as part of the effort
to subjugate their hunger-striking charges, CIA prison personnel injected
liquid protein into the bodies of prisoners via their anus. In 2023 testimony,
Dr. Sondra Crosby, a medical doctor and professor at Boston University
Schools of Medicine and Public Health, said that prisoners "experienced
it as a violent rape, a sexual assault," demolishing the paper-thin argument
that delivering food in this way was only to supply nutrition. "There is no

medical benefit ever to administering any form of nutrition through the rectum," she testified. Crosby helpfully explained that humans digest food through the stomach, and that "it cannot be done in reverse."

....

At the same time that force-feeding was taking place at Guantánamo, military authorities prevented some prisoners from fasting during the Muslim holy month of Ramadan, forcing them to break their religious vows and violate one of the basic premises of Islam. Mohamedou Ould Slahi is a former Guantánamo inmate who now lives in Mauretania. Slahi is a *hafiz*, someone who has memorized the Quran. It is a feat demanding both religious dedication and prodigious powers of memory, as the holy book comprises 77,430 words in Arabic. Slahi was never brought up on charges and was finally released in 2016 after spending more than fourteen years in jail. His torture was documented both in his bestselling book *Guantánamo Diary* and in the film *The Mauritanian*, which is based on his experiences. Slahi spoke to me from Dubai, where he was attending a conference. He said he remained mystified at his jailers' determination to keep him from fasting. There was "an effort at humiliation, an effort to cut the only spiritual connection that gives you strength," said Slahi. "I had these spiritual bonds through prayers and fasting, so then I was forbidden from praying and from fasting." He paused. "I think the point was that I should completely rely on them, that I was supposed to see them as the only escape. The basic thing they want you to see in your interrogators, your captors, is that they are the only way out, that they are the ones who give you food and help, that they are the source of everything, the source of your pain and your comfort."

....

Fasting in protest may be the last resource of the incarcerated, but people in all corners of the globe employ the tactic to defend old-growth forests, to protest school closings, to demand due process, to protest pollution, to demand reparations for slavery; in short, to amplify their voices and invoke the ancient right of *troscead/dharna*. The power of fasting-in-protest has even been employed to protect the rights of gardeners to use gasoline-powered leaf blowers, an issue not quite as frivolous as it may sound, because the gardeners in question were impoverished workers who were concerned their livelihoods were being threatened. (That weeklong hunger strike in January of 1998 ended with the Los Angeles city council saying that it would study the issue.)

A few more examples:

► Dick Gregory, the civil rights activist and comedian, first used fasting as a protest in 1967 against the Vietnam War. From Thanksgiving Day 1967 to January 9, 1968, he was said to have consumed only water and to have remained active, "traveling to fifty-seven cities and delivering sixty-three lectures." Later in 1968, after he was arrested and sentenced to three months in jail for participating in a "fish-in" in Washington State—which he had done to protest state laws restricting Native American fishing rights—he declared he would go on a bread-and-water fast in prison. On the thirty-ninth day of his fast, Gregory was sent to a hospital because of his deteriorating physical condition. He was released to serve the balance of his sentence at home. Over the years, Gregory went on dozens of hunger strikes to call attention to other issues ranging from the Equal Rights Amendment, South African apartheid, prison reform, oppressive drug laws, and police brutality, to fasting in support of singer Michael Jackson when Jackson was brought up on charges of sexual molestation in 2004.

► In December 1978, four Bolivian women from the Housewives Committee (*Comité Amas de Casa*)—Nelly de Paniagua, Angélica de Flores, Aurora de Lora, and Luzmila de Pimentel—initiated a fast in response to the Bolivian regime's harsh anti-union, anti-dissident policies. Organizers and other activists were routinely beaten and imprisoned or assassinated. The hunger strike gathered in scope, with fasts in solidarity occurring across Bolivia as church groups and women's rights organizations joined in. In the end, 1,380 people fasted for a total of twenty-two days. Although not all the demands of the women were met, the fast resulted in amnesty for nineteen thousand prisoners, exiles, and political refugees.

▶ Theresa Spence, chief of the Attawapiskat First Nation in northern Ontario, went on a six-week hunger strike beginning in December 2012 to force a meeting between Prime Minister Stephen Harper and First Nations leaders. "Right to the end, Spence has seemed remarkably buoyant for someone who has lived on fish broth and tea for forty-three days," reported the Canadian Broadcasting Corporation. "My heart is still good," Spence said at the strike's close. Although the PM didn't grant the meeting, media coverage of the strike was positive. The Assembly of First Nations, which according to the CBC "clos[ed] ranks" for the occasion, honored her for her activism, and a list of demands was presented to the government.

▶ Luaty Beirão, an Angolan rapper known by his stage name Ikonoklasta, was arrested in June 2015 after participating in a book club discussion of Gene Sharp's *From Dictatorship to Democracy*, a book about nonviolent resistance that includes an extensive discussion of fasting. After a hunger strike of thirty-six days, he was finally brought to trial. At first sentenced to five and a half years in prison, his sentence was reduced to house arrest, and he was subsequently released. "I kept testing my limits, seeing how strongly would I hold my convictions," he said. "I imagined the authorities would adopt the necessary measures for that not to [blow up] in their faces, but that's exactly what happened." It was only when Beirão was transferred to a hospital room and became aware of the extensive media coverage that the strike was receiving that he realized he wasn't protesting in vain.

▶ In the fall of 2019, Extinction Rebellion in the UK and activists in twenty-eight countries around the world (including the Sunrise Movement in the U.S.) undertook a limited hunger strike to protest the collapsing environment. Five hundred twenty people participated.

▶ Leyla Güven, an imprisoned deputy of the Peoples' Democratic Party in Turkey, began on November 8, 2018, what became a seventy-nine-day hunger strike, consuming only liquids and vitamins, in protest at the isolation of Abdullah Öcalan, the leader of the Kurdistan Workers'

Party. She was released on her own recognizance on January 25, 2019, and was arrested again shortly afterward on grounds that included, among other things, "matriarchal ideas." As of this writing, she remains in prison, this time under a sentence of eleven years and seven months, on charges of belonging to a terrorist organization.

▸ On January 29, 2020, Boston University professor Nathan Phillips began what became a two-week hunger strike to call attention to what he called a "public health emergency" in the planned construction of a nearby compressor station for natural gas. "The state basically rubber-stamped the project, so there was no [other way] to stop it," he said at the time. He ended his hunger strike once the state agreed to install permanent air monitors.

▸ For twenty-five days in the summer of 2020, hunger strikers in Louisville, Kentucky, demanded the three officers involved in the killing of Breonna Taylor be fired and stripped of their pensions, before converting their strike into a "rolling strike," inviting members of the community to join. "It is with full hearts and our heads held high that we end our hunger strike at 25 days. The passage of a recent ordinance denying protestors the right to create caravans and protest in the street ignited us enough to end our strike, gain our strength, and get back in the streets."

▸ Aleksei Navalny, the imprisoned leader of the Russian opposition, went on a three-week hunger strike in March to April 2021 to demand medical treatment for what he and others said was poisoning, the result of a failed assassination attempt. Navalny ended the strike when he said his demands were partly met. He said he had also ended his fast because "some supporters announced hunger strikes in solidarity and he did not want to risk their health."

▸ A seventy-three-year-old Chicago woman, Rachelle Zola, went on a forty-day hunger strike in the summer of 2021 to demand reparations for slavery. She didn't achieve her goal (passage of H.R. 40), but she received media attention and engaged Chicagoans who hadn't previously considered the matter. "My voice is just getting stronger," Zola told reporters.

▸ On February 1, 2022, two teachers announced they were going on a hunger strike of indefinite duration to protest the closing of their schools by the Oakland (California) Unified School District. The choir director of Westlake Middle School, André San-Chez, told the school board: "If I die, I want the board to know that my death was at your hands." San-Chez went on a liquid-only fast for a total of twenty days, and while he did not achieve his goals, the board postponed most of the school closings. "I believe this community has suffered enough, and I'm not sure people understand this suffering," he told me some months after the fast. "The idea popped into my head from thin air. . . . I knew something needed to be done." Like many hunger strikers, he was familiar with the work of Chavez and Gandhi—but additionally, San-Chez has a degree in musical theater, so he was, he said, comfortable with the idea of public engagement. The action wasn't done merely to get attention, he said. But "people don't necessarily understand [an issue] until they can see it, until it's physically manifested *in* something." His open display of vulnerability was meant to reach a wide audience. It did, although the school board ultimately refused to change its decision. While San-Chez told me that the exercise felt like a failure, "it also served as an empowerment tool, not only of myself, but hopefully for the community, because we only have ourselves. We have our voice, we have our body, and through some combination of those we have our actions. One individual can have a tremendous amount of power, and I wanted people to realize that."

▶ Alaa Abd El Fattah (sometimes spelled Abdel-Fattah), a blogger and software designer, became known for his writing during the 2011 Egyptian revolution and has served more than seven years in Egyptian jails. In April 2021, while incarcerated in Tora Maximum Security Prison No. 2 in Cairo, he began a hunger strike that lasted more than seven months, subsisting on tea with milk and honey. In December 2021 he was sentenced to an additional five years for "staging an illegal demonstration." As of this writing, the man sometimes referred to as "Egypt's most prominent political prisoner" is still not free, but in large part due to his hunger strike he has drawn international attention to his cause.

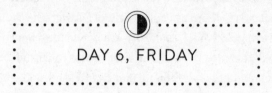

DAY 6, FRIDAY

Fasting, Frauds, and Faddism

Close to the final stretch, keen for this to be over. Uneven night last night. Felt weak and delicate this morning, better toward afternoon, but still jittery, much as I did on the second day. Perhaps it's just anticipation at ending the fast. Why do I want it to end? It's a deadline hanging over me, and I don't like boundaries, or deadlines. I like to be in the midst of a never-ending journey. Sipping diluted lemon juice and clear broth, found it delicious. A challenge to concentrate. There's the presence of an absence: I'm eager to fill the gap in my life that's left by not preparing meals, not going to restaurants, not nibbling a snack. Made a reservation at a restaurant for next week and for the first time, looking over menus and pictures of dishes, I really found myself longing for food. Korean dumplings: Why had I never before appreciated the paper-thin texture of the dough that envelops their chewy, moist fillings?

Mention "fasting" and people often react as though you plan to start sleeping on a bed of nails or let leeches suck your blood. By virtue of fasting's magical or spiritual dimension—its *weirdness*—it has long been associated with extremism. Cults, anti-science fanatics, and plain old fraudsters selling a cure are part of its fascinating history. For millennia, fasting was hailed as a way to open portals to another realm.

With the advent of the Christian ascetics it became a blade to flense away the unnecessary layers of one's own body.

Over the last several decades, what feminist Kim Chernin has memorably called the "tyranny of slenderness" has become a common topic, and justly so. When being slender is subverted by marketing, it becomes another mode of consumption, part of a social imperative, as Max Weber has argued. This drive to unattainable beauty benefits innumerable corporations and health practitioners. Lately, mere wellness is not enough: "hyper-wellness" and "hyper-growth," startling concepts that recall nothing so much as a human version of *Cocaine Bear*, are promoted by Restore Hyper Wellness, a corporation with close to two hundred franchises across the U.S. Its advertisements feature madly grinning clients, and an IV Drip of the Month may be had for under a hundred dollars.

The concept that the body can be restored to an Edenic state of perfect health goes back to one of the first self-help books, *Trattato de la vita sobria* (*Discourses on the Temperate Life*), written in 1558 by a Venetian nobleman, Luigi Cornaro, who was then in his eighties, in an epoch when it was a rarity to live past one's sixties. It is hard to overstate his importance to the modern understanding of fasting as a restorative practice: we can thank Cornaro for taking fasting out of the church and bringing it into the home. But he also set us on a course from which we still have not recovered, one that offers fasting as the miracle cure for just about every complaint.

Beset by numerous ailments and told by doctors that he was headed for an early grave, Cornaro self-diagnosed along Galenic principles that he suffered from an "exceedingly cold and moist stomach." By the age of forty, he had stopped relying on medicines and doctors, greatly reduced his intake of food and drink—restricting himself to one egg a day—and found he was revitalized. Eventually, he decided to share his formula for longevity with the world. His secret? Eating less is key to living well. No other special knowledge is required for good health. Also: avoid the medical profession. The book was an immediate success and launched a wave in publishing and commerce that hasn't subsided for more than 450 years. Its simple but democratic message remains part of its appeal. Three things keep us from paradise on earth, according to Cornaro: "Lutheranism," flattery, and intemperance. The intensity with which Cornaro launches his argument against gluttony might have, in fact, pleased Martin Luther:

> *O wretched and unhappy Italy! Do not you see, that intemperance murders every year more of your subjects than you could lose by the most cruel plague, or by fire and sword in many battles? Those truly shameful feasts, now so much in fashion, and so intolerably profuse, that no tables are large enough to hold the dishes, which renders it necessary to heap them upon one another; those feasts, I say, are so many battles: and how is it possible to support nature by such a variety of contrary and unwholesome foods?*

Left to its own devices, Cornaro's body healed itself, which he took to be a universal principle. This remains an attractive message to anyone who has suffered from the patronizing and often ill-informed advice of a self-important doctor.

> *Nay, by attending duly to what I have said, [any man] would become his own physician, and, indeed, the best he could have; since, in fact, no man can be a perfect physician to anyone but himself. The reason of which is, that any man may, by repeated trials, acquire a perfect knowledge of his own constitution, and the most hidden qualities of his body; and what wine and food agree with his stomach.*

With the passage of centuries, successive dieting enthusiasts elevated Cornaro to the level of a legendary hero. Even Benjamin Franklin, while a notorious gourmand himself, was an admirer. Franklin claimed that self-restraint enabled Cornaro to live to the age of 120; Cornaro actually died in 1566 at the still-impressive age of ninety-one.

Cornaro's concerns were taken up with passion by a member of the profession that he disdained. Santorio Santorio was an Italian physician who shared Cornaro's passion for regulating intake, and he did so with the obsessive focus of an alchemist. Santorio was consumed with quantification: by placing a graded scale behind a sealed thermoscope, he created the first sealed thermometer, and was able to measure both air and the human body. He also invented a wind gauge, a water current meter (hygrometer), a pulsilogium (for measuring pulse rates), and various other implements. He is credited with being one of the early proponents of scientific inquiry into the body's metabolism. His pulsilogium is said to have inspired his friend Galileo and to have set in motion many experiments in seventeenth-century Europe. But Santorio is most often cited for becoming the world's first compulsive weight watcher, thanks to his invention of an elaborate mechanism to weigh himself from one minute to the next: the steelyard chair, or medical balance. The chair was suspended from a weighing scale, and over the course of thirty years, Santorio regularly weighed himself and others. He reportedly collected ten thousand records, including those of Galileo. He weighed himself before and after meals, sex, bathroom visits, sleep, and exercise. The driven doctor determined that what Galen had called *perspiratio insensibilis* ("insensible perspiration") accounted for weight loss not measurable in normal bodily excretions. These subtle changes were a guide to

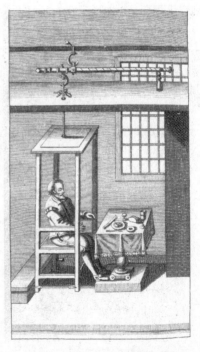

The weighing chair of Santorio Santorio. From *Medicina Statica: Being the Aphorisms of Sanctorious, Translated into English with Large Explanations*. Translated by John Quincy, 1718.

true health, or a lack thereof. With his discovery of the crucial role of this invisible diminution, the doctor had found his philosopher's stone, and he continued with his measurements until he died in his seventies of a urinary tract infection.

Santorio and Cornaro each represent what cultural historian Hillel Schwartz identified as one of the two tributaries of the mighty dieting river, the "dieting romance" and the "dieting ritual." With Cornaro, weight came to be connected with ideas of personal worth: he suffered his trials and emerged enlightened, entering a blissful realm of hyper-wellness that enabled him to live to a ripe old age with morals improved and faculties intact. For Santorio, a life in balance was all-important, and could be quantified by cutting-edge technology.

....

Fasting persisted past the age of miracles, although its transformative influence became more celebrated for its effect on the human machine than as a gateway to the spirit world. By the late seventeenth century, the emphasis was less on the sacred than the profane: the vicar Nathaniel Wanley's *The Wonders of the Little World: Or, a General History of Man* (1678), a sort of *Ripley's Believe It or Not!* of the period, is studded with fasting marvels. Fasters continued to be celebrated by the ballads of the time, venerated less for their divine insights than for being proof of the astounding new epoch. Fasting made the transition to the scientific age at first hesitantly and then emphatically, transformed from a predominantly devotional practice into one that came to be seen as an exemplary talent.

Crowds and scholars marveled at the extremes of fasting perpetrated by civilians outside the holy orders. These laypeople, for the most part young women or girls who sometimes showed signs of what we would now call anorexia, became celebrities of their time. They were visited by church leaders, clerics, and often skeptical scholars. A transitional example was the internationally celebrated "Dutch Virgin" Eve Fleigen/Eva

Vliegen (b. 1575), who for fourteen years lived off "th' scent of flowers" in Meurs, a town in what was then the Netherlands (and is now Germany). By some reports, Fleigen managed to deny the call of nature in any form:

Full strange it was to see, her belly was so flat,
The passages were shut, no entrance there was found,
She voyded nothing forth, nothing at all she ate
Her priuy parts were cleane, thence nothing fell to ground.

Fleigen's celebrity reportedly aroused the jealousy of some local nobles, who attempted to seduce her into "tasting exquisite fruits from nearby trees. But no sooner had Fleigen plucked a cherry, tasted, and ingested it than she became ill and nearly died." Wilhelm Fabry von Hilden, now known as the father of German surgery, paid her a respectful visit in 1612, describing her as pious but depressed. She persisted for thirty years convincing people she lived without food or drink, reaping contributions before the fraud was discovered after the smell of feces gave her away. She was sentenced to a public whipping, but received a royal pardon due to her advanced age.

The implication that physical improvement led to moral perfection was embraced by the same Lutherans that Cornaro had seen as

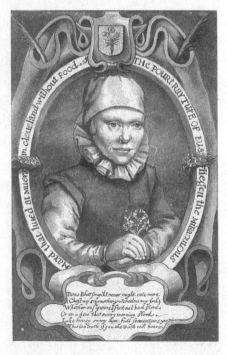

Eve Fleigen, a woman who lived off the smell of flowers. *Drawing after B. Flessiers.*

a threat to social morals. Cornaro's message of temperance found its most fervent adherents among the Protestant preachers of the seventeenth century, who linked spiritual health to physical health and for whom, after prayer, there was no better expression of holiness than fasting. This period saw the rise of what came to be known as "natural hygiene," which has origins in both Protestant elevation of common sense (versus the specialized, inaccessible knowledge reserved for elites) and in disgust at the degeneration of the self. "The seeds of Weakness and Pain, Sickness and Death, are now lodged in our inmost Substance. . . . The Heavens, the Earth and all Things contained therein conspire to punish the Rebels against their Creator," thundered the preacher John Wesley in the 1747 health book *Primitive Physick*. His appeal to "every man of common sense," along with his low regard for the medical community, marked him as a friend of the people. Sinners were sick, and the sick were sinners, and fasting (together with prayer) was the antidote. Wesley's tome, a guide for those who either could not afford physicians or did not trust them, was one of the most popular books published in eighteenth-century England. Thirty-six editions of the book were brought out in England by 1840. In America, a revised edition was published in Boston as late as 1858. The enduring appeal of Wesleyan Methodism lay in its fundamentally democratic outlook. Fasting was a means to bring the attention of sinners back to the divine. In a famous 1748 sermon ("Upon Our Lord's Sermon on the Mount"), Wesley specified that, while fasting "is not all" and it "is not the end, it is a precious means thereto."

....

Fraud and fasting are opposites and natural bedfellows. Although the number of holy fasters declined with modernization, fasting retained its association with miracle-working. The performative side of fasting together with its lingering air of the supernatural attracted fraudsters ready to bilk paying audiences. Extreme fasters brought fame and fortune to their families and even to their towns; they often attracted the attention and patronage of royals, as had Eve Fleigen. Extreme fasting was a tempting con, but any number of those condemned as fraudsters share characteristics with those whom we'd characterize today as anorexic.

Becoming famous by not eating was risky. If the discovery came that eternal fasters were actually eating, no matter how minimally, vindictiveness was guaranteed on the part of locals and the authorities. In 1512, for example, a miraculously fasting woman in Augsburg, Germany, initially hailed for her piety, was found to partake of earthly sustenance. She was summarily drowned. Another German, Margaretha Ulmer, faced similarly dire consequences after being exposed as a fraud in 1546: she was sentenced to life in prison after having her face pierced with a red-hot iron, while her mother was tortured and burned for complicity in the scheme.

While later "deceivers" received less severe punishments, they were at the very least sentenced to pay fines and serve prison time (as happened to Catherine of Veltlin in the mid-seventeenth century, who was sentenced to ten years in jail after claiming to have fed only on the Eucharist for twelve years). Some were forced to flee their homes, as happened to Ann Moore, "the Fasting Woman of Tutbury," in 1813. For a number of years she held that she "had not swallowed any kind of solid food, with the exception . . . of the inside of a few black currants." She underwent a supervised fast of sixteen days in 1808, which provided "conclusive evidence of her veracity." In that year she was inspired to stop drinking liquids as well. After numerous visitors flocked to Tutbury—many of them bearing gifts and donations—a commission composed of local dignitaries, clergy, and physicians was set up to examine her claims. The second supervised fast of one month in 1813 found that Moore had a "mind hardened in sin and moral insensibility" and that she had committed fraud by drinking tea with a bit of milk and sugar. She was made to sign a confession, which read in its entirety:

I, Ann Moore, of Tutbury, humbly asking pardon of all persons whom I have attempted to deceive and impose upon, and above all with the most unfeigned sorrow and contrition imploring the Divine Mercy

and Forgiveness of that God whom I have so greatly offended, do
most solemnly declare, that I have occasionally taken sustenance for
the last six years.

Several accounts of Ann Moore's deception were published, describing
her as "a notorious immoral character" who had profited off the credulity
of her visitors. The multiple editions of these pamphlets suggests that
they sold briskly.

In the case of the famous nineteenth-century Welsh "fasting girl"
Sarah Jacob, boys offered tourists their services as guides to visit her
home. Jacob ended by starving to death at the age of twelve while trying
to prove herself. She was caught between local pride at her "miracle"—
townspeople indignantly defended her honor—and diligent investigators.
Her parents were convicted of manslaughter.

By the mid-nineteenth century, fasting became less evidence of
sanctity than of desire or compulsion, and fasting-as-spectacle gained in
popularity, in many ways becoming the antithesis of what ancient spiritual-
minded fasters hoped to achieve. Ethics was now bound up with health.
For many, fasting was proof of mental prowess and the ability to conquer
natural impulses, but it also began to reflect a consumerist impulse. Fasting
with no purpose other than a stronger body becomes acquisition. The
surge in fasting in the latter part of the nineteenth century coincided
with mass industrialization. In a period when machinery became ever
more remarkable and inescapable, more people than ever hungered for
proof that their fellow humans could still astound. In breathless newspaper accounts, fasting reemerged as proof of humanity's—particularly
men's—magical ability to conquer nature.

....

In 1833, an English translation of Cornaro's book was accompanied by
an introduction from a Presbyterian minister, the same Sylvester Graham who invented the famous graham cracker. Even as Graham praised

Cornaro's abstinence, he condemned its precepts. "The whole system of governing the head by the stomach, instead of governing the stomach by the head, is absolutely wrong," he wrote. Graham was commonly known at the time as "Dr. Sawdust" for his Galenic insistence on bland, insipid foods. "Make your stomach the healthful minister of your body, and not your whole body the mere locomotive appendage of your stomach. Treat your stomach like a well governed child. . . ." Graham is often credited as having written the first modern diet book in 1837. He subsequently published the *Graham Journal of Health and Longevity*, which melded Protestant views on the inseparability of health and virtue. Gluttony was civilization's by-product, which seduced natural appetite. Hunger had less to do with the digestive juices of the stomach than with poor morals. Good, clean living—no spices, please—made for an even-tempered, courageous American man. Steering clear of man-made poisons and relying on the God-given, natural capacities of the body to right itself became the central maxims for the developing hygienist movement in America and Europe.

That "unnatural" methods should be avoided did not mean that people should do nothing in the event of disease. All true Christians recognized that the body was the soul's container. It followed that hygienic living and knowledge of physiology were moral obligations. But brands of physiology differed wildly. Some hygienists equated ingestion with the introduction of impurities to the God-given body, maintaining, as Graham did, that most foods were an impediment to physical and moral health. What further distinguished the hygienists from scientists was their disdain for empiricism, and what propelled the hygienists to the forefront of the American imagination was the work of Graham and another self-styled reformer, William Andrus Alcott, the "elder statesman of abstinence" (and cousin of writer Louisa May Alcott). For both these health reformers, America was facing a rapid decline.

Graham's teachings were spread by his disciple Isaac Jennings, an 1812 graduate of Yale Medical School, who took them to the next level. Like Graham, Jennings had no patience for conventional cures of the day—a not-unreasonable approach in a time before anesthetics or antibiotics, and when, for example, opium was commonly prescribed to prevent tuberculosis. Jennings decided that the best course was always to let the body cure itself. Stimulants of any kind, including medicinal drugs and spices, wore away vitality and corrupted the body. The best treatment was no treatment. In the middle of the century, Jennings put a name to the philosophy, and gave us what he called "orthopathy." In his 1867 treatise, *The Tree of Life, or, Human Degeneracy: Its Nature and Remedy*, he explained the appellation: "Right affection. From *orthos*, right, true, erect; and *pathos*, affection. Nature is always upright: moving in the right direction." With his conviction that "degenerate" humans could only be saved by a proper and meager diet, his rejection of organized medical treatment, and finally his invention of a new system of health care, Jennings opened the way to the later excesses of the alternative health movement.

....

While dieting became popularized in the United States after the Civil War, fasting as an antidote (and therefore a partner) to greed has been a recurrent boogeyman in the national psyche. The weird dyad of capitalism and Calvinism can never be reconciled. It's a familiar American trope that nothing is worthwhile unless it's expanding—progress above all else! The quintessential American holiday, Thanksgiving, exemplifies the dilemma: it is a bacchanal to commemorate the myth of the starving Puritans' rescue at the hands of kindly Native Americans; the moral feast where we stuff ourselves to the point of collapse. Maud Ellmann writes, "The emphasis on 'fiber' suggests that the failing *moral* fiber of America might be rescued by heroic mastication of the indigestible integuments of vegetables."

In 1866, a little-known freelancer for a California newspaper profiled survivors of the shipwreck of the *Hornet*, a catastrophe that resulted in an unintentional Biosphere 2–like fasting experiment. Decades after the incident, Mark Twain recalled the episode in his essay "My Début as a

Literary Person." A record-setting clipper ship on the circuit from New York City to San Francisco and back, the *Hornet* had rounded the tip of South America at Cape Horn and was sailing more than a thousand miles from land when it caught fire in the Pacific. The thirty-one-member crew piled into three small boats. Forty-three days and four thousand miles later, one longboat crammed with fourteen "lean and ghostly survivors" arrived in Hawaii. The men had survived on ten days' rations of food. Twain was in Honolulu at the time, bedridden with saddle sores. When he heard rumors of the saga, he realized its potential to make his career. He had himself carried down to the harbor on a stretcher to meet the arriving crew. Twain wrote some of his first dispatches about the disaster for the *Sacramento Daily Union*, later recycling the story that same year for *Harper's New Monthly Magazine* and then again for the *Century Illustrated Monthly Magazine* in 1899 and still again in his 1906 autobiography. What astounded Twain as much as the crew's survival, he wrote, was how after landing, the men "gathered strength fast, and were presently nearly as good as new." Wrote Twain (emphasis his):

> *A little starvation can really do more for the average sick man than can the best medicines and the best doctors. I do not mean a restricted diet; I mean* total abstention from food for one or two days. *I speak from experience; starvation has been my cold and fever doctor for fifteen years, and has accomplished a cure in all instances. . . . There were four sailors down sick when the ship was burned. Twenty-five days of pitiless starvation have followed, and now we have this curious record:* "All the men are hearty and strong; even the ones that were down sick are well," *except poor Peter* [a *Hornet* sailor who died]. *When I wrote an article some months ago urging temporary abstention from food as a remedy for an inactive appetite and for disease, I was accused of jesting, but I was in earnest.* "We are all wonderfully well and strong, comparatively speaking!" *On this day the starvation regimen drew its belt a couple of buckle holes tighter: the bread ration was reduced from the usual piece of cracker the size of a silver dollar*

to the half of that *and one meal was* abolished from the daily three. *This will weaken the men physically, but if there are any diseases of an ordinary sort left in them they will disappear.*

That Twain chose to avoid the word "fasting" was not an oversight. At the time, the word had a genteel connotation because of its association with organized religion and the "fasting girls" of the day. But to survive a starvation regimen was a physical feat worthy of any empire-building pioneer.

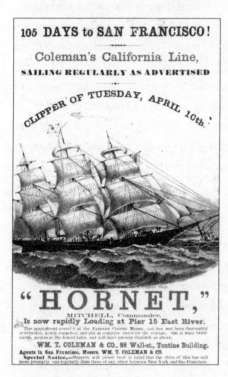

105 **DAYS** to **SAN FRANCISCO**!

Coleman's California Line,

SAILING REGULARLY AS ADVERTISED

CLIPPER OF TUESDAY, APRIL 10th.

" **HORNET,** "

MITCHELL, Commander.

Is now rapidly Loading at Pier 15 East River.

This magnificent vessel is of the EXTREME CLIPPER MODEL, and has just been thoroughly overhauled, newly coppered, and put in complete order for the voyage. She is WELL VENTILATED, dunnage at the lowest rates, and will have prompt dispatch as above.

WM. T. COLEMAN & CO., 88 Wall-st., Tontine Building.

Agents in San Francisco, Messrs. WM. T. COLEMAN & CO.

Special Notice.—Shippers will please bear in mind that the ships of this line sail more promptly and regularly than those of any other between New-York and San Francisco.

The *Hornet* burned at sea in 1866. As chronicled by Mark Twain, fourteen "lean and ghostly survivors" of the thirty-one-member crew arrived in Honolulu after a voyage of forty-three days in an open boat; they had survived on ten days' ration of food. The men "gathered strength fast, and were presently nearly as good as new."

Tapping into this growing trend of fasting-for-health was Dr. Edward Hooker Dewey, whose publications in the 1890s recycled Cornaro's case that nothing was so good for the body as starving it. Like Cornaro's screed, his books were based on personal experience and moral principles, all presented in a grand manner that obscured a lack of substance behind a lot of fluff, and in the words of one historian "allowed them to pass for elegant insights before the eyes of the uncritical." A veteran of the Civil War who saw firsthand that patients left untouched by the ministrations of physicians, including himself, were best off, he became a proselytizer for fasting and the "revolutionary" system of hygiene. The heart of Dewey's thesis was that disease came from the body's processes being overwhelmed by excess food. As with much in the hygienic movement, granules of scientific truth— eating too much is unhealthy, and incompetent treatment is worse than no treatment—became lost in a tsunami of overenthusiasm. In three publications totaling more than nine hundred pages, Dewey sermonized on behalf of his "No-Breakfast Plan," a *moral science* of digestive energy" that promised not only to strengthen American bodies but to heighten productivity, freeing American women to do more housework.

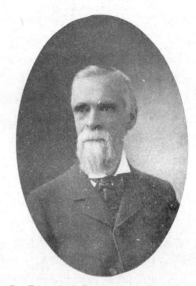

Dr. Edward H. Dewey, one of the first advocates in the Industrial Age of fasting for health. From the frontispiece to *The No-Breakfast Plan and the Fasting-Cure* (1900).

His conflation of good Christian morals with less eating or no eating became a guiding principle for the hygienic movement. Hygienic principles would set Americans apart from lesser cultures and peoples. Fasting, specifically, was "the long awaited key to perfect health, vitality, stamina, and longevity for the sick and the well alike."

....

Victorians regularly paid good money to attend a fasting spectacle, and extreme fasters of thirty days or more attracted paying audiences. These publicly feted "hunger artists" were almost always men. One of the first to showcase fasting machismo on a national scale was Dr. Henry S. Tanner, a graduate of the Eclectic Medical Institute in Cincinnati (class of 1859), who thrilled the New York City multitudes by not eating. His public performance in 1880 provided a model for professional fasters for generations to come. The action was sparked, Tanner said, by a gallant effort to defend the claims of another celebrated faster, Mollie Fancher, from a group of doctors led by Dr. William A. Hammond, the former surgeon general of the Union Army. Fancher's fasting, of course, took place in the respectable surroundings of the townhouse of a wealthy relative.

After a series of personal calamities that had resulted in paralysis and blindness, Fancher had been transformed into "the Brooklyn Enigma." She was compensated for "indescribable sufferings" by miraculous powers: she could read a book by passing her hand over its cover, foretell events, hear conversations fifty miles away, and occasionally could see through a portal in her forehead. Most crucially, she claimed she had lost her ability to swallow (although she could still speak) and therefore lived without eating or drinking. By 1879, she had supposedly lived this way for fourteen years. "She says she is a miracle, and I know she is one," declared a typical supporter.

In 1879, Hammond published *Fasting Girls: Their Physiology and Pathology*, in which he discussed a number of cases of famous fasters, among them Eve Fleigen, Ann Moore, and Sarah Jacob. The afflicted were first and foremost "girls"—what Hammond saw as society's weakest element. Although he cited as one of his examples of questionable fasting Nicholas of Flüe, men were exempt from Hammond's criticism: "I am not aware that this claim has been made in its fullest development for the male of the human species." Hammond held that long-term, complete abstinence was a matter of either self-delusion or fraud, although he also stated he was open to being shown proof that it was possible for humans to survive without food. At the time, the generally accepted limit for complete abstinence from food was fifteen days (today, a few weeks' abstinence from food is seen as the limit for most people, depending on their body type). Mollie Fancher was a particular focus of Hammond's ire, and in the appendix to his book he reprinted a December 1878 letter he had written to the *New York Daily Herald*, in which he presented two challenges to her: if she could read the bank information on a check "exceeding $1,000" (roughly the equivalent of $30,000 today) through a sealed envelope, he would sign it over to her; and if she would submit to monitoring of a monthlong fast by members of the New York State Neurological Society, he would give her another $1,000. Fancher declined to accept "for decency's sake." Henry Tanner stepped forward as her champion, declaring that he would fast for forty days and prove Hammond wrong. Hammond agreed to monitor the event assisted by his coterie of New York doctors, and the United States Medical College—a naturopathic institution with no connection to the government—stood by Tanner. The contest represented a clash of cultures—the populist, naturopathic rebels vs. the elite, "allopathic" establishment. The newspapers were enthralled by the prospect.

Several hundred people were on hand when Tanner began his fast on June 28, 1880, ready to witness what journalists hailed as an "extraordinary battle of a human will with a human stomach." Admittance was free at first, but after ten days, twenty-five cents was charged. "From the beginning it had attracted great attention, and in the eastern part of the United States it was nothing less than a sensation," wrote Herbert Asbury in the *New Yorker* more than half a century later. Tanner was receiving between three hundred and five hundred letters a day from around the country, accompanied by assorted gifts. A museum in Maine offered to stuff Tanner's body if he died during the contest. He was regaled by various admirers, and managed to rouse himself to applaud "the performance of a lady who had offered to entertain him by singing ballads with considerably more energy than the physicians who had evidently assembled to witness his death." A month into the fast, Hammond acknowledged its integrity and called on Tanner to relent, which he promised to do if he began to hiccup. He didn't hiccup, and so he continued to the fortieth day, when, wan but triumphant, he declared an end to the spectacle.

Doctors from all over the world wrote long letters telling him how to break his fast without harm to his stomach. One advised him to take five drops of milk and nothing more for twenty-four hours and another suggested that he smell a plate of buttered toast for half an hour before attempting to eat anything. . . . None of this advice was followed.

A small boy handed Tanner a peach, "which he held aloft for a moment and then ate with obvious relish." To resounding cheers, he subsequently consumed a half pound of steak together with copious amounts of fruit. He washed it all down with rice milk without a complaint or hint of refeeding syndrome. He continued binging for the rest of the day, and within three days regained ten of his thirty-six lost pounds. It would seem physiologically impossible to indulge in such a gargantuan feast after forty days of complete fasting—or at least to do so without suffering metabolic collapse in the form of refeeding syndrome, and indeed at the time there were accusations of fraud by members of the New York State Neurological Society. But Tanner shrugged off the critics. America was looking for a new hero (although Tanner had been born and raised in England), and his fans weren't concerned with whether or not he'd bent the rules. At the end, police were required to keep the boisterous crowd from pushing past the barricades to get a closer look, and it must have seemed as though, emerging from an ascetic interlude, Tanner had reaffirmed the American drive to consume. He had turned the fasting imperative inside out: it had become an endurance contest, not a space for contemplation or spiritual renewal. Here was proof of manliness and a hunger to consume on a colossal scale, worthy of ambitions of empire.

The small-minded scientific men had been defeated, Tanner had emerged victorious, and Mollie Fancher continued fasting and exercising her skills. She declined a request from P. T. Barnum to exhibit herself. A book detailing her amazing powers, including an account of her multiple personalities (Sunbeam, Idol, Rosebud, Pearl, and Ruby), was published in 1894, and she died in 1916, still busy fasting and mind-reading. Although Tanner's celebrity was fleeting, the water he drank during the fast came from a pool in Central Park that is known to this day as "Tanner's Spring." After the fast he put himself on exhibit for several weeks (admission fifty cents), and then little more was heard of him. Decades later, he popped up in the news again when he suggested that impoverished New Yorkers could survive winters by training themselves to hibernate.

In 1913, at the age of eighty-three, and by then a resident of Los Angeles, Tanner made a long-distance marriage proposal to the leading English suffragette and veteran hunger striker Emmeline Pankhurst (mother of Sylvia), apparently without having met her. Pankhurst spurned the stunt as "impudent and insulting."

Perhaps the world's most celebrated faster at the close of the nineteenth century was Giovanni Succi, an Italian from the Emilia-Romagna area of northern Italy whose career is now commonly accepted as the inspiration for Kafka's story "A Hunger Artist." In 1886, after several trips to "a remote village in Africa," where he claimed to have encountered a sorcerer who gave him a magical elixir, a few drops of which enabled him to survive without food for long periods, Succi began fasting publicly for weeks at a time. (It has been speculated that the "elixir" was some sort of opiate that suppressed hunger pangs.) Succi's fame grew as he traveled throughout Europe, putting on a fasting show in various cities and selling his potion. In Paris, he fasted for a month and received a prize of 15,000 francs, approximately $100,000 in today's dollars. Hailed as the "Fasting Man" in *Scientific American*, he arrived in Manhattan in 1890 to display his abilities of endurance. In New York, Succi performed at Koster & Bial's Music Hall, where he fasted for forty-five days, ending his ordeal on December 20. "He broke his fast with a cup of cocoa through an advertising arrangement with the manufacturer, and for a similar reason swallowed a cup of beef extract later." A portion of Koster & Bial's still stands at the corner of Sixth Avenue and Twenty-Fourth Street, where it was subsequently home to the storied Billy's Topless bar. Significantly, Succi's performance took place in Satan's Circus, the heart of the down-and-dirty neighborhood then known as the Tenderloin, a notorious red-light district where it was said that half the buildings were devoted "to some form of deviant behavior." Fasting had traveled a distance from the days of Anthony of the Desert. At least in the West, abstinence was now music hall entertainment—the domain of showmen, fraudsters, and the diseased.

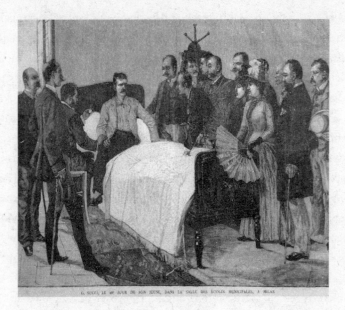

G. SUCCI, LE 28ᵉ JOUR DE SON JEUNE, DANS LA SALLE DES ÉCOLES MUNICIPALES, A MILAN

Giovanni Succi on the twenty-eighth day of a fast, 1886.

Succi was followed by a succession of fasters who offered themselves up in the name of commerce or science: in 1910, Clare de Serval, a rare female celebrity faster known as the "Apostle of Hunger," put herself on display in a glass box during her fast. In doing so, she foreshadowed the actions of the performer David Blaine, who in 2003 went on a water-only fast for forty-four days in a transparent box. The container was suspended from a crane placed near London's Tower Bridge, forty feet above often raucous crowds which perceived the action as a kind of provocation. People threw eggs, bottles, and bananas. They tried to hit the box with golf balls, banged drums to wake up the performer, and even tried to cut his water pipe. Blaine lost a quarter of his body weight during the fast and immediately went into a hospital with signs of hemoconcentration (highly concentrated blood, which can also be caused by hypothermia or extreme physical activity).

One of the last of the great fasting performers was Agostino Levanzin, a Maltese lawyer, novelist, pharmacist, newspaper publisher, social crusader, Esperanto enthusiast, and professional faster, who arrived in the United States in 1912. He intended to subsist two months without nutrition, drinking only distilled water. He would become, as he said, "a hero of science." His ability to endure a month or more without eating had previously been verified by Dr. Robert Samut (the composer of the Maltese national anthem), who had issued a certificate affirming Levanzin's mental and physical well-being. In the prestigious Nutrition Laboratory of the Carnegie Institution of Washington in Boston, Levanzin submitted himself to living in a "respiration calorimeter" which was described by a journalist as being "fitted with an ingenious mechanism so delicate that it records the effort expended in winking an eye, and thus discovers how much strength-giving quality there is in a food or how much energy the human machine consumes in work or leisure."

Levanzin's fasting trajectory will be familiar to students of the art: during the first three days of the fast, he complained of discomfort. "After that he said that he lost any desire for food and experienced a period of exhilaration," wrote a journalist. "He said his brain was clear and that he could think more rapidly and concisely." Levanzin terminated his fast after thirty-one days and sixteen hours without food, ending in "excellent health . . . with no decrease of his mental or physical powers." But he was reportedly upset at the doctors' insistence he end his fast before his "natural hunger" had manifested itself. Less than a week later, Levanzin abruptly changed his take on the matter, and told the press that he had been tortured, confined twelve hours a day to a "coffin-like affair . . . seven feet long, two feet wide, and one and one-half feet high. . . . In addition to the torture of being unable to move scarcely a muscle, a stethoscope was put over my heart. As the fast wore on the weight of the stethoscope was almost unbearable." When he was discharged, he was cast out into the street without the necessary oversight and without having gone through the careful refeeding process advisable for anyone emerging from a prolonged fast. Levanzin remained in the United States, eventually finding a position at the Los Angeles Chiropractic College. Among Maltese, he is revered to this day: in 2022, the Central Bank of Malta issued a ten-euro silver coin in his honor.

....

"I seemed to hollow out myself from head to toe," says Knut Hamsun's nameless protagonist in *Hunger* (1890), an autobiographical novel that is often cited as a classic of literary fasting. In the words of one critic, martyrdom is "a tempting pose" for a long-term faster, and Hamsun's hero revels in his slow degeneration and the tactile qualities of death by starvation. Deprived of food by his poverty—which makes the novel not so much about fasting as it is about involuntary starvation—the narrator links his creative powers with his deprivation, even as he desperately seeks sustenance. *Hunger* is a masochistic (albeit vividly depicted) celebration of suffering. It is perhaps relevant that the author was a crypto-fascist who celebrated Nazism over a period of many years.

According to Max Brod, Kafka was an admirer of Hamsun's work. But unlike Hamsun's hero, Kafka's fasters make a conscious, willful decision to set themselves apart. Just two years before his death, in 1922, Kafka published "A Hunger Artist." That same year, although he never released it for publication, he wrote "Investigations of a Dog." Fasting is the focal point of that marvelously meandering tale, in which the narrator dog's fascination with the provenance of his food—and by extension the limitations of his existence—culminates in his fasting. The narrator acknowledges that by freeing himself from the tyranny of the dog bowl, he upsets the order of things, presided over by a faceless "they": "They would rather do the impossible, that is, stop my mouth with food . . . than endure my questions." Food is a thought-stopper. With food in your jaws "your problems are over for the time being," and the narrator wants to be dissatisfied, to stay hungry. Unnamed instructors prohibit him from fasting, but he is a bad dog and refuses to obey, embracing dissatisfaction. "The way leads through starvation; the highest is only attainable through the most extreme privation, and for us this privation is voluntary fasting." The story ends inconclusively, with the protagonist separated from his fellow dogs by an "infinitely far distance," his senses "sharpened by hunger."

Kafka's disgust at his animalistic drive to eat is scattered throughout his diaries. Consumption of food was inversely connected with intellectual substance, as he made clear in an oddly boastful 1912 letter to his on-again, off-again fiancée, Felice Bauer: "Just as I am thin, and I am the thinnest person I know (and that's saying something, for I am no stranger to sanatoria), there is also nothing to me which, in relation to writing, one could call superfluous, superfluous in the sense of overflowing." Throughout his short life, he was obsessed with his body, alternately proud of his leanness and despairing at its scrawniness. Sustenance—and the option of its rejection—was in many ways central to Kafka's writing. Food was not a lifeline, but a distraction from meaning; at the same time, a superfluity of "lessness" inevitably leads to physical weakness.

As a follower of the *Lebensreform* movement ("life reform" or "life transformation"), a loose confederation of groups with roots in nineteenth-century German and Swiss reactions to industrialization, Kafka was a committed faster. Anticipating movements such as anthroposophy, the Bauhaus and, later, New Ageism, disciples of *Lebensreform* advocated a return to "natural" living in the form of simple clothing (no Victorian corsets!), outdoor sports, vegetarianism, pacifism, and fasting. *Lebendige Kraft* ("living power") came from sunlight, not food, inspiring breatharianism and related beliefs.

The intriguing idea that people can live off of air and perhaps a bit of sunshine has a long and distinguished history that persists to this day. Eve Fleigen was far from the first; Aristotle noted an adept who "neither ate nor slept and only lived on air," and the Roman historian Pliny the Elder is supposed to have referred to the Astomi, a people who lived on the banks of the Ganges, "who have no mouthes and are supported by the smell of roots, flowers, and wild apples." In the thirteenth century, the Franciscan philosopher Roger Bacon postulated that an Englishwoman, who had lived for twenty years without eating, was kept alive not thanks to divine intervention but to her ability to maintain her body in perfect Galenic equilibrium:

And some also lived a long time without nourishment, as in our times there was one woman in England in the diocese of Norwich, who did not eat for twenty years, and was fat and in good condition, emitting no excess from the body, as the bishop proved by a faithful examination. Nor was it a miracle, but the work of nature, for there was at that time a certain constellation capable of reducing the elements to a nearer degree of equality than they were before in her body; and because her combination was naturally proper to this constellation, and not so the combinations of others, therefore its alteration occurs in her body which does not occur in others.

Scientific advances in the late eighteenth century only served to boost the concept of inedia. Antoine Lavoisier, Joseph Priestley, and Carl Scheele all made discoveries related to the nature of the air, such as the existence of oxygen and the process of combustion, confirming that the air was filled with mysterious, nourishing qualities. Good-quality air, together with divine blessing, is apparently what kept long-term fasters such as the Swiss "tool of God" Christina Kratzer alive for three years without eating. Kratzer was a member of the Inspirationist Awakening, which was a Protestant movement linked to the Shakers and other Pentecostal communities. She inspired at least one book, *On the Impossibility and Possibility of Complete Abstinence of Food and Drink* (1737, by Johann Jacob Ritter). After having had a miserable childhood, during which she "lost her face" due to chicken pox, she became a fasting celebrity. Her advice was sought by royalty, including the Turkish sultan.

Inedia lives on in the persistent, anti-technocratic New Age movement known as the breatharians, who claim that they live on air and sunlight alone, and that prana, or "life force," sustains them. Their direct precedents lie in hucksters of previous centuries, as well as a few saints. The psychologist Carl Jung suggested that in the case of St. Nicholas of Flüe, "nourishment might have been effected by the passage of living molecules from one body to another." It is perhaps harsh but necessary to observe here that the movement is fraudulent. Breatharian teaching has been associated with several deaths around the world of people who became convinced that food and water are not necessary for human life. They are.

Purity in all forms, delivered individually via fasting and socially via quotas, had long been the obsession of antiestablishment health movements, for which a catchall term is "naturopathy." Somewhat cruelly dismissed by the late science writer Martin Gardner as "a worldwide medical cult," its many strands have origins in the eighteenth- and nineteenth-century European movements cited earlier. Naturopathy rests on the expulsion of unnatural poisons via fasting and enemas (and formerly via bloodletting). "The idea of detoxing, of cleansing your system, and withholding the intake of anything—social stimulation, food, water, drugs—is a big part of the naturopathic idea that your body can heal itself as long as you remove the external factors that are making you sick," Dr. Britt Marie Hermes tells me. Hermes is a former naturopathic doctor who became disillusioned with alternative medicine and subsequently earned a doctorate in evolutionary biology. Her specialty is the microbiome. "I knew too much" about naturopathy, she says. "I knew what my colleagues were doing, and I didn't want to be a part of it anymore." While there are almost as many definitions of naturopathy as there are credulous consumers—which is to say, a lot—most naturopaths share an antipathy to drugs as well as the contention that disease does not stem from genetic misfiring or germs and bacteria. Hundreds of strange therapies accrue to the naturopathic label, among them breatharianism, hydrotherapy, zone therapy (deafness, for example, requires a squeezing of the ring finger or the third toe), and iridiagnosis (ailments can be diagnosed by careful examination of the iris, one eye having different connotations than the other). As Hermes points out, there is a strange contradiction at the core of the philosophy: we need to return to the natural world and microbes don't make you sick, and yet the distinctly unnatural act of purging our insides via enemas, etc., is necessary for well-being. However, the naturopathic emphasis on listening to patients and expressing empathy, Hermes says, is something often lacking in mainstream medicine. It gives naturopathic practitioners tremendous influence over their patients.

....

Fasting's paradoxical relationship to the moneyed world was evident from its early commercialization by energetic American and European entrepreneurs. In Europe, Lebensreform combined with the influence of Edward Dewey to result in one of the lasting additions to the world of institutionalized fasting, the Buchinger Wilhelmi clinics, now being managed by the fourth generation of Buchingers in the business. Its two branches are located in the exclusive resort town of Marbella, Spain, and on the shores of Lake Constance, in Germany's Bodensee region. The first clinic was established in 1920 by a Quaker doctor, Otto Buchinger, who had emerged from the First World War stricken with rheumatoid polyarthritis. On the advice of a doctor who was steeped in Dewey's beliefs, Buchinger had started fasting and found himself miraculously cured. "The inflammation in his joints and nerves vanished entirely, and even before he completed his fast he was once more walking like a young man." Like Cornaro and countless other converts to fasting before and since, Buchinger decided that he would share his good news with the world. In 1935, at the height of the Nazi regime, he moved his business to Bad Pyrmont, a central German town famed for its healing waters. While "strongly anti-Nazi," Buchinger was not so strongly anti-Nazi that he avoided prospering through the Second World War—his book *Das Heilfasten* ("therapeutic fasting" or "fasting for health") was released in 1935 and was reprinted at least six times through 1942, at a time when Germany was experiencing a severe nationwide paper shortage and only Nazi-approved publications received permission to print—and his sanatorium and convictions have now been translated into ultra-luxury spas where guests pay upward of $10,000 a week for the privilege of having food withheld from them in pristine and luxurious surroundings.

Just two years after Kafka's death, Weimar Germany hosted what may have been the golden era of hunger artists, when fasting became synonymous with glamorous decadence. In 1926, six hunger artists in Berlin exhibited at the same time. One performance took place in a popular restaurant, where, in the middle of the hall under a glass bell, a man in a dinner jacket smoked cigarettes and sipped water. A nearby blackboard announced that he had not eaten for twenty-eight days. As one newspaper reported, "Around him corpulent gentlemen and fashionably dressed ladies are consuming Wiener Schnitzel with fried potatoes. They are discussing whether the hunger record will be broken this time."

While the largely unheralded writer of *The Metamorphosis* wrestled with his urges to consume, a celebrity journalist across the Atlantic exulted in his powers of self-control via fasting. Upton Sinclair is best known today for his first book, a fictionalized exposé of the meat industry that he wrote when he was twenty-six. *The Jungle,* based on a series Sinclair had published in the socialist magazine *Appeal to Reason* in 1905, became a bestseller the following year and was ultimately instrumental in the passage of the Pure Food and Drug Act as well as the Meat Inspection Act. But what works in journalism does not always translate to science. Despite Sinclair's reputation as a journalist, he confounded his personal impressions with impartial truth in much of his subsequent work. In 1911, he published *The Fasting Cure,* a distillation of essays he had written for *Cosmopolitan* magazine. The book became another bestseller. Several editions are still in print today. "I have written a great many magazine articles," Sinclair wrote in a typically self-satisfied passage, "but never one which attracted so much attention as this." As a younger man, he wrote, he was more inclined to listen to others; now he had access to direct truths: "In those days I believed something, because other people told me; today I know something else because I have tried it upon myself." A compilation of pseudoscientific, anecdotal observations that praise fasting for its purificative powers and "an automatic protection against disease," *The Fasting Cure* endures as part of an ineradicable trend of fasting-as-cure-all that some of us who advocate the practice would rather forget.

Upton Sinclair's preoccupation with purity also extended to blood and ancestry, as it does today with many health advocates. "Progressive hygienic ideology" reflected a common view that the human race was in a period of steep decline that could only be reversed by individual cleansing. A number of the health reformers who emerged in the nineteenth century had a particular focus on the purity of Anglo-Saxons in their writings. Hygienics promised to be the filter by which society could put itself back in order. All manner of waste and infection, whether moral, microbial, cultural, or racial, were the enemies in the Victorian "war on filth." American cities were dirty and getting dirtier, and with the steep increase in immigration that began in the late 1890s, principally from Southern and Eastern Europe, the wrong sort of immigrant was threatening to overwhelm the Anglo-Saxon bedrock. Even the unsullied natural environment was being corrupted by foreign elements: the chestnut blight of the early 1900s and, a few years later, Dutch elm disease were devastating the most magnificent specimens of the American forest. Both were the result of infection from imported fungi. Coinciding with a terrified reaction to recently freed enslaved people mixing with the general population, the result was a nationwide surge in bigotry justified by pseudoscience.

....

Horace Fletcher, the "Great Masticator," was another famous American naturopathic polymath, a businessman who had made a fortune by manufacturing printing ink. Fletcherism was an outgrowth of the hygienic mania that combined fasting with American efficiency. Around 1895, doctors told him that he had to lose weight, and Fletcher decided that the most direct way to do so was by fasting enforced by incessant chewing. Of everything: Milk had to be chewed. Soup had to be chewed. Liquids and low-fiber foods could be chewed lightly, but a dish of shallots, for example, could require seven minutes of diligent chewing. Refinement delivered via ritual chewing made for purity. The method for "attaining economic assimilation and immunity from disease" was within reach, Fletcher wrote in *The New Glutton or Epicure* in 1903. Weight loss was a social duty, and America would rise to greatness on the strength of "dietetic righteousness." "Efficiency" was the watchword of the day—after all, this was the era of Taylorism, the science of management that gave us the assembly line. Perfect chewing enforced perfect fasting, which thoroughly cleansed the body. Habitually dressed in white, Fletcher became a sought-after speaker and a bestselling author (*Fletcherism: What It Is, or, How I Became Young at Sixty* also referenced the ubiquitous and lightweight Cornaro). John D. Rockefeller was a passionate advocate, as was the philosopher William James, who along with his brother the novelist Henry James (who declared himself a "fanatic" of the practice), saw Fletcherism as a natural ally in achieving "healthy-mindedness" and ridding the body of evil.

With royalties earned from *The Jungle*, in 1906 Upton Sinclair founded a luxurious whites-only "cooperative colony" for himself and allied creative thinkers (professors, artists, and writers, among them Sinclair Lewis). It was presided over by a strict admissions committee to ensure that the enterprise "be open to any white person of good moral character"—that is, that it be closed to the rest of the population. Located outside Englewood, New Jersey, in an upscale former boys' school, Helicon Home Colony had a bowling alley, tennis courts, and an indoor swimming pool. Servants were relabeled "workers." The cooperative burned down the year after it was founded; Sinclair suspected arson.

Later that same year, Sinclair and his wife took refuge at a spa in Michigan founded by John Harvey Kellogg, a Fletcherite enthusiast and author of, among other things, the pamphlet *Tendencies Toward Race Degeneracy* (U.S. Government Printing Office, 1912). Kellogg's dedication to the cause was such that not only is he credited with coining the verb "to fletcherize" but he advocated grade school instruction "in the fine art of . . . fletcherizing" as one of his "suggestions toward checking race degeneration due to the conditions of school life."

Just as the American body politic was being polluted by waves of immigrants from unfamiliar cultures—accompanied by strange, pungent foods that often depended on fermentation—the individual American body was being assailed by all sorts of contaminants that came from something called autointoxication: poisoning induced by a clogged colon, in which alien bacteria thrived. It was our fault. We let them in, and now there was no more room in our collective, constipated bodies. Naturopathy had the answers.

Beginning in the late nineteenth century, health reformers began to highlight the dangers of newly discovered ammonia-derived compounds generically known as ptomaines, derived from the Greek for "corpse" or "one who has fallen." These included amines such as cadaverine and putrescine, which accompany putrefaction and were mistakenly believed to be the primary cause of food poisoning. (The minimally toxic amines coexist alongside highly toxic bacteria such as botulism and salmonella, which are the real culprits. The term "ptomaine poisoning" has now largely been discarded in favor of the term "food poisoning.") Obsession with foreign rot and the "impure" runs throughout Sinclair's *The Fasting Cure*:

> *The diseases for which fasting is most obviously to be recommended are all those of the stomach and intestines, which any one can see are directly caused by the presence of fermenting and putrefying food in the system. Next come all those complaints which are caused by the poisons derived from these foods in the blood and the eliminative organs. . . . Finally, there are the fevers and infectious diseases, which are caused by the invasion of the organism by foreign bacteria, which are enabled to secure a lodgment because of the weakened and impure condition of the blood-stream.*

Sinclair believed that foreign bodies had invaded the American gut and could be expunged by diligent fasts of two months or longer. All this advice was based on personal observations and anecdotes "which any one can see." Rigorous filtration of what Americans ingest—the most stringent kind of personalized immigration policy—was needed. Medical expertise was not needed. In his 1930 book, *Mental Radio: Does It Work, and How?*, Sinclair turned to exploring the telepathic abilities of his second wife, Mary Craig Kimbrough.

The Jungle was dedicated "To the Workingmen of America." *The Fasting Cure* is dedicated to Bernarr Macfadden, a spectacular showman/

entrepreneur in the great American tradition of P. T. Barnum. Like Barnum, Macfadden was an expert in the art of marketing. Macfadden was a fasting devotee and came of age at a time when Americans were reinventing everything—their bodies, their language, their histories. The scientific tradition was not immune. The plodding and frequently ineffective methods of medical doctors came under particular scrutiny. The profession did not help its cause by its resistance to new methods. Sir John Hall, the chief English physician during the Crimean War, typified the attitude of many doctors at the time when he wrote, in a swipe at anesthesia, that "the smart of the knife is a powerful stimulant and it is much better to hear a man bawl lustily than to see him sink silently into the grave." Reinvention was seen as a positively patriotic and Christian enterprise. Self-improvement was taking advantage of what God provided; it was Manifest Destiny on a personal scale. Alternative medicine—often simply made-up remedies heavily dosed with sedatives such as opium or laudanum—thrived. Osteopathy, with its whimsical belief in a "myofascial continuity" that linked the entire body, was developed in Missouri in the 1870s. Chiropractic medicine was invented in Iowa a decade later, and in 1891, Macfadden created "kinistherapy" out of nothing more than a desire to sell his services. But it led to so much else— not least of which, it seems

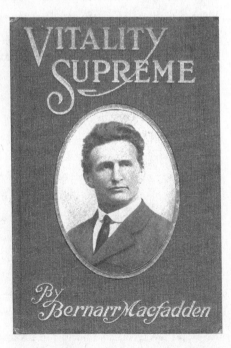

Bernarr Macfadden on the cover of his *Vitality Supreme* (1915).

likely, was pataphysics, "the science of imaginary solutions," the invention of Dr. Faustroll, who was himself the parodical creation of the French writer Alfred Jarry in 1898.

Like Sinclair, Macfadden was a fasting enthusiast who believed that a prolonged fast was a quick fix for just about anything wrong with the body. A self-promoter who would have put Galen to shame—in 1929 alone, he financed no fewer than three adulatory book-length biographies of himself—Macfadden was a passionate advocate of naturopathy. His was a classic rags-to-riches story, at least according to his own account. Born Bernard A. McFadden, he became an orphan at the age of eleven and a "bound boy" on an Illinois farm in his teens. He launched his career in St. Louis by selling the proceeds from a laundry that he co-owned. He rented space in a studio, and transformed his persona, starting with his name. He hung out a sign reading "Bernarr Macfadden—Kinistherapist—Teacher of Higher Physical Culture." His given name was too ordinary, he told a writer for the *New Yorker* in 1950. "I was starting out fresh. New business, new kind of culture, new name—the works." St. Louisans thronged the shop, "hoping to see some kind of peep show," and Macfadden explained that he would show paying customers how to get strong "according to a secret formula," a key component of which was fasting. The first visitors to his studio may not have been disappointed in their desire to catch an illicit thrill. At a time when a woman bearing her ankles or a shoulder was scandalous, and men went to the beach in suits that covered them from their neck to their feet, Macfadden made a habit of publicly displaying his finely toned, near-naked body to anyone ready to appreciate him. His genius lay in combining the thrill of the sideshow carnival with lectures on health and morality. It was physical—with an emphasis on the carnal—philosophy: and indeed his first magazine was called *Physical Culture*, the first American health periodical. "Medicine has had its day," he wrote in his publication in 1911. "It belongs to the ignorance of the distant past." The enemies were numerous: the "white bread curse," impurities in any form (he advocated the "eugenic improvement of the white race"), masturbation, and vaccines. "Weakness is a crime! Don't be a criminal!" Macfadden exhorted his readers.

Macfadden was generous with his output: he wrote more than a hundred tomes on health and nutrition and never hesitated to opine on a subject from the divine (he founded a religion, "Cosmotarianism," which concluded that people who took care of their bodies would go to heaven) to politics (he was a great admirer of Mussolini). The first true titan of the health industry, he started a chain of health restaurants and spas he called "healthatoriums," to distinguish them from his rival health entrepreneur Kellogg's "sanitariums."

At the core of Macfadden's health empire was the fundamentally democratic, Wesleyan concept that anyone could wrest control of his health from the medical establishment. "All types of disease" were susceptible to a regimen of "hygienic medicine" that combined fasting, unadulterated (and if possible uncooked) food, and regular exercise. Macfadden's advice on fasting was marginally better than his advice on a healthy diet: among other food substitutes, he recommended occasionally eating sand (his third wife, Mary Williamson, reported her surprise at seeing him eating handfuls of sand as they walked along the beach, and one of the columns he wrote for his magazine was titled "Sand Cleans Glass Bottles—Why Not Bowels?"). Throughout his career, he touted fasting as the One Sure Thing:

> In his advocacy of fasting, he made the considered declaration that it would "help and generally cure" asthma, epilepsy, bronchitis, constipation, heart disease, insomnia, paralysis, obesity, diabetes, impotence, dyspepsia, kidney ailments, bladder trouble, and seventeen other diseases, most of them serious.

This belief, along with many other spurious notions (for example, his firm belief that hair loss could be prevented by regular and emphatic tugging on one's hair), led to his being labeled a crackpot by some cynics. Fasting has not fully recovered from Macfadden's showy influence; a century later, its virtues are mired in association with various obsessions ranging from body-shaming to mysophobia (extreme fear of contamination) to fascism.

In Macfadden's aftermath, the leading modern proponent of modern fasting-as-cure-all was Herbert M. Shelton, who today may be better known than his irrepressible mentor. Shelton is cited as a distinguished forebear by everyone from the National Health Association (which he cofounded in 1948 as the American Natural Hygiene Society) to the highly successful TrueNorth Clinic in Santa Rosa, California. A graduate of Macfadden's College of Physcultopathy—where he studied "the complete instructions for the cure of all diseases"—Shelton in many ways personifies the most American aspects of the natural hygiene movement: homegrown, defiant of established medicine, and quick to dispense advice (he wrote dozens of books with titles such as *Fasting Can Save Your Life* and *The Science and Fine Art of Fasting*). Fasting was everything to him. At times sounding like a very slightly modified breatharian, Shelton contended that calories were largely irrelevant: they were the product of "fire-box dietetics." The body's energy somehow existed independently of food shoveled in. "Warmth, quiet (rest), and fasting, with a little water, as demanded by thirst, are the needs of a sick man or woman."

At least seven people died at "Dr. Shelton's Health School" in San Antonio, Texas, before it shut down in 1981 after fifty-four years, declaring bankruptcy in the face of several lawsuits. One lawsuit detailed the death of a man who had eaten nothing for a month and then died of bronchial pneumonia "brought on by his weakened condition." Shelton had a hand in the death of at least one more person not enrolled in his school: in 1964, the president of the San Diego chapter of the Natural Hygiene Society was convicted of involuntary manslaughter in the death of his seven-year-old daughter. After putting the girl on a liquid-only fast to cure her fever and cold, the father saw no signs of improvement. He consulted with Shelton, who advised him to stick to the treatment. After twenty-nine days, she died of bronchial pneumonia worsened by malnutrition. Yet people continue to swear by him.

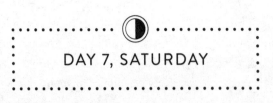

DAY 7, SATURDAY

Self-Cancellation

Uneven night. Woke up not feeling ravenous, but intensely curious, not driven by hunger, but eager for an escape from sensory deprivation. Went to the store. Had no problem sorting through produce, was musing on limits: in a real way this was about testing our limits by removing the eating diktats with which we largely define our lives. But the fast, of course, imposes new limits, those of the senses. It is intensely boring to be deprived of fat, sweet, tangy, and bitter flavors. And slippery pasta and the crevices of toast, the creamy sensation of a good cheese—different degrees of creaminess, too, of course. Very much looking forward to an end, and a return to decadence.

11:59 p.m.: Made it. Had a boiled egg, a couple of almonds, tea. Not what's recommended. What struck me most in these foods was the texture; I didn't close my eyes in ecstasy at flavors, in fact found the egg mildly disgusting (too meaty). The almonds inoffensive. What a relief not to feel I need to devour the contents of a refrigerator, almost as though I've gained some perspective on eating. I realize that even now I eat out of habit: it is something I am *supposed* to do. I am sure I felt more compulsion to eat pre-fast than I do just now. I don't imagine this feeling will stay with me for long, but at least now I reaffirmed that (1) I can comfortably last a week without eating, and (2) routine can be the enemy of rationality and self-control.

"Listen: a king sat upon his throne, surrounded by lofty and wonderfully beautiful columns ornamented with ivory, bearing the banners of the king proudly to all. Then it pleased the king to lift a small feather from the ground, and he commanded it to fly. Yet a feather does not fly because of anything, but because the air bears it along. Thus, I am a feather on the breath of God, not gifted with great powers or education, nor even with good health, but I rely completely on God."

—Hildegard of Bingen to Odo of Paris (1148 CE)

In Jainism, a religion that began about 2,500 years ago in India and that emphasizes the importance of regular fasting, the act of *sallekhana*— willfully starving to death—is not considered suicide. *Sallekhana* is a rite that takes place over many days or weeks. It has nothing about it of a crime of passion, and in fact is seen as a step toward becoming devoid of passion and ultimately attaining enlightenment. It is part of a drawn-out process that eliminates human emotion and karmic interference, thereby freeing the soul from the cycle of life, death, and reincarnation. Even partial fasting feeds the soul, as it starves the body, putting it on a path to salvation through renunciation.

....

I've known of two people, both bedridden and past ninety, who decided to take matters into their own hands by quietly refusing to eat. Neither was a big consumer of the planet's resources. One I knew personally: Mrs. X stood about five foot two, was careful in her movements and speech, what used to be described as "prim." She could have stepped out of a Jane Austen novel. She was not one to make any dramatic statements. Her voice was low and precise. When she was mobile, she favored kerchiefs over her hair, as though to complete her self-containment. At the end, when she couldn't leave her bed unassisted, with her world narrower than she had known it in many decades, she told her adult children of her determination to die. For her, a roving mind wasn't enough, or perhaps unabetted by the distractions of physical activity, it was too much. She had made a clear-eyed decision to spare herself (and her family) many weeks and possibly months of an agonizingly slow decline.

Most religions do not advocate suicide, and Judaism is no exception. But Mrs. Y had her rabbi's blessing to leave the planet with her dignity intact. After several false starts, she embarked on her final fast. Her rabbi called to see how she was doing, and she told him she was at peace. After they said a prayer together, at a loss for what else to say, the rabbi asked her what she had eaten as her last meal. She replied that she had eaten leftovers: a half sandwich from the deli that was in her refrigerator. The rabbi was surprised that she'd want to leave the earthly plane with such a humble repast as one of her last memories. Well, she told him, she didn't like to waste food.

By all accounts these deaths were quiet, gradual ones, like the dimming of a light. This is not to suggest that suicide is a good thing. But in the Stoic tradition it can be a wise and reasonable way to preempt a worse ending. Most of us would want to end the same way, but few among us has the courage to take that first, voluntary step along the road to oblivion, and then to commit to the path.

....

In the same period that men like Tanner, Succi, Levanzin, and others were achieving increasing fame for their "feats" of extreme fasting, women were similarly achieving notoriety for self-starvation. Their obsession was presented differently, as a symptom of feminine vulnerability. These fasters fed the great appetite for categorization as well as the drive to fill new hospitals. Six times as many Americans were labeled insane in 1880 as in 1850. But the fasting women required stern correction, not coddling. As A. R. Turnbull, the medical superintendent of Fife and Kinross District Asylum, wrote in 1895, in an article in the *Journal of Mental Science* advocating force-feeding: "Refusal of food may be due to mere stupidity, or to the restlessness and inattention of maniacal excitement; much more frequently it is seen in cases of melancholia, melancholic stupor or delusional insanity." If they were not charlatans, fasting women and girls were deemed mentally deficient and/or unstable. In what might have been wishful thinking on the part of male doctors, female anorexics were often determined to be suffering from "the repression of sexual desire."

Anorexia is an eating disorder that is difficult to cure and can be deadly. It hovers, or should hover, over every discussion of fasting. While relatively rare in the general population—a little over half of 1 percent receive the diagnosis—it occurs three times as often among women as men. Unlike a cause-and-effect disease like tuberculosis or even cancer, it is a malady with multiple origins that may be social, genetic, or some combination of the two. Anorexia may be ascribable to an emerging young adult's desire to conform to an unattainable ideal, and it may be a reaction to familial pressures and obligations presaging self-destruction. There is increasing evidence that shows there may be a genetic predisposition to the disease. Like fasting, it presents a paradox. The anorexic signals both a cessation of need and utter vulnerability: "I have no needs; take care of me." It is fasting with purpose, but with the added, insidious modifier of compulsion, of being convinced one is never thin enough, of being repulsed by food. It is distinct from other types of fasting in that the goal is fundamentally unattainable.

While many still characterize anorexia as a modern disease—a by-product of a combination of the patriarchy and capitalism—on closer inspection it seems to have always been with us. Perhaps the first recorded example of an anorexic, from the eighth century CE, is also one of the most revered saints of Hinduism, the poet Antal, a fifteen-year-old Tamil girl. She is the only woman among the Alvars, a dozen Tamil poet-saints who were devoted to Krishna, the blue-skinned avatar of the supreme being Vishnu. ("Al" means deep; it was a title given to the twelve saints who immersed themselves in their love of Vishnu.) Also known as Godadevi,

Antal was raised by a single father, himself one of the Alvars. Prefiguring the anorexic female saints of the European Middle Ages, Antal defiantly rejected the common notion in dharma that a woman's purpose was to get married and raise a family. She spurned all marriage proposals and sang of "her pallor and wasted body." In her classic poem "The Sacred Words of a Woman," Antal celebrates her emaciated self as proof of her devotion to what is holy:

> As part of my vow
> I eat just once a day.
> I neglect my body,
> it is not adorned.
> My hair is tangled in knots
> My lips are cracked . . .

Antal "disappeared in a blaze of glory" after declaring she could marry no one but Krishna.

The line between "healthy" fasting and pathological fasting constantly shifts, depending on the historical context. Pathological fasting, or fasting without end, became medicalized in the nineteenth century as anorexia. Like television and calculus, anorexia is often said to be a peculiar product of its era, a phenomenon that has come to be associated with some of the most visible elements of contemporary society, such as actors and influencers, and has thus acquired a sickly glamour. It is easy to tie the image of a waiflike artiste to cultural ancestors in the form of a Byron or Dickinson. But various scholars have made clear that what we now label anorexia has been around for a long time.

We need to want. Want, or perceived want, pushes us to sustain ourselves. Uncontrollable want tips over into disease. "I can't say that everyone who fasts has an eating disorder, but there is a relationship, and I think a lot of it has to do with the intention of the fast, its duration, and even how it's perceived by people around you," Kristen Portland, executive director of the National Association of Anorexia Nervosa and

Associated Disorders, told me. "Because if you are fasting and getting a lot of positive feedback, you're more likely to do it again, and that can be a road to an eating disorder." The anorexic becomes driven into perpetual dissatisfaction with the physical self, a situation only remedied by vigilance and continual, self-imposed discipline. A lack of control is despair-inducing, and in anorexia joy comes from never-ending control of the immediate, physical environment of the body. With the onset of the COVID-19 pandemic, Portland said calls to her organization's help line shot up by close to 50 percent.

And like television and calculus, anorexia is said to have been "discovered" by two different scientists working at the same time in rival nations. For calculus, it was Newton and Leibniz; for television, Zworykin and Farnsworth; and for anorexia, it was the English doctor Sir William Gull (1816–1890) and the French psychiatrist Ernest-Charles Lasègue (1816–1883). Gull and Lasègue were representative of the Western medical establishment at the time. Both were respected: Gull was Queen Victoria's adored personal physician, credited with having saved her son, the future Edward VII, from typhoid in 1871. By the time of Gull's death, he had amassed a considerable fortune (the equivalent of £56 million today); Lasègue was widely published and the clinical director of a prominent Parisian hospital for destitute women, Salpêtrière, which was founded in the seventeenth century and housed more than five thousand patients. Lasègue later became known for describing pathological instances of what he termed *folie à deux* (shared insanity) as well as exhibitionism. In 1873, Gull and Lasègue more or less simultaneously identified the disorder. Tellingly, they at first labeled it "anorexia hysterica," and saw it as symptomatic of uniquely feminine fallibility ("hysteria" comes from the Greek word for "womb"). There is some evidence that Gull claimed an inordinate amount of credit for the classification and may have lifted the very term "anorexia" from an article that Lasègue had published earlier; however, the word "anorexy" had been used to describe a ferocious lack of appetite in the early nineteenth century and for many years previous. As was pointed out a century later by the pioneering psychiatrist Hilde

Bruch, this term was a misnomer. People labeled as anorexic—"without appetite"—often retain an appetite. They can be "preoccupied with food and eating but consider self-denial and discipline the highest virtue and condemn satisfying their needs and desires as shameful self-indulgence."

Gull provided the medical establishment with three case studies of the disorder. Miss A, Miss B, and Miss C shared similar characteristics, and all were examples of unstable femininity. Miss A exhibited "some peevishness of temper and a feeling of jealousy. No account could be given of the exciting cause." Miss B displayed "a peculiar restlessness difficult, I was informed, to control"; and Miss C was possessed of a "mind weakened" and "temper obstinate." Gull wrote:

> *The want of appetite is, I believe, due to a morbid mental state. . . . That mental states may destroy appetites is notorious, and it will be admitted that young women at the ages named are specially obnoxious to mental perversity. . . . I have remarked above that these wilful patients are often allowed to drift their own way into a state of extreme exhaustion, when it might have been prevented by placing them under different moral conditions.*

Gull's and Lasègue's analysis of anorexia as being purely a mental disorder due to young women's particularly twisted nature is one that has persisted, despite increasing evidence of the biological and genetic origins of the disorder. For "most of these cases," Gull wrote in 1888, "perversions of the 'ego' [are] the cause." Lasègue had used exactly the same term in his 1873 description, adding that *perversion mentale* was characteristic of the disorder.

That this scientific competition occurred just as ideas were shifting about women's roles in politics and society is no coincidence. Both physicians were at the tail end of a long line of men of science who had, beginning in the early nineteenth century, alluded to the "hypochondriacal delirium" that seemed to afflict girls and young women almost exclusively. Ignoring readily available evidence to the contrary (such as childbirth), the accepted scientific dogma of the day held that women were frail and prone to suffer more from the ravages of industrialism and modernism. Just a few years previous, in 1869, New York physician George Beard had introduced the concept of "neurasthenia," or nerve exhaustion or weakness, as a by-product of modern society that might even be welcomed as a marker of advancement. The culmination of his thesis was the delightfully titled *American Nervousness: Its Causes and Consequences* (1881). That same year, Beard accompanied Dr. William Hammond, the author of *Fasting Girls: Their Physiology and Pathology*, in his examination of Mollie Fancher, who at that point claimed not to have eaten since 1864. Less delightful was his conviction that neurasthenia, like anorexia, was a disorder reserved almost exclusively for women. "In civilized lands," Beard wrote confidently, "women are more nervous, immeasurably, than men, and suffer more from general and special nervous diseases." The sickness was a regrettable by-product of the nation's destiny to lead, but its presence confirmed America's status as a modern country. The condition was exacerbated by overthinking. Men had a greater nervous reserve and could better withstand the rigors of deep thought. Since Beard concluded that nervousness was physical, not mental, it could be addressed by physical means. One of the recommended treatments was "franklinization," which involved "static discharge of sparks from the genitals and the passage of 'mild' currents through electrodes inserted into the urethra and rectum." At least this was a cure spared anorexics of the day. Thanks to Gull and Lasègue, anorexia was identified as psychosomatic, meaning a disease with purely mental roots. It was the corrupt mind infecting the vulnerable female body, and only occasionally a particularly feeble male one.

....

For decades, physicians agreed that anorexics were suffering from moral depravity or twisted family dynamics. Then, in 1914, a single autopsy by the German pathologist Morris Simmonds changed prevailing views: the emaciated corpse of a pregnant woman was found to have lesions in her pituitary gland, a part of the endocrine system that creates and releases hormones to help manage stress, growth, and metabolism. This disruption of the endocrine system was found to be the cause of the woman's wasting away, and for years psychological explanations for anorexia were set aside in favor of a diagnosis of "Simmonds' disease" (now known as Sheehan's syndrome). It was found, however, that most anorexic patients who received only body-focused (somatic) therapy for their symptoms relapsed, and that most patients suffering from pituitary insufficiency did not suffer emaciation and seemed well-nourished.

In the postwar period—particularly thanks to Hilde Bruch and Mara Selvini Palazzoli, both of whose work heavily influenced views on anorexia from the 1970s through to the present—the pendulum swung back. In what could be seen as a bridge from the medieval to the modern, Palazzoli, a famed psychiatrist and founder of the constructivist approach to family therapy, refused to go down what she called "the blind alley of moralistic psychiatry." She saw an anorexic as

> prey to a most disastrous Cartesian dichotomy: she believes that her mind transcends her body and that it grants her unlimited power over her own body and that of others. The result is . . . the mistaken belief that the patient is engaged in a victorious battle on two fronts, namely against: (1) her body; and (2) the family system.

Bruch's great contribution lies in her ability to popularize the anorexic predicament and take it out of the realm of shame. Her empathetic approach lifted the question of guilt from women. Women suffering from the disease, she wrote, were overwhelmed by "life choices" brought about by social change and family dynamics. A "disturbance of body image," according to Bruch, was both anorexia's root cause and the reason for its increase in the twentieth century. After Bruch, the common view was that anorexics were crushed by feelings of inadequacy, especially in the form of a "morbid dread of fatness," which was largely imposed by the multibillion-dollar fashion colossus. To this day, those suffering from the disorder are neatly packaged as victims of the fashion industry who starve themselves "because if thin is beautiful, skeletal must be gorgeous." But this explanation seems too pat, a modern version of the nineteenth-century view of anorexics as perverse, vulnerable "hysterics" particularly susceptible to corrupting outside influences.

It is true that women in particular suffer from an unending avalanche of exhortations to be thin, and that more people are exposed to the same trends due to the pervasive reach of mass media. The culture of slenderness can be condemned as both racist and sexist, as has been argued by an increasing number of anti-dieting movements such as "intuitive eating." Fat people, writes cultural critic Anna Mirzayan, are subjected to imperatives to "make themselves smaller, disappear or stop existing completely, by a populace that nonetheless needs fat bodies that exist in specific acceptable ways—as entertainment, moral analogue, before-and-after horror story, or as vehicles for humor." Prejudice against overweight people is rampant, particularly if they are women: research from America, Canada, Denmark, and the UK suggests they earn about 10 percent less than the nonobese.

A study of women's fashion magazines from 1909 to 1925 found a sudden predominance of "noncurvaceous figures (measured from bust-to-waist ratios)." The researchers quoted from a contemporary fashion arbiter: "The figures of our flappers . . . shall be slender and slinky and lath-like and the line of grace no longer the curve but the prolonged parallelogram." With the end of the 1920s and the beginnings of the Great Depression—and as famines took hold in Russia, Central Europe, and Asia—excess fat was even less fashionable. Endless brands touted slimming certainties. Lucky Strike cigarettes were there to help: "Modern way to diet! Light a Lucky when fattening sweets tempt you." There was reducing soap, a reducing brush, and Slends Fat Reducing Chewing Gum. Heroes (Charles "Slim" Lindbergh, Humphrey Bogart) were invariably slim. A number of the most successful comics—those with a sour, menacing undertone—were fat (Oliver Hardy, Fatty Arbuckle,

W. C. Fields). The socialite Wallis Simpson, whose marriage to King Edward VIII prompted his abdication in 1936, supposedly said that a woman "can never be too rich or too thin." And in tandem, accounts of anorexia were on the rise. The shift was notable even at the time: in 1939, British physician John Alfred Ryle predicted that anorexia nervosa would continue to increase, suggesting it would be driven by fashion mandates and heightened "emotionality" among young people. What is not certain is the degree to which media reflects trends, rather than creates them. What may have been changing was not growth of the phenomenon but recognition of its prevalence.

While few physicians would deny its psychological aspects, today anorexia is accepted as having a strong biological component. Eating disorders have many possible origins. They may even lie in sudden shocks to the system, including natural disasters.

In early January 1998, a sequence of devastating ice storms blasted through southern Québec. Over several days, snow, wind, and freezing rain brought down electric pylons and millions of trees. More rain fell in the Montréal metropolitan area than at any point since 1961. And then it froze. In the St. Lawrence River Valley around Québec City, up to four inches of solid ice accumulated. Tunnels and roadways in the province became impassable. At least thirty-four people died in the Great Ice Storm, and in some areas power and water was cut off for weeks. "I thought as a Canadian I'd seen everything winter can throw at you," one survivor told the magazine *Maclean's* later that same month. "But nothing prepares you for this."

People burned their furniture to stay warm. Five months after the storm, researchers at McGill University and the Canadian Institutes of Health Research contacted 244 women who had been pregnant at the time and lived in the hardest-hit areas. A follow-up study was done thirteen years later of fifty-four children of these same mothers. The scientists found that, irrespective of sex, the likelihood of adolescents' "disordered eating" was associated with the stress their mothers had experienced during the storms. "Genetic susceptibility can be activated by environmental exposures," Dr. Howard Steiger, one of the study's principal researchers, told me. "It's epigenetic. It's the mother's stress influencing gene expression. Every life experience, even prenatal events, contribute" to the presence of an eating disorder, he said. "Yes, family dysfunction can play a role, society plays a role, and everything else. But how does society get into your head? There is a pathway."

....

Accounts of anorexia mirabilis, "holy anorexia," increased in medieval times. Of the 261 "holy women" between the year 1200 and the present who are recognized by the Roman Catholic Church in the *Bibliotheca Sanctorum*, a good proportion displayed signs of anorexia; writes Rudolph Bell, the preeminent expert on the subject, "For several dozen the documentation is extensive and highly reliable." It doesn't take a Freudian student of the soul to make the connection between self-starvation (repression) and the sexual drive, but fasting just as evidently provided (and provides) a means to challenge, if not escape, the patriarchy of home and Church. For all those who fast, a fast becomes a test of willpower. What takes anorexics a step beyond is their determination "ultimately to obliterate" bodily desires.

One of the two patron saints of Italy (St. Francis of Assisi is the other), St. Catherine of Siena, born in 1347, was the best-known medieval practitioner of "miraculous lack of appetite." Her fasting may well have had its roots in protest against authoritarian dictates and in horror at the abuse of women she witnessed firsthand. Catherine was the twenty-third of twenty-five children, and the only one of her siblings who was breast-fed by her mother. As a six-year-old, she had observed one of her married sisters fasting in an attempt to change her husband's brutal behavior. Upon Catherine's sister's death, her parents declared their intention to marry Catherine off to the same widower. As the possibility of a lifetime of abuse and unceasing childbirths loomed before her, she was under-standably horrified. Catherine already had evinced "an abhorrence of being looked at by men." She undertook a fast in protest, declaring that she was wedded to Jesus (echoing Antal's devotion to Krishna). It was a rational response to what she had observed up to that point in her short life. In effect, Catherine rebelled against the notion of becoming food herself—as a warm resource for potentially many, many babies; as a resource in many respects for the man she was expected to marry.

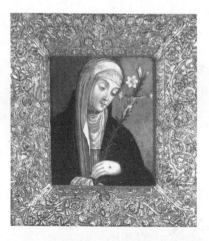

St. Catherine of Siena.
Unknown painter, seventeenth century.

As documented both by her confessor, Raymond, and in her own letters, Catherine felt that her revulsion toward eating was divine punishment for her sins. She also saw it as a route to salvation. What is divine must be perfect, and it follows that what is human is imperfect. Instead of embracing that imperfection, or being content with contemplating perfection from a distance, Catherine embraced absolute withdrawal. Devoting herself to God, she became a servant to no man—and sought to further suppress inclinations to any sustenance or pleasure other than the holy. She received her only nourishment from taking the Host. "If so much as a bean remained in Catherine of Siena's stomach, she vomited," writes Rudolph Bell. For her, as for many anorexics, the battle for purity was a constant one; to resume more conventional behavior would have been to concede defeat. Victory was achieved only with death. As she wasted away, she admonished others to "make a supreme effort to root out that self-love from your heart and to plant in its place this holy self-hatred. This is the royal road by which we turn our back on mediocrity, and which leads us without fail to the summit of perfection."

Among Catherine's distinctive traits was a particular fascination for the Eucharist, otherwise known among Christians as the Lord's Supper. One of her biographers admiringly wrote that "when Catherine advanced to receive holy Communion, her face was glowing with a deep color, and bathed in tears and drops of sweat. After receiving Our Lord, she fell into an ecstasy of great length, and when she recovered the use of her faculties, was unable to speak all that day." Catherine became a Dominican nun and committed herself to fasting for the rest of her life: when she was admonished that she was fasting to excess, she defiantly responded that "eating would kill her anyway, so she might as well die of starvation, and do as she wished in the meantime." She ended by starving to death at the age of thirty-three.

Beginning in the early sixteenth century, fasters became less associated with religion. They were distinct from the holy anorexics of earlier centuries in that they pursued their passions at home. Paulus Lentulus, a prominent Swiss doctor who documented dozens of fasting prodigies, was particularly fascinated with Apollonia Schreier, "a fasting virgin from the Bernese countryside" (*Virginis in agro bernensi, inedia*), who, at the time he visited her in 1604, had fasted continuously for three years. When she abruptly halted her fast in 1611, there was more than a note of disappointment among local notables and even foreign dignitaries who had come to visit. This sequence is characteristic of mystical fasters on display—when their fast comes to an end, unless its termination is due to death, onlookers and patrons seem bitterly disappointed. (See the contemporary example of Irom Sharmila, discussed in chapter 5. Worshipped as a goddess while she was fasting, when she halted her fast she was condemned by her former admirers.) Lentulus's work was widely disseminated in Europe, and George Hakewill's 1635 *Apologia; or, Declaration of the Power and Providence of God* relied heavily on its examples.

With fewer people believing in miracles and the possibility of women's suffering as a "vocation"—and as medicine became more evidence-based—physicians increasingly saw it as their duty to search for earthly causes of the compulsion. Richard Morton, a doctor who was one of the first to research pulmonary tuberculosis along modern lines, wrote the earliest clinical study of what is recognizably anorexia. In an early attempt at dispassionate scientific analysis, in his 1694 account,

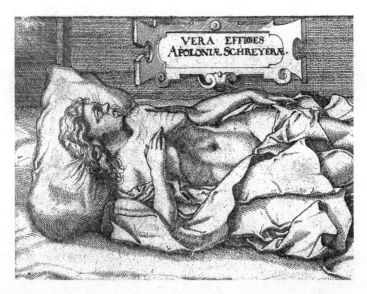

Apollonia Schreier. According to the 1604 account, her fast lasted ten years.

Phthisologia, or, a Treatise on Consumptions, he describes a girl who starved herself so that she looked like "a skeleton only clad in skin." Morton wrote that what he called "Nervous Consumption" was caused by "Sadness and Anxious Cares."

The fascination with holy fasting women who push their bodies to extremes persisted into the twentieth century. Therese Neumann von Konnersreuth, a Bavarian, supposedly lived without water from 1927 to 1962, only ingesting a small portion of the Eucharist. She nevertheless suffered no weight loss and also experienced miraculous, instantaneous healing of her ailments (and every Friday received the stigmata, resulting in blood-soaked images of her circulated to the faithful). Another such holy faster was Alexandrina Maria da Costa, a young Portuguese woman. In 1925, she leapt out a window to escape a trio of men attempting to rape her and became paralyzed. From 1942 until her death in 1955 she allegedly lived on the Eucharist alone, receiving many admiring visitors over the years. While the Church has not to date ruled on either of these women's sanctity, the Holy See's official account of da Costa, for example, writes that she suffered terribly over the years, but "little by little . . . God helped her to see that suffering was her vocation and that she had a special call to be the Lord's 'victim.'"

....

Despite its fairly recent incorporation into the medical lexicon, anorexia has been with us from the beginning of things, with anorexics themselves being hailed as very special humans whose behavior surpasses common understanding. Because the majority of its victims are women, that understanding has been delayed by fundamental prejudices in the medical field.

Whether sparked by social or genetic factors or some combination of the two, anorexia is a frequently lethal disorder related to, but distinct from, the hunger strike, fasting-as-spectacle, or deliberate fasting for purposes of self-improvement. It now appears to be a complex, heritable phenotype—a characteristic that depends both on genetic and environmental factors—which has both psychiatric and metabolic causes. It is real and dangerous, not simply a modern by-product of decadence or "nervous constitutions." But while we must be alert to its incidence, this disease should not keep us from exploring the gifts that fasting has to offer, in spiritual terms and very likely in physical ones as well.

Epilogue

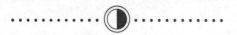

Fasting looks like something I am going to regularly turn to for the rest of my life. It takes me out of the stream of things. Always, in the aftermath of a weeklong fast, I feel refreshed. Now, when I close a fast, I feel it is not so much an end to hunger as an end to discipline. As with a virus that cannot be weighed and yet can kill millions, there can be power in nothing. When I am diminished, I feel part of something larger, a weird amalgam of a hippie pacifist and a marine who has survived basic training. That is the strange quality of fasting: its inside-out invertedness, the idea and the reality that cutting back can add, that diminishment can bring strength and a measure of serenity. And when implemented as a hunger strike, fasting amplifies resistance.

To consume is to annihilate, as both the radical atheist Jean-Paul Sartre and the radical mystic Simone Weil remind us. Consumption is necessary to life. It is not a bad thing as such, but there is no consumption without destruction. "Desire destroys its object," writes Sartre, quoting Hegel. It fractures. And Weil also highlights the inherent contradiction in desire: we are driven to consume, and yet the process can never fully satisfy. "All our desires are contradictory, like the desire for food. I want the person I love to love me. If, however, he is totally devoted to me, he does not exist any longer, and I cease to love him. And as long as he is not totally devoted to me he does not love me enough. Hunger and repletion."

In the aftermath of 9/11 and the death of more than three thousand people, President George W. Bush famously defended the rights of traumatized Americans "to go shopping," and urged a mourning nation to "go down to Disney World in Florida, take your families and enjoy life the way we want it to be enjoyed." Next to terrorism, nothing was as severe a threat to the American Way of Life as not buying things. When Bush issued his call to action, he was continuing a hallowed tradition of mixing consumerism with patriotism. Just as some of us compulsively down a pint of ice cream to soothe our nerves, consumption has been routinely offered up as an antidote to national anxieties in a time of crisis. The First World War—itself an unprecedentedly massive consumer of bodies, buildings, and cities—had been underway for two years when, at the World's Salesmanship Congress in Detroit in 1916, President Woodrow Wilson demanded that Americans not only consume but that they sell consumption. Failure to consume was not merely spurning the prerogatives of empire. It was shirking duty: "America, of all countries in the world, has been timid; has not until recently, has not until within the last two or three years, provided itself with the fundamental instrumentalities for playing a large part in the trade of the world." Wilson ended his lecture by exhorting listeners to "go out and sell goods that will make the world more comfortable and happy, and convert them to the principles of America."

Fasting itself can become a kind of consumption, an addiction. Guidelines on the point at which it becomes hurtful, or even if it can ever be helpful, are vague. Ideally, fasting signals a withdrawal from patterns of consumption. It allows us to reconsider our place in the world and enables reconsideration of "the deadening and cheapening influences of the forces that dominate the marketplace of products and ideas." But to do that, fasting must be employed in bursts.

In my research I came across very few spiritual traditions that do not incorporate fasting into their dogma. The few that explicitly reject fasting include Sikhism and Zoroastrianism. Zoroastrianism, which originated in Persia and is about three thousand years old, holds that the body's primary function is to battle evil, and therefore that any action that weakens the body is sinful: one Zoroastrian priest reportedly held that the only permissible fast is a fast from sin. Moderation in consumption is the ideal.

Disdain for fasting helps Sikhs assert their difference from competing religions. A declaration in the Guru Granth Sahib, the Sikh holy text—the book itself is regarded by observant Sikhs as the eleventh and final guru, which followed the ten human gurus of Sikhism—states: "I observe neither Hindu fasting nor the ritual of the Muslim Ramadan month.... From Hindus and Muslims have I broken free." An extended version of this defiant statement is frequently cited by Sikhs today as distinguishing the faith. And yet even Sikhs have turned to fasting-in-protest: in a famous incident in 1914, a cruel act of racism spurred a massive hunger strike by would-be Punjabi immigrants, for the most part Sikhs, aboard the passenger ship *Komagata Maru*. Refused entry to Vancouver, Canada, at a time when the Canadian government was accepting hundreds of thousands of European immigrants, the 376 passengers seized the vessel from its crew and then engaged in a hunger strike for several days. Two dozen were allowed to disembark, and then a British warship forced the vessel to turn back to India. After the boat reached Calcutta, twenty of the passengers were killed by police and many others were imprisoned. But public opinion, though glacially slow to recognize the injustice, came to side with the Sikhs. Just before the hundredth-year anniversary of the immigrants' forced return, a monument was erected to their memory overlooking Vancouver's Coal Harbor, a reminder of the arbitrariness and profound racism of the immigration laws.

....

Cuong Lu, a friend who is a former Buddhist monk and a current Buddhist teacher, recently spoke with me about fasting. Lu does not advocate the practice. He reminds me that after pursuing a fast to the point of near-death, Buddha turned away from fasting and began to develop the Middle Way. "Almost enough is enough," Cuong told me. "Stopping is a key to spiritual freedom." But I don't think I need to fast from fasting.

That is, I stop all the time; for me, fasting is the break, not the norm. I don't have anorexia, or literally "lack of appetite." I think that if done in limited amounts, fasting opens the way to growth.

A great part of fasting's attraction is its voluntary, private nature. Officially imposed abstinence subverts the notion of spiritual fasting and defeats its purpose: if anything, resentful, hungry people will be more likely to think of the here and now. An Irish delicacy, a cookie called the Connie dodger, illustrates the problem. His Most Reverend Excellency Cornelius "Connie" Lucey was the bishop of Cork, which was Terence MacSwiney's hometown. The bishop, whose rigid tenure lasted from 1952 to 1980, demanded that his parishioners adhere to a particularly strict form of fasting during Lent's forty days. The faithful were held to one meal a day, accompanied by two snacks, known as "collations," or cookies. As described by journalist Fintan O'Toole, this did not sit well even with traditional Catholics, and roused outrage instead of devotion in the Celtic soul. In a classic subversion, a local baker circumvented the spirit of the decree while remaining faithful to its letter: she sold customers giant cookies and christened them with the bishop's nickname. To eat a Connie dodger was to proclaim one's faith, one's status as a true Corkonian, and one's independence at the same time.

I find myself discussing the attributes of the Hindu god Shiva with Prem Krishnamurthy, a writer, designer, curator, and skilled archer. Krishnamurthy points out that Shiva, god of destruction and dissolution, is also the god of change. In that incarnation, Shiva becomes Nataraja, the divine cosmic dancer, who destroys the sun, earth, and moon, and then dances the world into being once more. "Transformation and destruction dance together as one," Krishnamurthy tells me. "Catastrophe also contains a seed: it is a position of loss or sudden change from which to lay new foundations." We are dependent on precarity. And so we come back to unexpected, unplanned progression—the *tzimtzum* of Isaac Luria, Simone Weil, and the *Zhuangzi*, as well as the "swerve" of Epicurus, which he deemed necessary to allow for free will in a cosmos ruled by atomic principles. The break in routine provided by fasting enables us to progress.

....

The first notion about refusing sustenance is that it is suicidal, a rejection of the impulse to live. And prolonged fasting, while to my mind life-affirming and an act of optimism, is paradoxically a flirtation with death. But its ultimate power lies in rejecting nonexistence and choosing to turn back to life. In its rejection of possession and of assimilation, limited fasting postpones destruction and invites creation.

One day early in September 2001, I was late for an appointment far downtown, at Manhattan's southern tip. It was a typically muggy New York City day, and I had been obliged to stuff myself into a jacket and tie and wasn't happy about it. I got off the subway, levels below the base of the World Trade Center, which back then was a maze of shops selling everything from junk food to fancy watches. I ran to my meeting, weaving through crowds of office workers and strolling tourists, bounding up escalators and rising toward the surface, where I entered onto a vast, antiseptic lobby. At some point, I sped around a corner. I remember a red carpet and sunlight streaming in. I stopped short at a singular sight: a group of Buddhist monks in scarlet and saffron robes had gathered around a large square table, perhaps fifteen feet on a side. There, a giant sand mandala was laid out. It was close to being finished. A monk was patiently tapping out a few grains of sand at a time from a handheld funnel to complete the intricate image. He focused laser-like on the two-dimensional world laid before him. People crowded around, most of them, like me, caught up in the minutiae of their daily lives. Brilliant reds, blues, and yellows depicted cavorting demons, deities, and monkeys dancing around elaborately detailed, crenellated buildings, all crafted grain by grain from the sand. In the background swirled the clouds of maya, the sea of illusion in which we swim. The table was filled from one edge to the other. The mandala was already a spectacular achievement and must have taken hundreds of hours to get to this point. Upon its completion, the monks intended to sweep away the sand and dump it all into the sea in a ritual reminder of our fleeting presence in the world. Memory says that this was a day or two before 9/11, but the only record I can find of a sand mandala at the World Trade Center was in 1994. Perhaps my memory, like the buildings and the mandala itself, has also been swept away.

It is one thing to disdain consumerism and to embrace less for a limited period. The advantages, both spiritual and material, are many. But go a bit further down that path and you encounter a treacherous intensity of the practice advocated by deluded fasting fanatics or self-righteous bigots like Jerome of Stridon and the poet Ezra Pound. In his determination to purge himself of materialism and the frantic pursuit of profit, Pound embraced fasting and fascism and worked long and hard for Mussolini's regime as a committed propagandist, spewing anti-Semitic rants for years before the fall of the Axis. And on the physical level, the damage that fasting can do to our delicate, immensely complicated organism is rarely assessed by uncritical fasting enthusiasts.

As we seek to reconsider what we consume, and if we should consume, a skeletal figure beckons. Complete abstinence is nothing to strive for. The ultimate faster was King Lear, who cast off everything: his power, his riches, his sanity. He pursued nothingness with addict-like intensity, until his kingdom was gone and his dead daughter lay in his arms. The trick works both ways: a bit of self-indulgence, if available, can teach us to appreciate absence as well. From emptiness, precarity shapes us. From that state of instability—with us always, but in our immediate purview exacerbated by rapidly mutating viruses, inscrutable world leaders, unpredictable natural disasters, financial euphoria, and financial miseries—we create and move ahead.

Acknowledgments

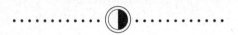

Any writer who attempts to unite Achilles, adenosine triphosphate, and Bobby Sands in one document must have patient and knowledgeable people to fall back on, and so it was in my case.

Without the inspiration of curator and critic Carin Kuoni, I would never have been able to finish this project. I thank her for her creative insight and rock-steady presence. Anna, Elias, and Nathaniel: a parent should not look to children for guidance, but you have been unceasingly supportive, and I am amazed by you and I thank you. My thanks go to my agent, Paul Bresnick, of the Bresnick Weil Literary Agency and my editor and publisher, Jofie Ferrari-Adler, at Avid Reader Press, who each took a flier on a first-time author. I am deeply grateful to both of them for their faith in me. My gratitude goes to assistant editor Carolyn Kelly, cover designer Alison Forner, rights director Paul O'Halloran, copyediting manager Jessica Chin, copyeditor Rob Sternitzky, and the entire team at Avid Reader Press, all of whom have made a challenging process as smooth as possible. It is one I know well, although until this book only from the other side of the desk. Katie Freeman has been instrumental in making sure this book is placed in the hands of people who might appreciate it.

Additional thanks go to the following, for their contributions to the book and/or their encouragement (at times unwitting): S. Anand, publisher of Navayana Books, New Delhi; Eric Banks; Helen Benedict; Rev. Dr. Michael Bos of the Marble Collegiate Church, New York City;

Rosanna Bruno; Paul Campion and the Sunrise Movement; Paul Chan; Bonnie Chau; Dr. Roy Christopher; Sue Coe; Prof. Simon Critchley, the New School; Prof. Laura Cronk, the New School; Prof. Faisal Devji, the University of Oxford; Fern Díaz; Dr. Luz Marina Díaz, director of religious education at the Church of St. Francis Xavier (New York City); Lisa Dierbeck; Barbara Epler; Farnaz Fatemi; Sahar Francis, director, Addameer Prisoner Support and Human Rights Association; Paul Friedman, research librarian in the General Research Division of the New York Public Library; Prof. Rubén Gallo, Princeton University; Roseanne Gerin, Radio Free Asia; Thomas H. Hartman; Dr. Britt Marie Hermes; Prof. Brooke Holmes, Princeton University; Shohret Hoshur, Radio Free Asia; Justin Humphries; Pat Irvin, Esq.; Jentel Arts; Miracle Jones; Prem Krishnamurthy, designer and curator; Rev. Wendell Lancaster, senior pastor, the Greater Hood Memorial A.M.E. Zion Church of New York City; Mike Levine; Richard Lipkin; Dr. Steven M. Lipkin, Weill Cornell Medicine; Margie Livingston; Prof. David B. Lombard, University of Michigan; Cuong Lu; Isaac B. Lustgarten, Esq.; Ru L. Marshall; Prof. Lucy McDiarmid, Montclair State University; Diane Mehta; Nathalie Miebach; T. D. Mitchell; Michael F. Moore; Sina Najafi; Haruko Nakamura, Japanese Studies Librarian, Yale University Library; Anne Nelson; the New York Public Library in general and the Wertheim Study in particular; Dr. Steven Novella, Yale School of Medicine; Christopher S. O'Brien; Steve Orfield, Mike Role, and Sherry Role at Orfield Labs; Dale Peck, whose admonitions on direct writing I have tried to keep in mind; Kristen Portland of ANAD; Prof. Claire Potter, the New School; Prof. Vyjayanthi Rao, CUNY; Sandy Restrepo, Esq., Colectiva Legal del Pueblo; Leslie Rogers; André San-Chez; Jacques Servin; Pat Sheehan of Sinn Féin; Larry Siems; Heidi Skolnik, the Women's Sports Medicine Center at the Hospital for Special Surgery; Mohamedou Ould Slahi; Dr. Howard Steiger, Douglas Mental Health University Institute and McGill University; Rabbi Michael Strassfeld; Prof. Radhika Subramaniam, Parsons School of Design, the New School; Prof. John M. Sullivan, Institut für Mathematik, Technische Universität Berlin; Pat

Thomas; Daniel Wakin, who, while speaking of another work, inspired me "not to bury the lede," which I hope I have not done; Shaykh Suhaib Webb; Rick Whitaker; Michael Z. Wise; the Yaddo Corporation; and Rabbi Eliezer Zalmanov, codirector of Chabad of Northwest Indiana.

Professional associations listed for ID purposes only.

A Sampling of Famous Fasters

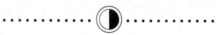

Achilles	Muhammad
Anthony of the Desert	Odin
Augustine of Hippo	Origen
Buddha	Sylvia Pankhurst
Byron	St. Patrick
John Cage	Alice Paul
Catherine of Siena	Plutarch
Cesar Chavez	Ezra Pound
Angela Davis	Bobby Sands
Emily Dickinson	Arthur Schopenhauer
Gandhi	Irom Chanu Sharmila
Dick Gregory	Upton Sinclair
Hildegard of Bingen	Socrates
Hippocrates	Doris Stevens
Thomas Jefferson	Tertullian
Jerome of Stridon	Tiberius
Jesus	Leon Trotsky
Franz Kafka	Mark Twain
Abraham Lincoln	George Washington
Maimonides	Simone Weil
Moses	John Wesley

Selected Books Related to Fasting

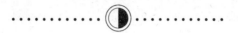

The following list focuses on my own areas of interest as they pertain to fasting. There are hundreds and perhaps thousands of titles related to "practical" fasting, and I did not come across a fasting guide that focuses purely on physical health that I would recommend. The books that I read in that area seemed to be all-out advocates for the practice largely devoid of nuance, in the Bernarr Macfadden/Herbert Shelton showman tradition of "fasting cures all your ills." (Chapter 3, "The Marvelous Machine," related to the biology of fasting, is based on interviews with medical professionals and articles in medical journals.) If you are planning a long-term fast from food, you would do well to first consult a nutritionist or other medical professional. Not all of us are comfortable with food fasting, but as I emphasize in this book there are many different avenues to accessing the insights and strengths that fasting can provide.

Rudolph M. Bell's research on medieval Italian fasting saints, *Holy Anorexia* (Chicago: University of Chicago Press, 1985), was the first in-depth modern study on anorexia and sainthood. A scholar of the Renaissance, Bell suggested connections between the oppression of women—or their liberation—and fasting.

Joan Jacobs Brumberg's comprehensive and nuanced history of anorexia nervosa, *Fasting Girls: The History of Anorexia Nervosa* (New York: Vintage, 2000), is essential to anyone interested in the phenomenon's evolution. She attempts to disentangle the strands of anorexia-as-disease and fasting-in-protest, which too often seem to be treated as one and the same. Unlike many scholars, she allows for the possibility of fasting by *choice*, as opposed to its being seen as resulting from manipulation by outside forces.

For a poetically written survey of a number of literary references to fasting, I recommend Maud Ellmann's highly readable *The Hunger Artists* (London: Virago Press, 1993). Particularly strong for its Anglo-Irish focus.

For an uncritical, fanboy account of Henry S. Tanner's celebrated, trendsetting, and possibly fraudulent fast, the biography by his ally Robert A. Gunn is the ticket: *Forty Days without Food!: A Biography of Henry S. Tanner, M.D., Including a Complete and Accurate History of His Wonderful Fasts* (New York: Albert Metz and Co., 1880). I recommend the book not as a model for a fasting regimen but as an example of "heroic" fasting in the late nineteenth century.

Peter Matthiessen's engaging profile of Cesar Chavez, an expanded version of what he had originally written for the *New Yorker*, takes a thoughtful, inspiring look at what is generally viewed as the dour business of hunger strikes: *Sal Si Puedes* (Berkeley: University of California Press, 2014).

The polymath Hillel Schwartz provides a far-ranging, well-researched, and opinionated history of the growing obsession with excess in *Never Satisfied: A Cultural History of Diets, Fantasies, and Fat* (New York: Anchor Books, 1990). A torrent of information on the subject of shifting views on weight.

Holy Feast and Holy Fast: The Religious Significance of Food to Medieval Women (Berkeley: University of California Press, 1988) by Caroline Walker Bynum predates Brumberg and is the source for many later works on the subject.

James C. Whorton's *Crusaders for Fitness: The History of American Health Reformers* (Princeton, NJ: Princeton University Press, 1982) is a lively and comprehensive history of the Americans who, stimulated both by nativism and pseudoscience, found that proselytizing for hygiene could be extremely profitable.

Asceticism (edited by Vincent L. Wimbush and Richard Valantasis; New York: Oxford University Press, 1995), a hefty (695-page) survey by academics for academics that contains arcana and insights. Its emphasis is on Western philosophy, but it contains a few worthwhile essays on other traditions.

From Feasting to Fasting: The Evolution of a Sin (London: Routledge, 1996) by Veronika E. Grimm is valuable for its chronicle of how Jerome's extremism and various obsessions, particularly his misogyny, gradually transformed the early Church.

A History of Force Feeding: Hunger Strikes, Prisons and Medical Ethics, 1909–1974 (London: Palgrave Macmillan, 2016) by Ian Miller provides an essential, unflinching account of the brutal response to hunger strikes by authorities.

It is hard to find a better guide for the perplexed than theoretical physicist Carlo Rovelli, whose calmness and intellectual vigor pervades *The Order of Time* (New York: Riverhead, 2019). Rovelli considers an unreasonable universe with a Buddha-like clarity.

Nayan Shah's *Refusal to Eat: A Century of Prison Strikes* (Oakland: University of California Press, 2022) is a good source for detailed, vivid accounts of hunger strikes in Ireland and India.

The classic guide by Gene Sharp, *The Politics of Nonviolent Action, Part Two: The Methods of Nonviolent Action* (Boston: Porter Sargent, 1973) has been the source of much trouble for those in power. It contains a long section on hunger strikes.

Walter Vandereycken and Ron Van Deth's book, *From Fasting Saints to Anorexic Girls: The History of Self-Starvation* (London: Athlone Press, 1994), provides a view of the historical span of fasting primarily as a phenomenon tied to femininity. A secondary source for some excellent anecdotes of fasters condemned as witches, it also has useful discussion of the Gull/Lasègue controversy.

Assembled from Simone Weil's notes after her death by her friend Gustave Thibon, *Gravity and Grace* (translated by Arthur Wills; Lincoln: Bison Books, University of Nebraska Press, 1997) is generally acknowledged to be one of the most important modern works in the mystical tradition.

Instructive, intriguing, and poetic, *The Complete Works of Zhuangzi* (New York: Columbia University Press, 2013) makes a perfect companion to a weeklong fast. Burton Watson's translation reads smoothly and, even if you're munching on a sandwich as you read, this little compendium of the third century BCE Taoist philosophy will not fail to inspire.

Notes

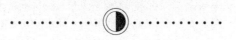

INTRODUCTION

vii *I decided to stop eating for seven days*: I was far from alone. As measured against its own historical popularity, Google searches for "fasting" saw a steady and rapid increase in the United States beginning in the spring of 2017, reaching an all-time high in January of 2020—by far the highest it had been since 2004, when Google started keeping track of such things. Post–January 2020, it showed an overall decline.

viii *he "is capable of watching and fasting"*: Simone Weil, *Gravity and Grace*, trans. Arthur Wills (Lincoln, NE: Bison Books, 1997), 103.

viii *it results from "self-hatred and desperation"*: Susan Bordo, "Anorexia Nervosa: Psychopathology as the Crystallization of Culture," in *Food and Culture: A Reader*, Carole Counihan and Penny Van Esterik, eds. (New York: Routledge, 1997), 226.

ix *they have been thoroughly discussed elsewhere*: See in particular Joan Jacobs Brumberg's comprehensive and nuanced history of anorexia nervosa, *Fasting Girls: The History of Anorexia Nervosa*, essential to anyone interested in the phenomenon's evolution. Rudolph M. Bell's research on medieval Italian fasting saints, *Holy Anorexia*, was the first in-depth modern study on anorexia and sainthood.

x *"It's dangerous and it's drastic"*: Michel Martin, "NYC Taxi Drivers Enter Day 11 of Hunger Strike for Medallion Debt Relief," *All Things Considered*, NPR, October 30, 2021, https://www.npr.org/2021/10/30/1050850701/nyc-taxi-drivers-enter-day-11-of-hunger-strike-for-medallion-debt-relief.

x *"As a person I'm really small"*: Molly Ball, "'What More Do We Need to Do to Win?' A Controversial Climate Group Rethinks Its Strategy," *Time*, March 17, 2022, https://time.com/6158322/sunrise-movement-climate-activism-struggles/.

x *"I'm always aware of being a flea"*: Salamishah Tillet and Elizabeth Paton, "A Hunger Strike Makes Headlines before Milan Fashion Week Begins," *New York Times*, February 13, 2023, https://www.nytimes.com/2023/02/13/fashion/stella-jean-diversity-milan-fashion-week.html/.

xi *breastfeeding mothers were instructed*: This advice was doomed to fail, and nursing mothers were blamed for their inability to breastfeed on schedule. See Molly Fischer, "Milking It," *New Yorker*, March 13, 2023, 30.

xii *"Work out your own salvation"*: Philippians 2:12, King James Version. All biblical quotes are from this translation.

xii *"Decay is inherent"*: See R. Raj Singh, *Bhakti and Philosophy* (Lanham, MD: Lexington Books, 2006), 47.

xii *"Two prisoners whose cells adjoin"*: Weil, *Gravity and Grace*, 200.

xii *"standing still"*: K. Wagtendonk, *Fasting in the Koran* (Leiden, Netherlands: E. J. Brill, 1968), 7.

xiii *"malnutrition and starvation are scourges"*: Eva Lerat and Sébastien Charbonnier, *Le jeûne: Une expérience philosophique* (Paris: Éditions Le Pommier, 2022), 108. My translation.

xiii *the largest single component of landfills*: "Sustainable Management of Food Basics," U.S. Environmental Protection Agency, https://www.epa.gov/sustainable-management-food/sustainable-management-food-basics.

DAY 1, SUNDAY

1 *falling out of an airplane*: Something I once did, accompanied by a parachute. Like fasting, the preparation was more stressful than the act, which was similarly freeing, but of briefer duration.

3 *During the third week of the 2022 invasion*: Eleonora Girotto, "Russian Police Arrest Demonstrator Protesting with Blank Sign," *Independent*, May 13, 2022, https://www.independent.co.uk/tv/news/russia-protest-war-blank-sign-ve9882053.

3 *Protesters held empty signs*: In Shanghai, some protesters said that the papers were inspired by an anecdote from the Soviet era, "in which a dissident accosted by the police for distributing leaflets in a public square reveals the fliers to be blank. When asked, the dissident replies that there is no need for words because 'everyone knows.'" See Chang Che and Amy Chang Chien, "Memes, Puns and Blank Sheets of Paper: China's Creative Acts of Protest," *New York Times*, November 28, 2022, https://www.nytimes.com/2022/11/28/world/asia/china-protests-blank-sheets.html.

3 *an empty sign instantly conveys*: A blank space has historically indicated mourning in Judaism. After the destruction of the first Temple in 586 BCE, Jewish leaders decided that the interiors of buildings should reflect purity and absence. Scholars decreed that walls in a home should be covered with mortar and painted only with lime, leaving an unpainted square directly opposite the entrance. (See Mishneh Torah, Fasts 5, https://www.sefaria .org/Mishneh_Torah%2C_Fasts.5?lang=bi.) The geometrically balanced space creates a window onto an unsullied new world.

4 *"That is not what I told them"*: Steve Orfield, interview with the author, October 19, 2021.

4 *"You can feel what's going on"*: Joseph Campbell (1904–1987), best known for his book *The Hero with a Thousand Faces* (1949).

5 *"Silence is suspect"*: Roy Christopher, "The Science of Sound and Silence," blog, issue #50, https://buttondown.email/roychristopher/archive/the-science-of-sound-and-silence/.

5 "living is loud and messy": Xochitl Gonzalez, "Let Brooklyn Be Loud," *The Atlantic*, September 2022, https://www.theatlantic.com/magazine/archive/2022/09/let-brooklyn-be-loud/670600/.

5 *According to one study, at the University of Virginia*: Timothy D. Wilson et al., "Just Think: The Challenges of a Disengaged Mind," *Science* 345, no. 6192 (July 4, 2014): 77.

6 *A recent article in* New Scientist: Kayt Sukel, "The Power of Quiet: The Mental and Physical Health Benefits of Silence," *New Scientist*, August 10, 2022, https://www.newscientist.com/article/mg25533990-700-the-power-of-quiet-the-mental-and-physical-health-benefits-of-silence/.

6 *"Rumination, stress and anxiety"*: J. P. Hamilton et al., "Default-Mode and Task-Positive Network Activity in Major Depressive Disorder: Implications for Adaptive and Maladaptive Rumination," *Biological Psychiatry* 70, no. 4 (August 15, 2011): 327–33.

6 *silence carries a mystery*: Rui Zhe Goh, Ian B. Phillips, and Chaz Firestone, "The Perception of Silence," *Psychological and Cognitive Sciences* 120, no. 29 (July 10, 2023).

6 *"To rest in a DreamSpace"*: Tricia Hersey, *Rest Is Resistance: A Manifesto* (New York: Little, Brown, 2022), 97.

7 *the elder Babylonian gods*: Hillel Schwartz, *Making Noise: From Babel to the Big Bang and Beyond* (New York: Zone Books, 2011), 18.

7 *"A constant sound"*: Roy Christopher, *The Medium Picture*, unpublished manuscript.

9 *"going from something towards nothing"*: John Cage, "Lecture on Something," in *Silence: Lectures and Writings* (Middletown, CT: Wesleyan University Press, 1961), 143.

9 *"What we require is silence"*: John Cage, "Lecture on Nothing," in ibid., 109.

10 *"The greater the distance, the clearer the view"*: W. G. Sebald, *The Rings of Saturn* (New York: New Directions, 1998), 19.

10 *Something and nothing need each other*: Cage, "Lecture on Something," 145.

11 *Literary scholar Maud Ellmann*: As quoted in Maud Ellmann, *The Hunger Artists* (London: Virago Press, 1993), 14.

11 *psychoanalyst Julia Kristeva's assertion*: Julia Kristeva, "Stabat Mater," trans. Arthur Goldhammer, *Poetics Today* 6, nos. 1–2 (1985): 135.

11 *"We hold that a friend"*: Aristotle, *Eudemian Ethics*, Book VII, 1.5, trans. and eds. Brad Inwood and Rachel Woolf (Cambridge, UK: Cambridge University Press, 2013), 121. I am indebted to artist Paul Chan for calling my attention to this passage, which he cited in "The Bather's Dilemma," at the Townsend Center for the Humanities annual "Una's Lecture," at the University of California, Berkeley, in October 2019.

12 *A UK study involving*: Chun Shen et al., "Associations of Social Isolation and Loneliness with Later Dementia," *Neurology* 99, no. 2 (July 2022): e164–e175.

12 *Prisoners kept in solitary*: Tiana Herring, "The Research Is Clear: Solitary Confinement Causes Long-Lasting Harm," Prison Policy Initiative, December 8, 2020, https://www.prisonpolicy.org/blog/2020/12/08/solitary_symposium/.

12 *drug overdoses reached record highs*: According to the Centers for Disease Control's National Center for Health Statistics, drug overdoses in the twelve-month period ending in April 2021 reached a record high of 100,431 deaths. See "Provisional Drug Overdose Death Counts," CDC, December 5, 2021, https://www.cdc.gov/nchs/nvss/vsrr/drug-overdose-data.htm. Again per the CDC, in 2020 mental-health-related emergency room visits for teens increased by a third over 2019. Suspected suicide attempts were more than 50 percent higher among girls age twelve to seventeen. See "Emergency Department Visits for Suspected Suicide Attempts among Persons Aged 12–25 Years before and during the COVID-19 Pandemic—United States, January 2019–May 2021," CDC, June 18, 2021, https://www.cdc.gov/mmwr/volumes/70/wr/mm7024e1.htm?s_cid=mm7024e1_w.

12 *To be conscious is*: The philosopher Noreen Khawaja expounds on this concept, key to asceticism, in *The Religion of Existence: Asceticism in Philosophy from Kierkegaard to Sartre* (Chicago: University of Chicago Press, 2016).

12 *Our inclination is anti-entropic*: See Carlo Rovelli, *The Order of Time* (New York: Riverhead, 2019).

13 *In chapter 4, "In the World of Men"*: Zhuangzi, *The Complete Works of Zhuangzi*, trans. Burton Watson (New York: Columbia University Press, 2013), 25.

14 *Confucius at last appears to approve*: Ibid., 26.

14 *Lord Wenhui marvels*: Ibid., 20.

15 *But there is no such thing as silence*: John Cage, "Composition as Process," *Silence: Lectures and Writings* (Middletown, CT: Wesleyan University Press, 1961), 51.

15 *In* Zero Decibels: George Michelsen Foy, *Zero Decibels: The Quest for Absolute Silence* (New York: Scribner, 2010), 176.

16 *longer periods derail us*: For example, after a six-month stint spent alone and underground at Midnight Cave in Austin, Texas, in 1972, French chrono-biologist Michel Siffre emerged deeply depressed. He had had minimal communication with the outside world.

16 *"Most of our lives"*: Steve Orfield, interview with the author, October 19, 2021.

16 *French philosophers Eva Lerat and Sébastien Charbonnier*: Lerat and Char-bonnier, *Le jeûne*, 105–6. See also Allan Snyder, "Explaining and Inducing Savant Skills: Privileged Access to Lower Level, Less-Processed Informa-tion," *Philosophical Transactions of the Royal Society* 364, no. 1522 (May 27, 2009): 1399–1405.

17 *even its root cause*: Timo Hener, "Noise Pollution and Violent Crime," *Journal of Public Economics* 215 (November 2022): 104748. See also I. Alimoham-madi et al. "Effect of Chronic Noise Exposure on Aggressive Behavior of Automotive Industry Workers," *International Journal of Occupational and Environmental Medicine* 9, no. 4 (October 2018): 170–75.

The writer George Prochnik quotes a Washington, D.C., police officer who specializes in resolving noise complaints. "You go into these houses where the couple, or the roommate, or the whole family is fighting and yelling and you've got the television blaring so you can't think, and a radio on top of that, and somebody got home from work who wants to relax or to sleep, and it's just obvious what they're actually fighting about," says the cop. "They're fighting about the noise. They don't know it, but that's the problem." From *In Pursuit of Silence: Listening for Meaning in a World of Noise* (New York: Knopf Doubleday, 2010), 18.

17 *Numerous studies draw a direct line*: See, for example, Jaana I. Halonen, "Road Traffic Noise Is Associated with Increased Cardiovascular Morbidity and Mortality and All-Cause Mortality in London," *European Heart Journal* 36, no. 39 (October 2015): 2653–61.

17 *the World Health Organization reported*: "Burden of Disease from Environmental Noise: Quantification of Healthy Life Years Lost in Europe" (Copenhagen: World Health Organization, 2011).

18 *used on prisoners in Guantánamo Bay*: "Blaring Music Used to Abuse War Prisoners," CBS News, December 9, 2008, https://www.cbsnews.com/news/blaring-music-used-to-abuse-war-prisoners/.

18 *one journalist present during Russian shelling*: Luke Mogelson, "Everyone Is a Target," *New Yorker*, July 23, 2022, https://www.newyorker.com/magazine/2022/08/01/the-desperate-lives-inside-ukraines-dead-cities.

18 *report of the U.S. Senate Select Committee on Intelligence*: U.S. Senate Select Committee on Intelligence, "Committee Study of the Central Intelligence Agency's Detention and Interrogation Program," Executive Summary, 55. Approved December 13, 2021.

19 *"In order to make a signal clear"*: Steve Orfield, interview with the author, October 19, 2021.

19 *he documents the* yamabushi: Donald Frederick Lach and Edwin J. Van Kley, *Asia in the Making of Europe*, vol. 3, book 4 (Chicago: University of Chicago Press, 1965), 1832.

19 *Buddhist ascetics practiced sokushinbutsu*: Iwahana Michiaki, "'Sokushinbutsu': Japan's Buddhist Mummies," Nippon.com, January 26, 2022, https://www.nippon.com/en/japan-topics/g02008/.

19 *Japanese followers of Tendai Buddhism*: "Japanese Monk Completes Feat of Extreme Fasting, First in 8 Years," *San Diego Union Tribune*, October 21, 2015, https://www.efe.com/efe/english/life/japanese-monk-completes-feat-of-extreme-fasting-first-in-8-years/50000263-2743587. Depending on environmental conditions and the subject, most people die after four days without food or water.

20 *passage in chapter 19*: Zhuangzi, *The Complete Works*, 152–53.

21 *"They said of one old man"*: Owen Chadwick, ed., *Western Asceticism* (London: SCM Press, 1958), 108.

21 *muses that he "should"*: Ibid., 109.

DAY 2, MONDAY

25 *"slaughter and blood and the rattle"*: *The Iliad of Homer* (19.214), trans. Samuel Butler (London: Jonathan Cape, 1923), 314.

25 *in eleventh-century Japan*: As quoted in William E. Deal, "The Lotus Sūtra and the Rhetoric of Legitimization in Eleventh-Century Japanese Buddhism," *Japanese Journal of Religious Studies* 20, no. 4 (December 1993): 279.

26 *The idea that the senses are a distraction*: Hannah Arendt, "Thinking and Moral Considerations: A Lecture," *Social Research* 38, no. 3 (Autumn 1971): 420.

26 *"the most beautiful part of justice"*: Porphyry, *Select Works of Porphyry*, trans. Thomas Taylor (London: Thomas Rodd, 1823), 93.

27 *only moderation precents depletion*: Herodotus, active a generation after Pythagoras, is most commonly cited as a referent for fasting in the modern era. But the many aphorisms and prescriptions attributed to him were likely put together by a broad swath of different physicians. One thing Herodotus almost certainly would have advocated is moderation: holding back, both in terms of abstention and in terms of indulgence, is consistent with what we can glean of his worldview. See Helen Morales, *Antigone Rising: The Subversive Power of the Ancient Myths* (New York: Hachette, 2020).

28 *in the fifth century BCE*: Robert A. F. Thurman, "Tibetan Buddhist Perspectives on Asceticism," in *Asceticism*, eds. Vincent L. Wimbush and Richard Valantasis (New York: Oxford University Press, 1995), 111.

28 *the extreme asceticism current at that time*: Bellanwila Thera Wimalaratana, "Buddhism and the Brahma Concept," BuddhaSasana, August 31, 2005, https://www.budsas.org/ebud/ebdha321.htm.

29 *The earliest Buddhist images*: Vidya Dehejia, "Aniconism and the Multivalence of Emblems," *Ars Orientalis* 21 (1991): 45–66.

29 *"God has no hand"*: Jacques Derrida, *Of Grammatology*, trans. Gayatri Chakravorty Spivak (Baltimore: Johns Hopkins University Press, 2016), 280. In less mystical terms than Weil, Derrida speaks here of the power of smallness: a disruptive energy that "produces a revolution out of nothing... A nearly nil force is a nearly infinite force when it is strictly alien to the system it sets going." (Ibid., 280.)

29 *In a stunning break with Vedic Hindu tradition*: Gail P. Corrington-Streete, "Trajectories of Ascetic Behavior," in *Asceticism*, eds. Vincent L. Wimbush and Richard Valantasis (New York: Oxford University Press, 1995), 121.

30 *Buddha's first followers*: Wimalaratana, "Buddhism and the Brahma Concept."

30 *As Buddha's followers gained in number*: Thurman, "Tibetan Buddhist Perspectives on Asceticism," 112.

31 *the Christian Orthodox Hesychast movement*: For more on Hesychast principles, see Metropolitan Kallistos (Ware) of Diokleia, "Praying with the Body: The Hesychast Method and Non-Christian Parallels," Bogoslov.ru, July 11, 2012, https://bogoslov.ru/article/2671134. Compare this statement with one by T'ien-T'ai Chih-i (538–597 CE), the first teacher associated with what came to be known as Lotus Sutra Buddhism: "At such times [of

distraction] it is advisable to focus attention on the navel, which tends to unify the mind and prevent confusion." (Lectures given by Grand Master Chih-chi of Tien-tai Mountains, at the Shiu-ch'an Temple; "Dhyana," in *A Buddhist Bible*, ed. Dwight Goddard [New York, E. P., 1938].)

31 *Hesychasm persists in Christian Orthodox monasteries*: For more on Buddhist influences on other religions, see, for example, Ahmad Faizuddin Ramli, Jaffary Awang, and Zaizul Ab Rahman, "Muslim Scholars' Discourse on Buddhism: A Literature on Buddha's Position," *SHS Web of Conferences* 53, nos. 2–3 (January 2018): 04001.

31 *the legend of Barlaam and Josaphat*: Nathan H. Levine, "Barlaam and Josaphat," *Brill's Encyclopedia of Buddhism*, vol. 2 (Leiden, Netherlands: Koninklijke Brill NV, 2019), 43.

32 *"While the soul is infected"*: Plato, *Phaedo*, in *The Dialogues of Plato*, vol. 2, trans. Benjamin Jowett (New York: Macmillan, 1892), 205.

33 *admired Socrates's "hardiness" and "impassivity"*: Diogenes Laërtius, *Lives of the Eminent Philosophers*, book 6, passage 3, ed. James Miller, trans. Pamela Mensch (Oxford, UK: Oxford University Press, 2020), 192.

33 *"To someone praising luxury, he said"*: Ibid., book 6, passage 8, 194.

33 *the Confucian* Analects *provide the same message*: Diana Lobel, *Philosophies of Happiness* (New York: Columbia University Press, 2017), 79.

34 *a short poem to the memory of Antisthenes*: Diogenes Laërtius, *Lives of the Eminent Philosophers*, book 6, passage 19, 198.

35 *lived as a stray in the streets*: And in fact, Diogenes the Cynic was dismissed as "someone whose sanity sounds shaky at best" by the English writer Sarah Bakewell: "Lives of the Philosophers, Warts and All," *New York Times*, January 20, 2011, https://www.nytimes.com/2011/01/23/books/review/Bakewell-t .html. The poet and activist Eileen Myles explored the concept of living within society, but not as a conventionally functioning part of it, in 2012 and again in 2016, when as part of a "Zen Street Retreat," she took up living on the streets of New York City for several days and begged for food. See Shelly Marlow, "Why Eileen Myles Spent a Week Living on the Streets of New York," *Hyperallergic*, September 23, 2016, https://hyperallergic.com/324819/why-eileen-myles -spent-a-week-living-on-the-streets-of-new-york/.

37 *Pleasure was divided into two main classes*: Alan Neuringer and Walter Englert, "Epicurus and B. F. Skinner: In Search of the Good Life," *Journal of the Experimental Analysis of Behavior* 107, no. 1 (January 2017): 27.

37 *"The origin and root of everything good"*: Athenaeus, *The Learned Banqueters: Vol. VI: Books 12–13.594b*, ed. and trans. S. Douglas Olson (Cambridge, MA: Harvard University Press, 2006), 179.

37 *Epicurus was a committed atomist*: Neuringer and Englert, "Epicurus and B. F. Skinner," 23.

38 *"man stands by his desires fiercely"*: Jean-Paul Sartre, *Being and Nothingness*, trans. Sarah Richmond (New York: Routledge, 2018), 158.

39 *To Romans such as Cicero*: Catherine Edwards, *The Politics of Immorality in Ancient Rome* (Cambridge, UK: Cambridge University Press, 1993), 81.

39 *he engaged in spirited attacks*: J. M. Rist, *Epicurus: An Introduction* (Cambridge, UK: Cambridge University Press, 1972), 5.

41 *as historian Eliezer Diamond has pointed out*: Eliezer Diamond, *Holy Men and Hunger Artists: Fasting and Asceticism in Rabbinic Culture* (Oxford, UK: Oxford University Press, 2003), 14.

41 *asceticism recurrent throughout*: Joseph Tamney, "Fasting and Modernization," *Journal for the Scientific Study of Religion* 19, no. 2 (June 1980): 136–37.

42 *in the words of behavioral psychologist B. F. Skinner*: Neuringer and Englert, "Epicurus and B. F. Skinner," 26.

DAY 3, TUESDAY

44 *In Europe, the notion*: Brooke Holmes, "Aelius Aristides' Illegible Body," in *Aelius Aristides between Greece, Rome, and the Gods*, eds. Brooke Holmes and William V. Harris (New York: Columbia University Press, 2009), 89.

45 *classics scholar Brooke Holmes*: Ibid., 86.

45 *the revelation of things*: This tendency perhaps reached its height or depths in the late nineteenth century, with the incarceration of the female form under what philosopher Martha Nussbaum described as "billowing petticoats that made women seem vaguely like mermaids, human on top and some hidden uncleanness below." See Martha Nussbaum, "Man Overboard," *New Republic*, June 22, 2006, https://newrepublic.com/article/64199/man-overboard.

46 *"Hopdance cries in Tom's belly"*: *King Lear*, act 3, scene 6. Untamable appetite is "the swollen shadow." It is always with us, the "stupid clown of the spirit's motive," as the doomed poet Delmore Schwartz wrote at the age of twenty-five in "The Heavy Bear Who Goes with Me." The poem's title perfectly evokes Schwartz's sense of a dual self, cogently expressing the push-me-pull-you struggle we all experience daily to various degrees. The cryptic epigraph Schwartz placed at the work's beginning, "the withness of the body," is a reference to the work of Alfred North Whitehead, another philosopher whose outlook suggests Epicurean roots. Whitehead argued that our perception and understanding of the world is both limited and

made possible by our physical boundaries. Our senses are the conduit to our feelings: our eyes convey images and we derive meaning from what we see. Our ears hear something that we interpret, and so on. The "withness" is the incarnation of an uneasy alliance, a rickety partnership in which our fleshy self has glommed onto the spirit.

46 *Certain of the tiny animals*: M. Srivastava et al., "The Trichoplax Genome and the Nature of Placozoans," *Nature* 454 (August 2008): 955–60.

46 *a microbiologist working at the Argonne National Laboratory*: Stephen Miller, "Charles F. Ehret (1923–2007): Scientist Offered Solution to Victims of Jet Lag," *Wall Street Journal*, March 10, 2007, https://www.wsj.com/articles /SB117349084761632907.

47 *A 2008 study conducted by doctors*: P. M. Fuller, J. Lu, and C. B. Saper, "Differential Rescue of Light- and Food-Entrainable Circadian Rhythms," *Science* 320, no. 5879 (May 23, 2008): 1074–77.

47 *"We discovered that a single cycle"*: Bonnie Prescott, "Study Identifies Food-Related Clock in the Brain," *Harvard Gazette*, May 19, 2008, https:// news.harvard.edu/gazette/story/2008/05/study-identifies-food-related -clock-in-the-brain/.

48 *lightning-fast signaling node*: Benjamin U. Hoffman and Ellen A. Lumpkin, "A Gut Feeling" *Science* 361, no. 6408 (September 21, 2018): 1208.

50 *backed up by a five-year study*: E. G. Neal et al., "The Ketogenic Diet for the Treatment of Childhood Epilepsy: A Randomised Controlled Trial," *Lancet Neurology* 7, no. 6 (June 7, 2008): 500–506.

50 *some studies show that ketone bodies*: "Although nutritional ketosis is widely assumed to be a safe metabolic condition, proper consideration has not been given to the fact that ketones are reactive toward proteins through the same mechanisms as glucose." See Mark J. Burkitt, "An Overlooked Danger of Ketogenic Diets: Making the Case That Ketone Bodies Induce Vascular Damage by the Same Mechanisms as Glucose," *Nutrition* 75–76 (February 2020): 110763. See also Ira J. Goldberg et al., "Ketogenic Diets, Not for Everyone," *Journal of Clinical Lipidology* 15, no. 1 (January–February 2021): 61–67.

50 *"Ketone bodies are not just fuel"*: Rafael de Cabo and Mark P. Mattson, "Effects of Intermittent Fasting on Health, Aging, and Disease," *New England Journal of Medicine* 381, no. 26 (2019): 2541–51.

50 *the Okinawa Centenarian Study*: D. C. Willcox et al., "Caloric Restriction and Human Longevity: What Can We Learn from the Okinawans?" *Biogerontology* 7, no. 3 (June 2006): 174–75.

51 *The trick is calorie restriction*: The same study noted that "a modestly low energy

intake (85% of group mean) had the lowest risk for all-cause mortality (Willcox et al. 2004). There was higher mortality risk when caloric intake dropped below 50% of the group mean. This is consistent with previous animal findings that show decreased risk for mortality from age associated diseases and increased life span under a CR regimen of up to 50% restriction." (Ibid., 174.)

51 *a fifth of the American population*: "2021 Profile of Older Americans," Administration for Community Living, U.S. Department of Health and Human Services, November 2022.

51 *In the 1950s, it was discovered that*: Antidepressants such as Zoloft, Prozac, and Paxil are supposed to work by preventing serotonin from being re-absorbed into the system, thereby increasing serotonin levels. Whether that is indeed how they work to fight depression is a matter of increasing debate. The connection between low levels of serotonin and depression is not universally accepted: a July 2022 study published in *Molecular Psychiatry* examined seventeen separate studies of the hormone and could only conclude that the evidence was inconclusive. See J. Moncrieff et al., "The Serotonin Theory of Depression: A Systematic Umbrella Review of the Evidence," *Molecular Psychiatry* 381 (July 2022): 1–14.

52 *Higher levels of endocannabinoids*: I. Matias et al., "Endocannabinoids Measurement in Human Saliva as Potential Biomarker of Obesity," *PLoS One* 7, no. 7 (2012): e42399.

52 *There is more to the ketone cocktail*: This link seems to have first been posited by Andrew J. Brown in 2007: "Low-Carb Diets, Fasting and Euphoria: Is There a Link between Ketosis and Gamma-Hydroxybutyrate (GHB)?," *Medical Hypotheses* 68, no. 2 (2007): 268–71. Many studies have since affirmed the connection: see, for example, Yifan Zhang et. al., "The Effects of Calorie Restriction in Depression and Potential Mechanisms," *Current Neuropharmacology* 13, no. 4 (July 2015): 536–42, https://www.ncbi.nlm.nih.gov/pmc/articles/PMC4790398/; and Stephen Malunga Manchishi et al., "Effect of Caloric Restriction on Depression," *Journal of Cellular and Molecular Medicine* 22, no. 5 (May 2018): 2528–35.

52 *Recently, ketones fueling the brain*: Jip Gudden, Alejandro Arias Vasquez, and Mirjam Bloemendaal, "The Effects of Intermittent Fasting on Brain and Cognitive Function," *Nutrients* 13, no. 9 (September 2021): 3166.

53 *As BDNF increases, so does NGF*: Abdolhossein Bastani, Sadegh Rajabi, and Fatemeh Kianimarkani, "The Effects of Fasting during Ramadan on the Concentration of Serotonin, Dopamine, Brain-Derived Neurotrophic Factor and Nerve Growth Factor," *Neurology International* 9, no. 2 (June 23, 2017): 7043.

53 *Low BDNF has also been connected*: For more about how fasting affects synaptic plasticity and may protect the aging brain, see, for example, Elif Tugce Karoglu-Eravsar, Melek Umay Tuz-Sasik, and Michelle M. Adams, "Short-Term Dietary Restriction Maintains Synaptic Plasticity Whereas Short-Term Overfeeding Alters Cellular Dynamics in the Aged Brain," *Neurobiology of Aging* 106 (October 2021): 169–82.

53 *In one small study presided over*: G. Komaki et al., "Orexin-A and Leptin Change Inversely in Fasting Non-Obese Subjects," *European Journal of Endocrinology* 144, no. 6 (June 2001): 645–51.

53 *In other research that took place in Saudi Arabia*: A. S. Almeneessier et al., "The Effects of Diurnal Intermittent Fasting on the Wake-Promoting Neurotransmitter Orexin-A," *Annals of Thoracic Medicine* 13, no. 1 (January–March 2018): 48–54.

53 *The most prominent animal study*: S. A. Deadwyler et al., "Systemic and Nasal Delivery of Orexin-A (Hypocretin-1) Reduces the Effects of Sleep Deprivation on Cognitive Performance in Nonhuman Primates," *Journal of Neuroscience* 27, no. 52 (December 26, 2007): 14239–47.

54 *In a conversation with the novelist Peter Matthiessen*: Peter Matthiessen, *Sal Si Puedes* (Berkeley: University of California Press, 2014), 187.

54 *As the body runs out of carbohydrates*: See Anna Perrone et al., "Advanced Glycation End Products (AGEs): Biochemistry, Signaling, Analytical Methods, and Epigenetic Effects," *Oxidative Medicine and Cellular Activity* 2020, no. 3 (March 2020): 1–18.

55 *Acidosis occurs when excessive amounts*: B. Bashir et al., "Non-Diabetic Ketoacidosis: A Case Series and Literature Review," *Postgraduate Medical Journal* 97, no. 1152 (October 2021): 667–71.

55 *Severely malnourished patients near death*: D. Rigaud et al., "A Paradoxical Increase in Resting Energy Expenditure in Malnourished Patients Near Death: The King Penguin Syndrome," *American Journal of Clinical Nutrition* 72, no. 2 (August 2000): 355–60.

56 *Translated into English as* Hunger Disease: Myron Winick, *Hunger Disease: Studies by the Jewish Physicians in the Warsaw Ghetto* (New York: John Wiley & Sons, 1979), 15.

56 *"Gradually youth was drained"*: Ibid., 43. There is no end of horrible events in human history, but surely the creation of the Warsaw ghetto in 1940, when 380,000 people were corralled into a confined space and left to die, ranks among the worst. Out of that misery came one of the most important studies on malnutrition, one that is still cited by researchers. Jewish doctors under the direction of Dr. Israel Milejkowski, the chief health official within

the ghetto, meticulously documented the effects of involuntary long-term starvation on 140 people, including 40 children, who were patients of the Jewish Hospital in Czyste. The study ran from February until July 22, 1942, when deportations to the concentration camps of Treblinka and Majdanek began and, in the words of Milejkowski, "the hospitals and laboratories were destroyed, and, most important, the human element, our workers and the subject of our work, was gone" (Ibid., 3). At that point, the research was compiled into one manuscript and smuggled out of the ghetto. Milejkowski committed suicide before he could be deported.

56 *the longest recorded hunger strike*: Peter Taylor, "Bobby Sands: The Hunger Strike That Changed the Course of N Ireland's Conflict," BBC News, May 1, 2021, https://www.bbc.com/news/stories-56937259.

56 *In 2020, the Turkish lawyer Ebru Timtik*: "Turkish Lawyer Dies after 238-Day Hunger Strike," Agence France Presse, August 28, 2020, https://www.france24.com/en/20200828-turkish-lawyer-dies-after-238-day-hunger-strike.

57 *A study headed by de Cabo*: Andrea Di Francesco et al., "A Time to Fast," *Science* 362, no. 6416 (November 16, 2018): 770–75.

57 *Coming out of a long fast can be dangerous*: H. M. Mehanna, J. Moledina, and J. Travis, "Refeeding Syndrome: What It Is, and How to Prevent and Treat It," *BMJ* 336, no. 7659 (June 28, 2008): 1495–98.

58 *a study of Muslim soccer players*: Eduard Bezuglov et al., "Running Performance during the Holy Month of Ramadan in Elite Professional Adult Soccer Players in Russia," *International Journal of Environmental Research and Public Health* 18, no. 21 (November 2021): 11731.

59 *one 2014 paper detailed the experiences*: Mohamed Fenneni et al., "Effects of Ramadan on Physical Capacities of Boys Fasting for the First Time," *Libyan Journal of Medicine* 9, no. 1 (September 24, 2014): 25391.

59 *but if monitored over time*: Bruce R. Bistrian, "Clinical Use of a Protein-Sparing Modified Fast," *Journal of the American Medical Association* 240, no. 21 (November 17, 1978): 2299–2302.

59 *A three-month-long University of California study*: D. A. Lowe et al., "Effects of Time-Restricted Eating on Weight Loss and Other Metabolic Parameters in Women and Men with Overweight and Obesity: The TREAT Randomized Clinical Trial," *JAMA Internal Medicine* 180, no. 11 (November 1, 2020): 1491–99.

59 *The results of a year-long study in 2022*: Deying Liu et al., "Calorie Restriction with or without Time-Restricted Eating in Weight Loss," *New England Journal of Medicine* 386 (April 2022):1495–1504.

59 *In one recent U.S. study*: K. Cuccolo et al., "Intermittent Fasting Implementation and Association with Eating Disorder Symptomatology," *Eating
Disorders: Journal of Treatment and Prevention* 30, no. 5 (September–October
2022): 471–91.

60 *The truth is that most people*: J. R. Thorpe, "Research Shows Intermittent
Fasting Has Some Health Benefits—But Experts Say the Risks Aren't
Worth It," *Bustle*, August 31, 2019, https://www.bustle.com/p/intermittent
-fasting-can-be-dangerous-according-to-experts-18700817.

60 *Obesity rates have escalated sharply*: See "The State of Obesity: Better Policies for a Healthier America 2022," Trust for America's Health, September
2022, https://www.tfah.org/wp-content/uploads/2022/09/2022Obesity
Report_FINAL3923.pdf.

60 *estimated by the* Wall Street Journal: Andrea Petersen, Rolfe Winkler, and
Sara Ashley O'Brien, "The $76 Billion Diet Industry Asks: What to Do
about Ozempic?" *Wall Street Journal*, April 10, 2023, https://www.wsj
.com/articles/ozempic-wegovy-mounjaro-weight-loss-industry-89419ec
b?mod=Searchresults_pos1&page=1.

60 *make people become more food-obsessed*: P. S. Maclean et al., "Biology's
Response to Dieting: The Impetus for Weight Regain," *American Journal
of Physiology* 301, no. 3 (September 2011): R581–600, https://www.ncbi
.nlm.nih.gov/pmc/articles/PMC3174765/.

60 *an American Heart Association study*: "Yo-Yo Dieting May Increase
Women's Heart Disease Risk," American Heart Association, March
7, 2019, https://newsroom.heart.org/news/yo-yo-dieting-may-in
crease-womens-heart-disease-risk; also https://www.sciencedaily.com
/releases/2019/03/190307161902.htm.

60 *"If you were to come to me"*: Dr. Howard Steiger, interview with the author,
April 3, 2022.

61 *fasting to improve your health*: Australian journalist John Macgregor assembled a brief survey of longevity experts who seemed to have a marked
tendency to die ahead of the average. Among them were Paavo Airola
(*How to Get Well* and *How to Keep Slim, Healthy and Young with Juice
Fasting*), who died at the age of sixty-four; Nathan Pritikin (*The Pritikin
Program for Diet & Exercise*, founder of Pritikin Longevity Centers), who
committed suicide at sixty-nine; T. C. Fry (*The Life Science Health System*,
etc.), who was a leader of the natural hygiene movement and a fruitarian,
and who died at seventy; and J. I. Rodale, founder of *Prevention* magazine,
who died of a heart attack during a taping of *The Dick Cavett Show* at the
age of seventy-two. "During the interview he stated his intention to live

to 100. The talk show host thought he had dozed off in his chair." John Macgregor, "No Recommendation for the Good Life," *Sydney Morning Herald*, March 21, 2001, 15.

61 *Genetic differences determine*: See, for example, Claude Bouchard, "Genetics of Obesity: What We Have Learned over Decades of Research," *Obesity* 29, no. 5 (May 2021): 802–20, https://onlinelibrary.wiley.com/doi/10.1002/oby.23116.

61 *Neurobiologist Stephan Guyenet*: In conversation with Ezra Klein, "Our Brains Weren't Designed for This Kind of Food," *The Ezra Klein Show*, podcast transcript, *New York Times*, February 28, 2023, https://www.nytimes.com/2023/02/28/opinion/ezra-klein-podcast-stephen-guyenet.html.

61 *what behavioralists call "sensory specific satiety"*: See, for example, Barbara J. Rolls, Edward A. Rowe, and Edmund T. Rolls, "How Sensory Properties of Foods Affect Human Feeding Behavior," *Physiology & Behavior* 29, no. 3 (September 1982): 409–17.

61 *chronicles in* The Psychology of Overeating: Kima Cargill, *The Psychology of Overeating: Food and the Culture of Consumerism* (London: Bloomsbury Academic, 2015), 87.

62 *the number one cause of death*: "The Top 10 Causes of Death," World Health Organization, December 9, 2020, https://www.who.int/news-room/fact-sheets/detail/the-top-10-causes-of-death.

62 *A 2014 study by the USC Longevity Institute*: Susanne Wu, "Fasting Triggers Stem Cell Regeneration of Damaged, Old Immune System," USC News, June 5, 2014, https://news.usc.edu/63669/fasting-triggers-stem-cell-regeneration-of-damaged-old-immune-system/.

62 *Otto Warburg was a quirky physiologist*: For more on Warburg, see Sam Apple, *Ravenous: Otto Warburg, the Nazis, and the Search for the Cancer-Diet Connection* (New York: Liveright, 2021).

63 *It was something shameful*: Barbara Ehrenreich, "Welcome to Cancerland," *Harper's Magazine*, November 2001, 45.

63 *A characteristic of carcinomas*: Giovanna Bianchi et al., "Fasting Induces Anti-Warburg Effect That Increases Respiration but Reduces ATP-Synthesis to Promote Apoptosis in Colon Cancer Models," *Oncotarget* 6, no. 14 (May 20, 2015): 11806–19.

63 *This state, in which normal cells are protected*: Fan Xing et al., "The Anti-Warburg Effect Elicited by the cAMP-PGC1α Pathway Drives Differentiation of Glioblastoma Cells into Astrocytes," *Cell Reports* 18, no. 2 (January 10, 2017): 468–81.

63 *Fasting further suppresses the growth*: Russel J. Reiter, Ramaswamy Sharma,

and Sergio Rosales-Corral, "Anti-Warburg Effect of Melatonin: A Proposed Mechanism to Explain Its Inhibition of Multiple Diseases," *International Journal of Molecular Sciences* 22, no. 2 (January 2021): 764.

64 *"genome within the metagenome"*: Alessio Fasano and Susan Flaherty, *Gut Feelings: The Microbiome and Our Health* (Cambridge, MA: MIT Press, 2021), 48.

65 *these notorious proteins*: See for example: Y. Zhu et al., "Metabolic Regulation of Sirtuins upon Fasting and the Implication for Cancer," *Current Opinion in Oncology* 25, no. 6 (November 2013): 630–36.

65 *All that has been documented for certain*: Wioleta Grabowska, Ewa Sikora, and Anna Bielak-Zmijewska, "Sirtuins, a Promising Target in Slowing Down the Ageing Process," *Biogerontology* 18, no. 4 (2017): 447–76.

66 *Seventy-five years after McCay's findings*: Roger B. McDonald and Jon J. Ramsey, "Honoring Clive McCay and 75 Years of Calorie Restriction Research," *Journal of Nutrition* 140, no. 7 (July 2010): 1205–10, https://www.ncbi.nlm.nih.gov/pmc/articles/PMC2884327/.

66 *As Dr. Richard Weindruch*: Richard Weindruch, "Calorie Restriction and Aging," *Scientific American*, December 1, 2006, https://www.scientificamerican.com/article/calorie-restriction-and-aging/.

66 *This ability to delay aging*: D. E. Harrison and J. R. Archer, "Natural Selection for Extended Longevity from Food Restriction." *Growth, Development, and Aging Journal* 53, nos. 1–2 (Spring–Summer 1989): 3.

67 *Ancel Keys was a world-roving adventurer*: For more on the amazing career of Ancel Keys, see Todd Tucker's *The Great Starvation Experiment: Ancel Keys and the Men Who Starved for Science*, rev. ed. (Minneapolis: University of Minnesota Press, 2007).

67 *Keys's subjects battled with their intensifying*: Elke Eckert et al., "A 57-Year Follow-Up Investigation and Review of the Minnesota Study on Human Starvation and Its Relevance to Eating Disorders," *Archives of Psychology* 2, no. 3 (March 2018): 9, https://www.researchgate.net/publication/324507398.

68 *In the first half of the experiment*: Tucker, *The Great Starvation Experiment*, 102.

69 *A mere 42,000 Americans were COs*: Sharman Apt Russell, *Hunger: An Unnatural History* (New York: Basic Books, 2005), 115–16.

69 *Almost sixty years after Keys's project ended*: Elke Eckert et al., "A 57-Year Follow-Up Investigation and Review of the Minnesota Study on Human Starvation and Its Relevance to Eating Disorders," *Archives of Psychology* 2, no. 3 (March 2018), https://www.researchgate.net/publication/324507398.

71 *still being cited by researchers*: See, for example, Leanne M. Redman, "Caloric Restriction in Humans: Impact on Physiological, Psychological, and Behavioral Outcomes," *Antioxidants and Redox Signaling* 14, no. 2 (January 2011): 257–87.

71 *"Their blood pressure, blood sugar"*: "Roy Walford, 79; Eccentric UCLA Scientist Touted Food Restriction," *Los Angeles Times*, May 1, 2004, https://www.latimes.com/archives/la-xpm-2004-may-01-me-walford1-story.html.

72 *Twenty-five percent was settled upon*: Luigi Fontana, "The Scientific Basis of Caloric Restriction Leading to Longer Life," *Current Opinion in Gastroenterology* 25, no. 2 (March 2009): 144.

72 *The lower range was determined*: Jon Gertner, "The Calorie-Restriction Experiment," *New York Times*, October 7, 2009, https://www.nytimes.com/2009/10/11/magazine/11Calories-t.html.

72 *"Aging and chronic diseases are often viewed"*: Fontana, "The Scientific Basis of Caloric Restriction Leading to Longer Life."

73 *A follow-up study ten years later*: L. M. Redman et al., "Metabolic Slowing and Reduced Oxidative Damage with Sustained Caloric Restriction Support the Rate of Living and Oxidative Damage Theories of Aging," *Cell Metabolism* 27, no. 4 (April 3, 2018): 805–15.e4.

73 *Based on studies on animals*: Gertner, "The Calorie-Restriction Experiment."

73 *In one study, in 2022*: See, for example, Anastasia V. Shindyapina et al., "Rapamycin Treatment during Development Extends Lifespan and Healthspan of Male Mice and Daphnia Magna," *Science Advances* 8, no. 37 (September 2022), https://doi.org/10.1101/2022.02.18.481092.

74 *"I think aging is a program"*: Clare Ainsworth, "Growing Younger: Radical Insights into Ageing Could Help Us Reverse It," *New Scientist* April 27, 2022, https://www.newscientist.com/article/mg25433843-000-growing-younger-radical-insights-into-ageing-could-help-us-reverse-it/.

DAY 4, WEDNESDAY

75 *Too easily we get diverted*: Exactitude can have the opposite effect and bring understanding of a complex system to what the casual observer takes for chaos. Swarms of midges have recently been shown to exhibit "collective correlation," and this was determined only through painstaking observation and calculations. See Alessandro Attanasi et al., "Collective Behaviour without Collective Order in Wild Swarms of Midges," *PLoS Computational Biology* 10, no. 7 (July 2014): e1003697.

76 *Materialism is as useful to advocates*: Sartre, *Being and Nothingness*, 752.

76 *For Romans, profligacy*: Catherine Edwards, *The Politics of Immorality in Ancient Rome* (Cambridge, UK: Cambridge University Press, 1993), 185.

76 *virtuous self-deprivation has played*: Veronika Grimm, *From Feasting to Fasting: The Evolution of a Sin* (London: Routledge, 1996), 28.

77 *some scholars warned*: Babylonian Talmud 11a, "attributed to Samuel, a Babylonian first generation *amora*" [from the Aramaic, meaning "scholar"], as quoted in Grimm, *From Feasting to Fasting*, 28.

77 *"You shall eat bread with salt"*: Diamond, *Holy Men and Hunger Artists*, 5.

77 *"In general," writes Boyarin*: Daniel Boyarin, *Unheroic Conduct: The Rise of Heterosexuality and the Invention of the Jewish Man* (Berkeley: University of California Press, 1997), 53.

78 *"Man's lack of power to moderate"*: As noted in Nancy Levene, *Spinoza's Revelation: Religion, Democracy and Reason* (Cambridge, UK: Cambridge University Press, 2004), 22. Spinoza here makes an oblique reference to Medea's self-critical assessment in Ovid's *Metamorphoses*: "I see and approve the better, but follow the worst."

78 *Moses fasted for forty days*: As it is on much else, the Bible is confusing if not contradictory on the fasting habits of Moses: some scholars read Exodus as indicating that he fasted for forty days on three different occasions.

79 *anarchist Emma Goldman*: Candace Falk, "Emma Goldman," Shalvi/Hyman Encyclopedia of Jewish Women, The Jewish Women's Archive, https://jwa.org/encyclopedia/article/goldman-emma.

79 *Similarly, Elijah, having busied himself*: 1 Kings 19:7–8.

80 *"A certain man clothed in linen"*: Daniel 10:5–6.

80 *"When we fast, we have the chance"*: Lerat and Charbonnier, *Le jeûne*, 109. My translation.

81 *The Catholic scholar John Dominic Crossan*: Alicia von Stamwitz, "John Dominic Crossan on What We Get Wrong about Easter," March 31, 2020, https://broadview.org/john-dominic-crossan-interview/.

81 *"The relevant biblical passage says"*: Rabbi Michael Strassfeld, interview with the author, May 26, 2021.

81 *"You don't rend garments on fast days"*: Ibid.

82 *"He must increase, but I must decrease"*: John 3:30.

82 *"I am God's abdication"*: Simone Weil, *First and Last Notebooks*, trans. Richard Rees (Eugene, OR: Wipf and Stock, 2015), 213.

82 *"the unrestricted existence and assertion"*: Arthur Schopenhauer, *The World*

as Will and Idea, vol. 1 (London: Kegan, Paul, Trench, Trübner, 1891), 515. Schopenhauer, like Buddha, held that suffering pervades life. Asceticism, he argued, was a means to attempt to redirect the drive of the will to live. Renunciation, while not a solution, freed people from useless striving.

83 *"patron saint of twentieth-century anorexics"*: Francine du Plessix Gray, "On Thin Ice," in *Going Hungry: Writers on Desire, Self-Denial, and Overcoming Anorexia*, ed. Kate M. Taylor (New York: Anchor Books, 2008), 64.

83 *"this continuous process of consuming and being consumed"*: Sebald, *The Rings of Saturn*, 23.

83 *Almost all of us participate in the process of avoidance*: For more on this topic, see Hannah Arendt, "Thinking and Moral Considerations: A Lecture," *Social Research* 38, no. 3 (Autumn 1971): 417–46.

84 *Jehoshaphat also called for a fast*: 2 Chronicles 20.

84 *"The Bible doesn't tell us why"*: Rabbi Michael Strassfeld, interview with the author, May 26, 2021.

84 *the intellectual aspect of "sacrifice"*: Grimm, *From Feasting to Fasting*, 25.

85 *On Tish'ah b'Av*: Mishneh Torah, Fasts 5, https://www.sefaria.org /Mishneh_Torah%2C_Fasts.5?lang=bi.

85 *"all the people go out to the cemetery"*: Mishneh Torah, Fasts 4, https://www .sefaria.org/Mishneh_Torah%2C_Fasts.4?lang=bi.

85 "When there is peace in the world": The William Davidson Talmud (Koren-Steinsaltz), Rosh Hashonah 18b, https://www.sefaria.org /Rosh_Hashanah.18b.1?lang=bi.

86 *A quote from Talmudic literature*: Grimm, *From Feasting to Fasting*, 26.

87 *The Jewish sect seemed uncomfortably close*: André Dupont-Sommer, *The Essene Writings from Qumran*, trans. G. Vermes (Cleveland: Meridian Books, 1962), 13.

88 *who praised the Epicureans*: Richard P. Jungkuntz, "Christian Approval of Epicureanism," *Church History* 31, no. 3 (September 1962): 279.

88 *"food destroys or damages all discipline"*: Grimm, *From Feasting to Fasting*, 129.

88 *"An emaciated body will more readily pass"*: Walter Vandereycken and Ron Van Deth, *From Fasting Saints to Anorexic Girls* (London: Athlone Press, 1994), 515.

88 *"It is easier for a camel"*: Matthew 19:24.

88 *"The character of the soul"*: Teresa M. Shaw, "Practical, Theoretical and Cultural Tracings in Late Ancient Asceticism," in *Asceticism*, eds. Vincent

L. Wimbush and Richard Valantasis (New York: Oxford University Press, 1995), 77.

89 *notes food historian Ken Albala*: Ken Albala, "Historical Background to Food and Christianity," in *Food and Faith in Christian Culture*, eds. Ken Albala and Trudy Eden (New York: Columbia University Press, 2011), 14.

89 *it was during dinner, Origen wrote*: Origen, Book 32.1–140, in *Origen*, ed. Joseph W. Trigg (New York: Routledge, 1998), 215.

90 *"Who could ever thirst"*: Origen, "Commentary on John, Book 13.3–192," in ibid., 153.

90 *He believed that the Bible was full*: Ibid., 62.

91 *The Greeks left, "astonished"*: In Plato's *Phaedrus*, Socrates quotes a legend concerning an Egyptian pharaoh who is approached by the god Thoth, the scribe of the gods and the god of scribes, with various gifts that Thoth explains should be shared with the people. After going through a lengthy catalog of wonders, finally he presents the king with his greatest gift: something that will be an "elixir of memory and wisdom." The gift, of course, is writing. The king demurs: whether out of error or malice, Thoth has ascribed to letters "a power the opposite of that which they really possess. For this invention will produce forgetfulness in the minds of those who learn to use it, because they will not practice their memory." (Plato, *Phaedrus*, trans. Harold N. Fowler [New York: G. P. Putnam's Sons, 1923], 563.) Words never precisely describe a thought or an occurrence: they convey an approximation. Until Zeno of Elea (fl. fifth century BCE), Greek philosophers conveyed their arguments via poetry, which may be a more effective means of transmitting complex ideas.

91 *Writing is at the mercy of its author*: "Writing is the lesser of the two sons of understanding: compared with 'living and animate speech' which is 'written on the soul of the hearer together with understanding,' writing is but a shadow." (Geoffrey Galt Harpham, *The Ascetic Imperative in Culture and Criticism* [Chicago: University of Chicago Press, 1987], 7.) A more nuanced view comes from the poet Anne Carson, who suggests in *Eros the Bittersweet* that writing is more in line with ascetic principles. Writing is indirect, but it involves discipline and strictures. "As an individual reads and writes he gradually learns to close or inhibit the input of his senses, to inhibit or control the responses of his body, so as to train energy and thought upon the written words. He resists the environment outside him by distinguishing and controlling the one inside him." Anne Carson, *Eros the Bittersweet* (Princeton, NJ: Princeton University Press, 1986), 44. Writing is to communication what the monastery is to asceticism.

91 *ascetic discipline was "a science of imitation"*: Harpham, *The Ascetic Imperative in Culture and Criticism*, 13.

91 *unusual devotees such as Simeon the Stylite*: "He watched his foot as it rotted and its flesh decayed. And the foot stood bare like a tree beautiful with branches. He saw that there was nothing on it but tendons and bones." *Homily on Simeon the Stylite* by Jacob of Serug, a fifth century CE theologian cited in Kallistos Ware, "The Way of the Ascetics: Negative or Affirmative?" in *Asceticism*, eds. Vincent L. Wimbush and Richard Valantasis (New York: Oxford University Press, 1995), 4.

91 *when Macarius of Alexandria*: Vandereycken and Van Deth, *From Fasting Saints to Anorexic Girls*, 22.

91 *Palladius, estimated that the number of women*: Laura Swan, *The Forgotten Desert Mothers: Sayings, Lives and Stories of Early Christian Women* (Mahwah, NJ: Paulist Press, 2001), 3.

92 *The historian Susanna Elm*: Susanna Elm, *Virgins of God: The Making of Asceticism in Late Antiquity* (Oxford, UK: Clarendon Press, 1994), 85.

92 *These Desert Mothers had shattered*: Ibid., 89.

92 *Amma Theodora of Alexandria*: John Sanidopoulos, "Saint Theodora of Alexandria, Who Struggled in the Guise of a Man," Orthodox Christianity Then and Now, September 11, 2015, https://www.johnsanidopoulos .com/2015/09/saint-theodora-of-alexandria-who.html.

92 *"Once some travelers heard"*: Vandereycken and Van Deth, *From Fasting Saints to Anorexic Girls*, 22.

93 *As Susanna Elm observes*: Elm, *Virgins of God*, 267.

93 *He was a fanatical proponent of fasting*: Grimm, *From Feasting to Fasting*, 160.

93 *His exhortations are couched in loathing*: Ibid., 164.

94 *Jerome was both fascinated and repulsed by women*: Trigg, *Origen*, 64.

94 *In Origen's extensive analysis*: Ibid., 62.

94 *"antics of the lower body"*: Daniel Boyarin, *Socrates and the Fat Rabbis* (Chicago: University of Chicago Press, 2009), 4.

95 *Jerome had convinced Blaesilla*: Finley Hooper and Matthew Schwartz, *Roman Letters: History from a Personal Point of View* (Detroit: Wayne State University Press, 1991), 206.

95 *"Letter to Laeta"*: Jerome, "Letter CVII to Laeta," Umilta, http://www .umilta.net/jerome.html.

96 *The sayings of the desert sages*: Chadwick, *Western Asceticism*, 40–44 passim.

96 *The fifth-century philosopher John Cassian*: Ibid., 196.

97 *"Ascetic practices commonly"*: Caroline Walker Bynum, *Holy Feast and Holy*

Fast: The Religious Significance of Food to Medieval Women (Berkeley: University of California Press, 1988), 210.

97 *Sumptuary laws were enacted*: Johanna B. Moyer, "The Food Police: Sumptuary Prohibitions on Food in the Reformation," in *Food and Faith in Christian Culture*, eds. Ken Albala and Trudy Eden (New York: Columbia University Press, 2011), 60. As luxuries became more common and trade essential to people's well-being, around the time of Luther sumptuary laws began to focus more on food and less on clothing and other accessories. Examining this period's legislative records, historian Johanna B. Moyer discerns a distinction between Christian schools of thought: Catholics were prone to focus on the specifics of what was eaten, and Protestant lawmakers were concerned with the quantity of food eaten—and its cost. Thrift was good housekeeping and also kept believers clear of the sin of overindulgence. (Moyer, 63–64.)

98 *In his* Summa Theologica: Thomas Aquinas, *Summa Theologica*, question 148, article 4.

98 *Gelassenheit, or "letting-go"*: Sometimes translated as "serenity," but the element of actively opening up is present in the word.

98 *it is only through emptying oneself*: Meister Eckhart, *Meister Eckhart: The Essential Sermons, Commentaries, Treatises and Defense*, trans. Edmund Colledge and Bernard McGinn (Mahwah, NJ: Paulist Press: 1981), 91.

98 *"No cask can hold two different kinds of drink"*: Ibid., 220.

99 *He abjures us to leave*: Dietmar Mieth, "Self-Transcendence in Meister Eckhart," in *Religious Individualisation: Historical Dimensions and Comparative Perspectives*, vol. I (Berlin: De Gruyter, 2019), 75.

99 *"brides of Christ"*: Bynum, *Holy Feast and Holy Fast*, 62.

99 *"For a man to conceive God in himself"*: Eckhart, *Meister Eckhart*, 178.

99 *eroded by the image of Jesus himself*: Bynum, *Holy Feast and Holy Fast*, 289.

99 *Similarly, argues Caroline Walker Bynum*: Ibid.

100 *was a confidante of Pope Gregory XI*: Rudolph M. Bell, *Holy Anorexia* (Chicago: University of Chicago Press, 1985), 52.

100 *Nicholas of Flüe*: Centuries later, Nicholas was mocked by no less a personage than Mark Twain, himself a dedicated faster as well as a bon vivant—he solemnly declared he was moderate in his cigar consumption because he only smoked one at a time. Twain mixed up his St. Nicholases by confusing the Swiss saint with the fourth-century St. Nicholas of Myra, often credited with being the inspiration for Santa Claus. Wrote Twain in *A Tramp Abroad* (1880), after visiting a shrine to the Swiss ascetic:

This was the children's friend, Santa Claus, or St. Nicholas. There are some unaccountable reputations in the world. This saint's is an instance. [Nicholas of Flüe] has ranked for ages as the peculiar friend to children, yet it appears he was not much of a friend to his own. He had ten of them, and when fifty years old he left them, and sought out as dismal a refuge from the world as possible in order that he might reflect upon pious themes without being disturbed by the joyous and other noises from the nursery, doubtless (p. 325).

100 *accused of being fed by devils at night*: Vandereycken and Van Deth, *From Fasting Saints to Anorexic Girls*, 35.

100 *Witches were held to be part*: Ibid., 37.

101 *the "weighing test"*: Ibid., 38.

101 *Since suicide or self-harm was a mortal sin*: Albala, "Historical Background to Food and Christianity," 15.

102 *"So any one of you who sees in that month should fast"*: The Quran, Surah Al-Baqarah 2:185, trans. M. A. S. Abdel Haleem (Oxford, UK: Oxford University Press, 2004).

103 *Within a thirty-three-year cycle*: See Wagtendonk, *Fasting in the Koran*, 1.

103 *Shaykh Suhaib Webb*: Suhaib Webb, interview with the author, May 25, 2021.

104 *In the Xinjiang Uyghur Autonomous Region*: Shohret, Hoshur, "Chinese Officials Restrict Number of Uyghurs Observing Ramadan," English version by Roseanne Gerin, Radio Free Asia, April 1, 2022, https://www.rfa.org/english/news/uyghur/ramadan-restrictions-04012022173039.html.

104 *"Fasting in the eyes of the Chinese [government]"*: Shohret Hoshur, personal correspondence with author, August 29, 2022.

105 *Increasingly, the Catholic hierarchy*: Moyer, "The Food Police: Sumptuary Prohibitions on Food in the Reformation," 75.

105 *The Cambridge academic Thomas Cartwright*: Martha L. Finch, "Pinched with Hunger: Partaking of Plenty," in *Eating in Eden: Food and American Utopias*, eds. Martha L. Finch and Etta Madden (Lincoln: University of Nebraska Press, 2006), 39.

105 *"that like children newe come into the worlde"*: T.C., *The Holie Exercise of a True Fast, Described out of God's Word* (London: John Harison and Thomas Man, 1580), 10–11.

106 *inveighing against the "Popish"*: Finch, "Pinched with Hunger: Partaking of Plenty," 39.

106 *In 1604, Englishman Nicholas Bownde*: Ibid.

106 *"Half-naked" and "full of sadness"*: Ibid., 35.

107 *"The Fatter the Soil, the Ranker the Weeds"*: As quoted in Hillel Schwartz, *Never Satisfied: A Cultural History of Diets, Fantasies and Fat* (New York: Anchor Books, 1990), 117.

107 *The Reverend Cotton Mather*: Joan Jacobs Brumberg, *Fasting Girls: The History of Anorexia Nervosa* (New York: Vintage, 2000), 54. The 1692–93 witch trials resulted in the execution of nineteen innocent men and women. In the aftermath, the Mathers simultaneously tried to defend the rulings and to distance themselves from the hysteria they had helped to incite, arguing that "spectral evidence" was not admissible in court. Perhaps as a sort of atonement for his pivotal role in the trials, in the years that followed, Cotton Mather devoted himself to chronicling New England's history and natural world and became one of the first advocates of the smallpox vaccine. Many of his fellow Protestants felt that epidemics were God's way of punishing humanity, and man's hubris at struggling against fate in the form of vaccines would not help and would likely worsen the situation. After being used in China, Turkey, and Africa for centuries, vaccines had first been introduced on a wide basis in the West in Boston in 1721. That same year, in a remarkable foreshadowing of what the world has endured with the controversy over COVID-19 vaccines, a lit grenade was thrown through Cotton Mather's window. (See John B. Blake, "The Inoculation Controversy in Boston: 1721–1722," *New England Quarterly* 25, no. 4 [December 1952]: 489.) That Mather had been introduced to the concept of inoculation by Onesimus, an African enslaved person, and openly acknowledged the fact, animated the racist diatribes of anti-vaccine propaganda circulating at the time. See Margot Minardi, "The Boston Inoculation Controversy of 1721–1722: An Incident in the History of Race," *William and Mary Quarterly* 61, no. 1 (January 2004): 47.

107 *"A day of fasting, humiliation, and prayer"*: Harry M. Ward, *The War for Independence and the Transformation of American Society* (London: UCL Press, 1999), 15; see also Eugene R. Sheridan, *Jefferson and Religion* (Charlottesville, VA: Thomas Jefferson Memorial Foundation, 1998).

107 *a sort of American Protestant mantra*: It also appears in *Moby-Dick* (1851), chapter 16, in which the wise and talented harpooner and former cannibal Queequeg goes on "a day of fasting, humiliation, and prayer" before the voyage.

107 *The Continental Congress*: Hezekiah Niles, *Principles and Acts of the Revolution in America* (New York: A. S. Barnes & Co., 1876), 396.

108 *President James Madison decreed*: Gerhard Peters and John T. Woolley, "Zachary Taylor, Proclamation—Day of Fasting, Humiliation, and Prayer, July 3, 1849," American Presidency Project, https://www.presidency.ucsb.edu/node/351943.

108 *In March 1863*: Abraham Lincoln, "A Proclamation for a National Day of Humiliation, Fasting, and Prayer!" Library of Congress, https://www.loc.gov/resource/lprbscsm.scsm0265/.

108 *In 1899, the newly formed Afro-American Council*: Shawn L. Alexander, "Vengeance without Justice, Injustice without Retribution: The Afro-American Council's Struggle against Racial Violence," *Great Plains Quarterly* 27, no. 2 (Spring 2007): 119.

108 *Richard J. Foster*: Richard J. Foster, *Celebration of Discipline: The Path to Spiritual Growth* (New York: HarperCollins, 1998), 147.

109 *Dr. Michael Bos*: Michael Bos, interview with the author, June 15, 2021.

DAY 5, THURSDAY

110 *the Middle Way of Nagarjuna*: Nagarjuna was an Indian Buddhist philosopher active in the second century CE, known for his writings on emptiness and the emptiness of emptiness. Among other things, he posited that things are not autonomous, they exist only in relation to one another, that this pervasive relationship is constantly changing, and that recognition of interconnectedness brings a sense of liberation. Nagarjuna's concept of a lack of stable, permanent identity in people, or *sunya*, also came to refer to the new idea of the number zero. In Mahāyāna Buddhism, Śūnyakarā, or "emptiness," is one of the four marks of existence (together with impermanence, suffering, and selflessness).

112 *anti–Vietnam War activist William Gamson*: See William A. Gamson, *The Strategy of Social Protest* (Homewood, IL: Dorsey, 1975), and "Reflections on the Strategy of Social Protest," *Sociological Forum* 4, no. 3 (1989): 455–67.

112 *the praiseworthy concept of* prāya: John Nemec, "Dying to Redress the Grievance of Another: On Prāya/Prāyopaveśa(na) in Kalhana's Rājatarangini," *Journal of the American Oriental Society* 137, no. 1 (January–March 2017): 43.

112 *The routines of the Knights Templar*: See Judith Mary Upton-Ward, ed., *The Rule of the Templars* (Martlesham, UK: Boydell Press, 1997).

113 *Self-harm or suicide from despair*: E. Washburn Hopkins, "On the Hindu Custom of Dying to Redress a Grievance," *Journal of the American Oriental Society* 21 (1900): 147.

113 *Sanskrit scholar John Nemec*: Nemec, "Dying to Redress the Grievance of Another," 44.

113 *In one episode in the saga, Brahmans*: Ibid., 49.

114 *referred to as being "besieged"*: "With Manmohan Singh's United Progressive Alliance (UPA) government besieged by hunger strikers and charges of corruption on the one hand, and an EU beleaguered by fiscal crises and internecine squabbling amongst member states on the other, the India-EU FTA appears to have run out of political steam." Pallavi Aiyar, "Utopia Lacks Sponsors: FTA Talks with EU Resume without Drive," *Business Standard*, September 13, 2011.

115 *Wrote the historian Tacitus*: Tacitus, *The Annals of Tacitus*, trans. Alfred John Church and William Jackson Brodribb (London: Macmillan, 1876), 129.

115 *Similarly, Marcus Cocceius Nerva*: Ibid., 166.

116 *In Ireland, the history of fasting in protest*: Dorothy Whitelock, Rosamund McKitterick, and David Dumville, eds., *Ireland in Early Medieval Europe: Studies in Memory of Kathleen Hughes* (Cambridge, UK: Cambridge University Press, 1982), 169.

116 *According to the* Senchus Mór: *Ancient Laws of Ireland: Introduction to Senchus Mór, and Achgabail, or Law of Distress, as Contained in the Harleian Manuscripts*, vol. 1, Published Under the Direction of the Commissioners for Publishing the Ancient Laws and Institutes of Ireland (Dublin: Alexander Thom, 1865), 113.

116 *"fasting illegally" merited a fine*: Ibid., 87. Even the Irish days of the week reflect fasting's importance: Wednesday, *Dé Céadaoin*, in English means "first fast of the week" and Thursday, *Déardaoin*, means "between two fasts." Friday is *Dé hAoine*, the "day of fasting."

117 *At the age of twenty-three*: George T. Stokes, *Ireland and the Celtic Church* (London: Society for Promoting Christian Knowledge, 1907), 44.

117 *Máel Ruain, a bishop and saint*: John Joseph O'Kelly, *Ireland: Elements of Her Early Story* (Dublin: M. H. Gill and Son, 1921), 97.

118 *dharna was suppressed by the British*: H. R. Fink, "The Hindu Custom of 'Sitting Dharna,'" *Calcutta Review*, vol. LXII, ed. E. Lethbridge (Calcutta: Thomas S. Smith, 1876), 47.

118 *"If she was force-fed through her nose"*: Michael Safi, "How Love and a Taste of Honey Brought One Indian Woman's 16-Year Hunger Strike to an End," *Guardian*, November 11, 2018, https://www.theguardian.com/world/2018/nov/11/irom-sharmila-love-story-worlds-longest-hunger-strike.

119 *Sharmila was held in isolation*: Nayan Shah, *Refusal to Eat: A Century of Prison Hunger Strikes* (Oakland: University of California Press, 2022), 237.

119 *Always alone, she "rose"*: Safi, "How Love and a Taste of Honey."

119 *As long as she was fasting, Sharmila's*: Ibid.

119 *in southern India in the spring of 2022*: "Mamata Banerjee Sits on Dharna against EC Campaign Ban; Paints Picture at Protest Site," India Today video, YouTube, n.d., https://www.youtube.com/watch?v=-L5LMKCe J4Y&ab_channel=IndiaToday.

120 *"Those Englishmen who know something"*: R. D. Collison Black, "Economic Policy in Ireland and India in the Time of J. S. Mill," *Economic History Review* 21, no. 3 (August 1968): 321–36.

120 *massive, prolonged famines under English*: Mark Thornton, "What Caused the Irish Potato Famine?" *Free Market* 16, no. 4, April 1998, https://mises .org/library/what-caused-irish-potato-famine.

120 *The widely reviled administrator*: Charles Trevelyan will forever be remembered for revealing his profound bigotry in a letter he wrote in 1847—by which time the Famine had been underway for the better part of two years—urging that relief efforts not attempt to contravene the will of God, which was "to teach the Irish a lesson." Wrote Trevelyan: "The real evil with which we have to contend is not the physical evil of the Famine but the moral evil of the selfish, perverse and turbulent character of the people." (As quoted in Thomas Keneally, *Three Famines: Starvation and Politics* [New York: Public Affairs, 2011], 65.) Trevelyan was later knighted for his efforts.

121 *The tactic was first given a name*: Nemec, "Dying to Redress the Grievance of Another," 57.

121 *Shops refused to serve Boycott*: James Quinn, "Boycott, Charles Cunningham," *Dictionary of Irish Biography*, last revised October 2009, https://www.dib .ie/biography/boycott-charles-cunningham-a0825.

121 *Boycott alerted the English press*: This pattern with boycotts, where its targets claim the mantle of victim because they have no other moral recourse, echoes the perception of assault-by-hunger-strike and continues much the same today. During the grape boycott, then governor of California Ronald Reagan made a point of sympathizing with the growers by eating grapes in public and declared the boycott "immoral." More recently, the nonviolent "Boycott, Divest and Sanction" (better known as BDS) movement, founded by Palestinians to draw attention to civil rights violations by the Israeli government, has been accused of anti-Semitism, and laws have been passed in the United States and Germany to stifle the boycott.

122 *One abolitionist account from 1836*: Lydia Maria Francis Childs, *Appeal in Favor of That Class of Americans Called Africans* (New York: John S. Taylor, 1836), 21.

122 *What one scholar has termed "subtle resistance"*: Antonio T. Bly, "Crossing the Lake of Fire: Slave Resistance during the Middle Passage, 1720–1842," *Journal of Negro History* 83, no. 3 (Summer 1998): 181.

122 *After the death of Hu Yaobang*: "Timeline: What Led to the Tiananmen Square Massacre," *Frontline*, June 5, 2019, https://www.pbs.org/wgbh/frontline/article/timeline-tiananmen-square/.

123 *the poet Liu Xiaobo*: Liu Xiaobo et al., "Tiananmen Square Hunger Strike Declaration," trans. Chong-Pin Lin, *World Affairs* 152, no. 3 (Winter 1989–90): 148–49.

123 *As the struggle for constitutional representation*: See, for example, Leo Deutsch's *Sixteen Years in Siberia* (1903) and Vera Figner's *Memoirs of a Revolutionist* (1927).

124 *The prisoners called their self-starvation*: Kevin Grant, "British Suffragettes and the Russian Method of Hunger Strike," *Comparative Studies in Society and History* 53, no. 1 (2011): 117.

124 *In 1906, the American journalist George Kennan*: Shah, *Refusal to Eat*, 31.

124 *In 1878, political prisoners in St. Petersburg*: The strikes ended "in the death of one woman after she was flogged and in five suicides by female and male political prisoners," who reportedly poisoned themselves. Grant, "British Suffragettes and the Russian Method of Hunger Strike," 113–14.

125 *After his 1902 escape from Siberia*: Issac Deutscher, *The Prophet Armed: Trotsky: 1879–1921* (New York: Oxford University Press, 1963), 40–41, as cited in Gene Sharp, *The Politics of Nonviolent Action, Part Two: The Methods of Nonviolent Action* (Boston: Porter Sargent, 1973), 365.

125 *The "Russian method of the hunger strike"*: Grant, "British Suffragettes and the Russian Method of Hunger Strike," 114.

125 *The first use of the word "suffragette"*: *Oxford English Dictionary*, 2nd ed., vol. XVII (Oxford, UK: Clarendon Press, 1989).

125 *English suffragette Sylvia Pankhurst*: E. Sylvia Pankhurst, *The Suffragette Movement* (London: Virago, 1977), 92.

126 *The first voting rights advocate*: The Irish poet W. B. Yeats claimed to have been the first to resurrect the idea of the hunger strike, in his 1903 play *The King's Threshold*, in which the poet Seanchan fasts on the king's doorstep after having been forbidden to dine with the court. Yeats wrote that when he created the scene, "neither suffragette nor patriot had adopted the hunger strike, nor had the hunger strike been used anywhere, so far as I know, as a political weapon." (As quoted in Ellmann, *The Hunger Artists*, 59–60.) However, even leaving aside the prior fasting-in-protest by Russian revolutionaries, the use of a hunger strike in Yeats's play is very different from

Wallace-Dunlop's application of it: Seanchan pursues his own interests (he has personally been denied access to the court) and he does so in a free environment. He is unconfined; other options are available to him (he could simply walk away). Wallace-Dunlop adopted the hunger strike on behalf of a political cause while a disenfranchised prisoner of the state. The entire prison system is designed to deprive those convicted of certain rights, and the imprisoned hunger striker defiantly asserts rights, demanding dialogue in the face of a structure that is meant to isolate and overwhelm. Yeats's play itself was based on a fourteenth-century saga that was translated into English in the mid-nineteenth century.

126 *A veteran suffragette, in 1909*: In 1899 she had published a tale for children, *The Magic Fruit Garden*, in which a young girl is guided by fairies to a magic garden. "I am getting very hungry," she says at one point. "I wonder if I shall starve, and then I shall never reach the garden at all." She perseveres and reaches the garden. As cited by Joseph Lennon, "Fasting for the Public: Irish and Indian Sources of Marion Wallace Dunlop's 1909 Hunger Strike," in *Enemies of Empire: New Perspectives on Imperialism, Literature and History*, eds. Eóin Flannery and Angus Mitchell (Dublin: Four Courts Press, 2007), 28.

126 *She was in the midst of stenciling*: Ibid., 22.

126 *Wallace-Dunlop later said*: Shah, *Refusal to Eat*, 27.

126 *"I wondered what I could do"*: Ibid.

127 *Already a patient in the prison hospital*: Ibid., 30.

128 *Philippe Pinel*: Ian Miller, *A History of Force Feeding: Hunger Strikes, Prisons and Medical Ethics, 1909–1974* (London: Palgrave Macmillan, 2016), 63.

128 *Asylum doctors quickly embraced*: Ibid., 38.

128 *But force-feeding is physically*: Wrote physician Frank Moxon in his 1914 pamphlet "What Forcible Feeding Means": "The Government and the law officers pursue this policy because they know that the alternative to torture is that the law would utterly break down before the just demands of these women. Now it perhaps does seem a difficulty to some that men like these prison doctors should be placed in such a position, but their duty is perfectly clear. They have nothing whatever to do with the Government's difficulties. They are, or should be, solely concerned with the health of their patients. . . ." Frank Moxon, *What Forcible Feeding Means* (London: Woman's Press, 1914), 12.

128 *or the rectum to convey nutrients*: It has long been established that a feeding tube inserted into the rectum provides little if any nutrition. See, for example, N. Mutch and J. H. Ryffel, "The Metabolic Utility of Rectal Feeding," *BMJ* 1, no. 2716 (January 18, 1913): 111–12.

128 *although liberated concentration camp inmates*: Tucker, *The Great Starvation Experiment*, 194.

129 *As one doctor pointed out*: See Moxon, *What Forcible Feeding Means*.

129 *"During this operation"*: "Alice Paul Describes Force Feeding," Miller NAWSA Suffrage Scrapbooks, 1897–1911, Library of Congress, https://www.loc .gov/resource/rbcmil.scrp6014301/.

129 *In the span of just six months*: Chloe Bowerbank, "'How Long Will It Go On?'—Sylvia Pankhurst and the Hunger Strike," UKVote100, September 27, 2017, https://ukvote100.org/2017/09/27/how-long-will-it-go-on-syl via-pankhurst/.

129 *An outcry arose as details*: With World War I's outbreak in 1914, English activists for women's suffrage changed their tactics and became less militant, not wanting to be seen as unpatriotic. But their cause received a boost when it was supported in the Irish rebels' Proclamation of the Republic during the 1916 Easter Rising. Two years later, the Representation of the People Act gave the vote to women thirty years or older, as long as they owned property (propertyless women had to wait another decade), as well as to all men over twenty-one. In the United States, the Nineteenth Amendment to the Constitution, which guarantees women the right to vote, was ratified in 1920.

130 *hundreds of members of the IWW staged*: Shah, *Refusal to Eat*, 41.

130 *The first to use a hunger strike*: George Sweeney, "Irish Hunger Strikes and the Cult of Self-Sacrifice," *Journal of Contemporary History* 28, no. 3 (July 1993): 424.

131 *Doris Stevens, an American leader*: Doris Stevens, *Jailed for Freedom: American Women Win the Vote* (New York: Liveright, 1920), 130.

131 *And so at first it aroused*: Ibid., 184.

132 *The first to revive the tradition*: Tomás Mac Conmara, "The Hunger Strike of 1917 and the Death of Thomas Ashe," The Irish Story, https://www .theirishstory.com/2017/12/10/we-had-to-go-forward-the-mountjoy -hunger-strike-of-1917/#_edn33.

132 *Between 1913 and 1923*: Michael Biggs, "The Rationality of Self-Inflicted Suffering: Hunger Strikes by Irish Republicans, 1916–1923," *Sociology Working Papers*, no. 3 (2007), 1–24.

132 *in 1916, a doctor*: Miller, *A History of Force Feeding*, 145.

132 *Thomas Ashe, a thirty-five-year-old*: Sweeney, "Irish Hunger Strikes and the Cult of Self-Sacrifice," 426.

132 *The revolutionary leader Michael Collins*: Miller, *A History of Force Feeding*, 96.

133 *the Lord Mayor of Cork, Terence MacSwiney*: Peter Berresford Ellis, *A History of the Irish Working Class* (New York: George Braziller, 1973), 254.

134 *Bonar Law, Conservative leader*: Sharp, *The Politics of Nonviolent Action, Part Two*, 366.

134 *Even the Catholic chaplain at Mountjoy Prison*: As quoted in Sweeney, "Irish Hunger Strikes and the Cult of Self-Sacrifice," 426–27.

134 *sannyasi (male) and sannyasini (female)*: Vasudha Narayanan, "Renunciation and Gender Issues in the Sri Vaisnava Community," in *Asceticism*, eds. Vincent L. Wimbush and Richard Valantasis (New York: Oxford University Press, 1995), 445.

135 *"For modern Hinduism"*: Faisal Devji, interview with the author, May 12, 2021.

135 *"stymies the speech acts"*: Gilles Deleuze, *Essays Critical and Clinical*, trans. Daniel W. Smith and Michael A. Greco (Minneapolis: University of Minnesota Press, 1997), 73.

136 *the "responsive awareness"*: M. Lacertosa, "Sense Perception in the *Zhuangzi* 莊子," *Philosophy Compass* 17, no. 1 (January 2022): e12798.

136 *Hindu fast days such as Ekadashi*: Ekadashi is a fast day that occurs twenty-four times a year in accordance with the waxing of the moon. It is a period of rejuvenation devoted to Krishna, god of compassion, one of the avatars of Vishnu.

137 *"The idea," says Faisal Devji*: Faisal Devji, interview with the author, May 12, 2021.

137 *one must not "play religion"*: Lerat and Charbonnier, *Le jeûne*, 105.

137 *Gandhi saw both fasting*: Mohandas K. Gandhi, *Satyagraha in South Africa*, trans. Shri Valji Desai (1928; Ahmedabad, India: Navajivan, 1972), xi, xvi.

137 *The boycotting activists were*: Mahatma Gandhi, speech made at the Sabarmati sands in Ahmedabad, India, March 11, 1930, on the eve of the Dandi Satyagraha (also known as the "Salt March"), https://www.mkgandhi.org/speeches/dandi_march.htm.

137 *"I was familiar with the old tradition"*: Pat Sheehan, interview with the author, August 17, 2022.

138 *Humphrey Atkins, the British secretary of state*: Shah, *Refusal to Eat*, 204.

139 *Thatcher told a radio interviewer*: Rushworth M. Kidder, "Thatcher Says She's Sorry about Hunger Strikes, but She Won't Yield," *Christian Science Monitor*, December 4, 1980, https://www.csmonitor.com/1980/1204/120446.html.

139 *As "officer commanding"*: Ed Moloney, *Voices from the Grave: Two Men's War in Ireland* (London: Faber & Faber: 2010), 104.

139 *a kind of "post-mortem ventriloquism"*: Alexandra Poulain, "The King's Threshold, Calvary, The Death of Cuchulain: Yeats's Passion Plays," *Yeats's Mask: Yeats Annual No. 19*, eds. Margaret Mills Harper and Warwick Gould (Cambridge, UK: Open Book, 2013), 49–63.

139 *the BBC called Sands's death*: Peter Taylor, "Bobby Sands: The Hunger Strike That Changed the Course of N Ireland's Conflict," BBC News, May 1, 2021, https://www.bbc.com/news/stories-56937259.

139 *in October 1988, the British government*: Knight-Ridder, "British Ban IRA Remarks from TV, Radio," *Chicago Tribune*, October 20, 1988, https://www.chicagotribune.com/news/ct-xpm-1988-10-20-8802080976-story.html.

140 *Angela Davis, was arrested*: George Jackson, a Black Panthers official and a founder of the Black Guerilla Family, was one of the three Soledad Brothers accused of killing a guard at Soledad Prison in 1970 in retaliation for the killing of Jackson's mentor, W. L. Nolen, by another guard.

140 *to "dramatize the situation"*: Angela Davis, *Angela Davis—An Autobiography* (Chicago: Haymarket Books, 2022), 37.

140 *she had "persuaded [her]self"*: Ibid., 42.

140 *the annual fast known as Black August*: "Black August: A Celebration of Freedom Fighters Past and Present," Center for Constitutional Rights, August 10, 2021, https://ccrjustice.org/black-august#:~:text=Black%20August%20began%20in%20the,of%20the%20Black%20freedom%20struggle.

140 *"a constant reminder of the conditions"*: Bilal Ali, "Resistance: The Meaning of Black August," *Street Sheet*, August 15, 2017, https://www.streetsheet.org/resistance-the-meaning-of-black-august/.

140 *"to honor and stand in solidarity"*: TysonJXN, "The Origins of Black August," Black with No Chaser, August 1, 2022, https://blackwithnochaser.com/the-origins-of-black-august/.

141 *Robinson, a champion athlete*: Victoria Wolcott, *Race, Riots, and Roller Coasters* (Philadelphia: University of Pennsylvania Press, 2014), 70.

141 *Arrested for nonpayment of taxes*: "Rose Robinson Tells of Her Arrest and Prison Experiences," *Catholic Worker* XXVII, no. 1 (July 1, 1960): 8.

141 *In 2014 at the Northwest Detention Center*: Shah, *Refusal to Eat*, 275.

142 *"We have a profound respect for food"*: J. Cipriano et al., *The Hunger Strikers' Handbook*, NWDC Resistance, 2017.

142 *Sandy Restrepo, an immigration attorney*: Sandy Restrepo, interview with the author, May 2, 2023.

142 *The week after the strike ended*: Tess Owen, "Hundreds of Immigrants

Detained in a Private Prison Have Gone on Hunger Strike," *Vice*, April 14, 2017, https://www.vice.com/en/article/5958m5/hundreds-of-immigrants-detained-in-a-private-prison-have-gone-on-hunger-strike.

143 *twenty-four-year-old Paul Campion*: Paul Campion, interview with the author, February 26, 2021.

144 *Sahar Francis, the director*: Sahar Francis, interview with the author, August 21, 2022. Under Article 111 of the Israeli constitution, the military can arrest and detain people for up to one year without providing a rationale, although prisoners are routinely held far longer. Since 1967, around one-fifth of the Palestinian population has been arrested. See Rory McCarthy, "Israel Releases 198 Palestinian Prisoners," *Guardian*, August 26, 2008, https://www.theguardian.com/world/2008/aug/26/israelandthepalestinians1.

144 *Almost every Palestinian in Israeli prisons*: Stephen Erlanger, "Palestinians on Fast in Israeli Jails Struggle for Attention," *New York Times*, August 28, 2004, https://www.nytimes.com/2004/08/28/world/palestinians-on-fast-in-israeli-jails-struggle-for-attention.html.

144 *Khader Adnan, a baker*: "Israel/OPT: Death of Khader Adnan Highlights Israel's Cruel Treatment of Palestinian Prisoners," Amnesty International, May 3, 2023, https://www.amnesty.org/en/latest/news/2023/05/israel-opt-death-of-khader-adnan-highlights-israels-cruel-treatment-of-palestinian-prisoners/.

145 *His death led to international*: Dov Lieber, "Gaza Militants Fire Rockets at Israel after Palestinian Hunger Striker Dies," *Wall Street Journal*, May 2, 2023, https://www.wsj.com/articles/palestinian-militant-dies-in-israeli-prison-after-hunger-strike-ba90907d.

145 *In his memoir,* To Build a Castle: Vladimir Bukovsky, *To Build a Castle: My Life as a Dissenter*, trans. Michael Scammell (New York: Viking, 1978), 394.

145 *"Prison governors had grown terrified*: Luke Harding, "Vladimir Bukovsky Obituary," *Guardian*, October 28, 2019, https://www.theguardian.com/world/2019/oct/28/vladimir-bukovsky-obituary.

146 *In 1968, Chavez undertook his first*: Susan Ferriss and Ricardo Sandoval, *The Fight in the Fields: Cesar Chavez and the Farmworkers Movement* (New York: Harcourt Brace, 1997), 142.

147 *In Peter Matthiessen's profile*: Matthiessen, *Sal Si Puedes*, 190.

148 *To call this fast a "punishment"*: See Jason Pierce, "César Chávez, Dolores Huerta, and the United Farm Workers," Bill of Rights Institute, https://

billofrightsinstitute.org/essays/cesar-chavez-dolores-huerta-and-the
-united-farm-workers.

148 *"a defining moment for the union"*: Ferriss and Sandoval, *The Fight in the Fields*, 143.

148 *Chavez was consciously echoing*: Ibid., 141.

149 *"A fast is first and foremost personal"*: Cesar Chavez, *The Words of Cesar Chavez*, eds. John C. Hammerback and Richard J. Jensen (College Station: Texas A&M University Press, 2002), 169.

150 *Bioethicist Jacob M. Appel*: Jacob M. Appel, "Beyond Guantanamo," *Huffington Post*, March 18, 2010, https://www.huffpost.com/entry/beyond-guanta namo-torture_b_360082.

150 *In 2023 testimony, Dr. Sondra Crosby*: Carol Rosenberg, "Doctor Describes and Denounces C.I.A. Practice of 'Rectal Feeding' of Prisoners," *New York Times*, February 24, 2023, https://www.nytimes.com/2023/02/24/us /politics/cia-torture-guantanamo-nashiri-doctor.html.

151 *Slahi spoke to me from Dubai*: Mohamedou Ould Slahi, interview with the author, November 18, 2021.

152 *to protect the rights of gardeners*: Matea Gold and Jim Newton, "Fast Ends with Accord on Leaf Blowers," *Los Angeles Times*, January 10, 1998, https:// www.latimes.com/archives/la-xpm-1998-jan-10-me-6884-story.html.

152 *Dick Gregory, the civil rights activist*: Clovis E. Semmes, "Entrepreneur of Health: Dick Gregory, Black Consciousness, and the Human Potential Movement," *Journal of African American Studies* 16, no. 3 (September 2012): 537–49.

152 *In December 1978, four Bolivian women*: Elena McGrath, "Housewives against Dictatorship: The Bolivian Hunger Strike of 1978," Nursing Clio, December 29, 2016, https://nursingclio.org/2016/12/29/housewives-against-dictatorship-the-bolivian-hunger-strike-of-1978/.

152 *In the end, 1,380 people*: Svevo Brooks et al., "A Guide to Political Fasting," Nonviolent Tactics Development Project, 1981, 8.

153 *Theresa Spence, chief of the Attawapiskat First Nation*: "Chief Theresa Spence to End Hunger Strike Today," CBC News, January 23, 2013, https:// www.cbc.ca/news/politics/chief-theresa-spence-to-end-hunger-strike -today-1.1341571.

153 *Luaty Beirão, an Angolan rapper*: Ricardo Miguel Vieira, "Angolan Awak-ening: Ikonoklasta Doubles Down in His Fight for Change," OkayAfrica, https://www.okayafrica.com/angolan-awakening-ikonoklasta-doubles-down-in-his-fight-for-change/.

153 *In the fall of 2019, Extinction Rebellion*: Jane Dalton, "Extinction Rebellion:

Four Climate Activists Take Hunger Strike into Second Week," *Independent*, November 24, 2019, https://www.independent.co.uk/climate-change/news/extinction-rebellion-hunger-strike-protest-climate-activists-global-parties-a9215411.html.

153   *Leyla Güven, an imprisoned deputy*: "Turkey Court Frees Hunger-Strike Kurdish MP Leyla Guven," BBC News, January 25, 2019, https://www.bbc.com/news/world-europe-46999128.

154   *She was released on her own*: "Kurdish Politician Leyla Güven Sentenced to More Than Eleven Years in Prison," ANF News, October 17, 2022, https://anfenglishmobile.com/women/kurdish-politician-leyla-guven-sentenced-to-more-than-eleven-years-in-prison-63127.

154   *On January 29, 2020, Boston University*: Jessica Colarossi, "Why BU Environmental Researcher Nathan Phillips Is on a Hunger Strike," Brink, February 5, 2020, https://www.bu.edu/articles/2020/environmental-researcher-nathan-phillips-hunger-strike/.

154   *For twenty-five days in the summer*: "Hunger Strikers for Breonna," Facebook, https://www.facebook.com/hungerstrikersforbreonna.

154   *Aleksei Navalny, the imprisoned leader*: Andrew E. Kramer, "Navalny, Putin's Nemesis, Ends Hunger Strike in Russia," *New York Times*, April 23, 2021, https://www.nytimes.com/2021/04/23/world/europe/russia-naval-ny-putin-hunger-strike.html.

154   *A seventy-three-year-old Chicago woman, Rachelle Zola*: Molly Morris, "73-Year-Old Chicago Woman Completes a 40-Day Hunger Strike," *News Tribune*, July 8, 2021, https://www.newstribune.com/news/2021/jul/08/73-year-old-chicago-woman-completes-a-40-day/.

154   *On February 1, 2022, two teachers*: Bob Nesbitt and Sara Stinson, "Hunger Strike, Protest Planned to Pressure Oakland Unified School District against Closures," KRON4, February 2, 2022, https://www.kron4.com/news/bay-area/oakland-staff-go-on-hunger-strike-to-protest-school-closures/.

155   *"I believe this community has suffered"*: André San-Chez, interview with the author, June 29, 2022.

155   *Alaa Abd El Fattah*: Jennifer Holleis, "Egypt: New Push to Free Activist Alaa Abdel-Fattah," Deutsche Welle, March 18, 2023, https://www.dw.com/en/egypt-alaa-abdel-fattahs-sister-re-starts-freealaa-campaign-after-cop27-silence/a-65023873. See also Vivian Yee, "Prominent Egyptian Political Prisoner Ends Hunger Strike, Family Says," *New York Times*, November 15, 2022, https://www.nytimes.com/2022/11/15/world/middleeast/egypt-alaa-abd-el-fattah-hunger-strike.html.

DAY 6, FRIDAY

157 Trattato de la vita sobria: Maria Patrizia Carrieri and Diego Serraino, "Longevity of Popes and Artists between the 13th and the 19th Century," *International Journal of Epidemiology* 34, no. 6 (December 2005): 1435–36.

157 *Beset by numerous ailments*: Lewis Cornaro [sic], *Discourses on a Sober and Temperate Life*, trans. and intro. Sylvester Graham (New York: Mahlon Day, 1833), 23.

157 *The book was an immediate success*: In 1986, Hillel Schwartz recorded that *Trattato de la Vita Sobria* had been made available in "at least three Swedish editions, four Dutch, four German, seven Latin, eleven French, twelve Italian: it reached its fifty-third English edition by 1826 and has had thirty-three American editions." (Hillel Schwartz, *Never Satisfied: A Cultural History of Diets, Fantasies and Fat* [New York: Anchor Books, 1990], 347.) In *Morton's Medical Bibliography*, it is unaccountably listed as "the best treatise on personal hygiene and the simple life in existence."

158 *"O wretched and unhappy Italy!"*: Cornaro, *Discourses on a Sober and Temperate Life*, 19.

158 *"Nay, by attending duly to what I have said"*: Ibid., 52.

158 *Franklin claimed that self-restraint*: Schwartz, *Never Satisfied*, 14.

159 *His pulsilogium is said to have inspired*: F. Bigotti, D. Taylor, and J. Welsman, "Recreating the Pulsilogium of Santorio: Outlines for a Historically-Engaged Endeavour," *Bulletin of the Scientific Instrument Society* 133 (June 30, 2017): 30–35.

160 *cultural historian Hillel Schwartz*: Schwartz, *Never Satisfied*, 10.

160 *"Dutch Virgin" Eve Fleigen/Eva Vliegen*: Also sometimes written "Eve Fliegen" (Hyder E. Rollins, "Notes on Some English Accounts of Miraculous Fasts," *Journal of American Folklore* 34, no. 134 [October–December 1921]: 364–71) or "Eva Fillgen" ("Feats of the Fasters," *The Illustrated American*, January 10, 1891, 285). Fliegen/Vliegen/Fleigen/Fillgen's supposed anthophilia, whereby the perfume of flowers alone was enough to keep her alive, preceded by just a few years the height of the region's Tulip Craze, which, according to numerous accounts, by 1610 had reached proportions such that a single tulip bulb could buy a house.

161 *"Full strange it was to see"*: Rollins, "Notes on Some English Accounts of Miraculous Fasts," 367–68.

161 *Fleigen's celebrity reportedly*: Brumberg, *Fasting Girls*, 50.

161 *Wilhelm Fabry von Hilden*: Vandereycken and Van Deth, *From Fasting Saints to Anorexic Girls*, 63.

162 *"The seeds of Weakness and Pain"*: Samuel J. Rogal, "Pills for the Poor: John Wesley's Primitive Physick," *Yale Journal of Biological Medicine* 51, no. 1 (January–February): 82. Many of Wesley's recommendations came from medical tracts of the day, such as his prescription for "raving madness": shave the head and wash it with vinegar. Another standout is his recommendation for cure from colic: place a live puppy on the afflicted person's stomach (Rogal, 87), which echoes Hildegard of Bingen's cure for jaundice: she recommended tying a live bat to a sick person's stomach. For centuries, the idea that an animal could transfer its health-giving qualities to a person via skin-to-skin transmission over the belly had been accepted as solid advice. Certainly it would distract from whatever ailments the afflicted currently suffered from.

162 *Extreme fasters brought fame*: Vandereycken and Van Deth, *From Fasting Saints to Anorexic Girls*, 50.

163 *In 1512, for example, a miraculously fasting woman*: W. Morgenthaler, "Eine Hysterika zu Beginn des 17. Jahrhunderts," *Archiv für Geschichte der Medizin* 18, no. 2 (June 15, 1926): 200.

163 *Another German, Margaretha Ulmer*: Vandereycken and Van Deth, *From Fasting Saints to Anorexic Girls*, 56.

163 *Catherine of Veltlin in the mid-seventeenth century*: Ibid., 28.

163 *Ann Moore, "the Fasting Woman of Tutbury"*: Legh Richmond, *A Statement of Facts, Relative to the Supposed Abstinence of Ann Moore, of Tutbury, Staffordshire* (London: J. Croft, 1813), 45.

164 *"a notorious immoral character"*: J.L., *An Account of the Extraordinary Abstinence of Ann Moor [sic], of Tutbury, Staffordshire, Who Has for More Than Two Years, Lived Entirely without Food* (Uttoxeter, UK: R. Richards, 1809), 10.

164 *Welsh "fasting girl," Sarah Jacob*: William Hammond, *Fasting Girls: Their Physiology and Pathology* (New York, G. P. Putnam's Sons, 1879), 28.

164 *a Presbyterian minister, the same Sylvester Graham*: Graham notes in Cornaro, *Discourses on a Sober and Temperate Life*, 4–5.

165 *Graham is often credited*: Schwartz, *Never Satisfied*, 25.

166 *Jennings decided that the best course*: James Whorton, *Crusaders for Fitness: The History of American Health Reformers* (Princeton, NJ: Princeton University Press, 1982), 136.

166 *Jennings put a name to the philosophy*: Isaac Jennings, *The Tree of Life: Or, Human Degeneracy, Its Nature and Remedy* (New York: Miller, Wood, 1867), 118.

166 *"The emphasis on 'fiber'"*: Ellmann, *The Hunger Artists*, 10.

167 *the men "gathered strength fast"*: Mark Twain, *The Man That Corrupted*

Hadleyburg, and Other Essays and Stories (New York: Harper and Brothers, 1898), 87.

167 *"A little starvation can really do more"*: Ibid., 106.

168 *"allowed them to pass for elegant"*: Whorton, *Crusaders for Fitness*, 264.

169 *In three publications totaling more*: Ibid., 263–64.

169 *"the long awaited key"*: R. Marie Griffith, "Apostles of Abstinence: Fasting and Masculinity during the Progressive Era," *American Quarterly* 52, no. 4 (December 2000): 604.

169 *Dr. Henry S. Tanner*: According to his authorized biography, Tanner, who had started life as a carriage maker in rural southeastern England, had immigrated to Ohio, where he reinvented himself and enrolled in the Eclectic Medical School after being dissatisfied with "the intolerance of the old-school societies." (Robert A. Gunn, *Forty Days without Food! A Biography of Henry S. Tanner, M.D., Including a Complete and Accurate History of His Wonderful Fasts with Valuable Deductions* [New York: A. Metz, 1880], 8.) One barrier to being tolerated by the old school might have been his incipient breatharianism: Tanner maintained that life was sustained by "the electricity of the atmosphere." (Ibid., 9.) Years later, Tanner explained to the *New York Times* that "the body is fed and nourished through the lungs which supply the principal vital forces, the stomach being only a secondary consideration." ("AT 81 STARTS 80-DAY FAST. Dr. Tanner Says People Eat Too Much, and Essays to Prove It," *New York Times*, February 9, 1911, 1.)

170 *Fancher's fasting, of course, took place*: Daily, *Mollie Fancher*, 111.

170 *"She says she is a miracle"*: Ibid., 211.

170 *"I am not aware that this claim"*: Hammond, *Fasting Girls*, 1.

171 *"From the beginning it had attracted"*: Herbert Asbury, "That Was New York: Forty Days and Forty Nights," *New Yorker*, April 27, 1934, 70.

171 *Tanner was receiving between*: Schwartz, *Never Satisfied*, 121.

171 *He was regaled by various admirers*: "A Stomach in Open Revolt: Tanner Declines to Treat with the Thing," *New York Times*, July 31, 1880, 2, https://timesmachine.nytimes.com/timesmachine/1880/07/31/98549901.html?pageNumber=2.

171 *A month into the fast, Hammond*: Asbury, "That Was New York," 78–79.

172 *there were accusations of fraud*: On the tenth day of the fast, at midnight, "Dr. Bradley leaped to his feet and accused Frost Johnson, a Medical College watcher, of passing something surreptitiously to Dr. Tanner. The faster promptly became hysterical and screamed that Johnson had only handed

him a sponge. 'Soup!' cried Dr. Bradley. 'Full of soup! What do you want with a sponge?' 'I like sponges,' said Dr. Tanner, greatly upset. Repeating his accusation that the sponge had been dripping with soup, Dr. Bradley ordered the watchers of the Neurological Society to leave the Hall, and declared that the Society would have nothing further to do with the experiment. A few hours later both Johnson and Dr. Tanner formally denied, in writing, that the sponge had contained food, and said that Dr. Tanner had used it to wipe his face." (Ibid., 76.)

172 *She declined a request from P. T. Barnum*: Daily, *Mollie Fancher*, 112.

172 *After the fast he put himself on exhibit*: Asbury, "That Was New York," 79.

173 In 1913, at the age of eighty-three: "Dr. Tanner Gets Mitten," *New York Times*, November 13, 1913, 1, https://timesmachine.nytimes.com/times machine/1913/11/13/104788718.html?pageNumber=1.

173 *commonly accepted as the inspiration for Kafka's story*: See, for example, Mark Christian Thompson, *Kafka's Blues: Figurations of Blackness in the Construction of an Esthetic* (Chicago: Northwestern University Press, 2016), 122. Thompson notes that Kafka would have had the opportunity to read accounts of Succi's escapades in 1896, in a five-part illustrated series in *Das interessante Blatt* and then again in 1917, when Succi performed in Vienna. By that time, Succi's celebrity had waned, and he was earning a fraction of what he had commanded in previous years.

173 *In 1886, after several trips*: Ennio Ferretti, "Giovanni Succi, il digiuna-tore di Cesenatico che ispirò Kafka," Giannella Channel, https://www.gi annellachannel.info/giovanni-succi-il-digiunatore-di-cesenatico-che-ispiro -kafka/.

173 *Succi's fame grew and he traveled*: "Feats of the Fasters," 286.

173 *A portion of Koster & Bial's*: "Koster and Bial's Music Hall," NoMad, September 25, 2015, https://experiencenomad.com/koster-and-bials-music-hall/.

174 *in 1910, Clare de Serval*: Sharman Apt Russell, *Hunger: An Unnatural History* (New York: Basic Books, 2005), 53–54.

174 *the performer David Blaine*: "Above the Below," London, 2003. Blaine's symptoms were detailed in "Refeeding David Blaine—Studies after a 44-Day Fast," *New England Journal of Medicine*, November 24, 2005, https:// www.nejm.org/doi/full/10.1056/nejm200511243532124.

174 *Agostino Levanzin, a Maltese lawyer*: Lino Bugeja, "Agostino Levanzin: Man for Reasons," *Times of Malta*, July 14, 2012, https://timesofmalta.com /articles/view/Agostino-Levanzin-man-for-all-reasons.428703.

175 *"After that he said that he lost"*: "Breaks 31 Days' Fast," *New York Times*,

May 15, 1912, https://www.nytimes.com/1912/05/16/archives/breaks
-31-days-fast-levanzin-lost-weight-but-felt-better-mentally.html.

175 *But he was reportedly upset*: Schwartz, *Never Satisfied*, 132.

175 *Less than a week later, Levanzin abruptly*: "Levanzin's New Charges," *New York Times*, May 21, 1912, https://www.nytimes.com/1912/05/22/archives/levanzins-new-charges-fasting-professor-says-he-was-nearly-killed.html; see also "Torture in Starving Test," *New York Times*, May 20, 1912, https://www.nytimes.com/1912/05/21/archives/torture-in-starving-test-levanzin-complains-of-treatment-at.html.

176 *"I seemed to hollow out myself"*: Knut Hamsun, *Hunger*, trans. Robert Bly (New York: Farrar, Straus and Giroux, 1986), 33.

176 *martyrdom is "a tempting pose"*: Dale Peck, correspondence with the author, June 13, 2023.

176 *"They would rather do the impossible"*: Franz Kafka, *Investigations of a Dog and Other Creatures*, trans. Michael Hoffmann (New York: New Directions, 2017), 158.

176 *"your problems are over"*: Ibid., 174.

176 *"The way leads through starvation"*: Ibid., 181.

177 *Kafka's disgust at his animalistic drive*: For example: "If I see a sausage labeled as an old hard Hauswurst, I bite into it in my imagination with all my teeth and swallow quickly, regularly and heedlessly like a machine. The despair that this act even in the imagination has as an immediate result increases my haste. I shove the long rinds of rib meat unbitten into my mouth and then pull them out again from behind tearing through my stomach and intestines. I eat dirty grocery stores completely empty." October 1911 entry in *The Diaries of Franz Kafka*, trans. Ross Benjamin (New York: Schocken, 2022), 107.

177 *"Just as I am thin"*: Franz Kafka, *Letters to Felice*, eds. Erich Heller and Jürgen Born, trans. James Stern and Elisabeth Duckworth (New York: Schocken Books, 2016), 21.

177 *Aristotle noted an adept*: James Caulfield and Henry Wilson, *The Book of Wonderful Characters* (London, Chatto & Windus, 1869), 249.

178 *"And some also lived a long time"*: My translation of Rollins, "Notes on Some English Accounts of Miraculous Fasts," 360.

178 *the Swiss "tool of God" Christina Kratzer*: Vandereycken and Van Deth *From Fasting Saints to Anorexic Girls*, 106.

178 *After having had a miserable childhood*: "Werkzeuge," Inspirationist Archive, https://inspirationistarchive.org/zeugnisse-testimonies/who-were-the-werkzeuge/.

178 *The psychologist Carl Jung*: Vandereycken and Van Deth, *From Fasting Saints to Anorexic Girls*, 108.

179 *"a world-wide medical cult"*: Martin Gardner, *Fads and Fallacies in the Name of Science* (New York: Dover, 1957), 191.

179 *"The idea of detoxing"*: Britt Marie Hermes, interview with the author, March 24, 2023.

179 *Hundreds of strange therapies accrue*: Naturopathic remedies led to the death of the socialist leader Eugene V. Debs, who in 1926 went on a fasting "cure" in a naturopathic sanatorium to address the lingering effects of his multiyear imprisonment in the Atlanta federal penitentiary. A family member had asked a local physician to check on Debs, who was found in a coma. "His body was badly dehydrated. Being unconscious, he had not asked for a drink in two days, and so no one had given him one." (Gardner, *Fads and Fallacies in the Name of Science*, 197.) Debs died shortly thereafter of heart failure. (The common naturopathic response in such instances is that the subject had a preexisting condition.)

180 *The first clinic was established in 1920*: Steve Hendricks, *The Oldest Cure in the World: Adventures in the Art and Science of Fasting* (New York: Abrams, 2022), 177.

180 *In 1935, at the height of the Nazi regime*: "History," Buchinger Wilhelmi Clinics, https://www.buchinger-wilhelmi.com/en/geschichte/.

180 *While "strongly anti-Nazi"*: Michael H. Kater, *Doctors under Hitler* (Chapel Hill: University of North Carolina Press, 2005), 54.

180 *In 1926, six hunger artists*: Vandereycken and Van Deth, *From Fasting Saints to Anorexic Girls*, 89.

181 *"I have written a great many"*: Upton Sinclair, *The Fasting Cure* (1911; Carlisle, MA: Applewood Books, 2022), 5.

181 *As a younger man, he wrote*: Ibid., 7.

181 *praise fasting for its purificative powers*: Ibid., 25.

182 *a nationwide surge in bigotry*: As Edwin Black and others have established (see his *War against the Weak: Eugenics and America's Campaign to Create a Master Race* [New York: Four Walls Eight Windows, 2003]), American eugenic principles provided the basis for much of Nazi ideology.

182 *Horace Fletcher, the "Great Masticator"*: Schwartz, *Never Satisfied*, 125.

182 *The method for "attaining economic"*: James C. Whorton, "'Physiologic Optimism': Horace Fletcher and Hygienic Ideology in Progressive America," *Bulletin of the History of Medicine* 55, no. 1 (Spring 1981), 59.

182 *Taylorism, the science of management*: Frederick W. Taylor (1856–1915) was one of the first to analyze factory workflows in an attempt to minimize waste

and maximize efficiency. First employed in the 1880s at a Pennsylvania steel mill, Taylor's theories of scientific management received broad attention with the publication of his *Principles* in 1911.

183 *Habitually dressed in white*: Schwartz, *Never Satisfied*, 126.

183 *saw Fletcherism as a natural ally*: See James's 1901–1902 lectures, *The Varieties of Religious Experience*, in which he expounds on "the religion of healthy-mindedness" and cites Fletcher as an exemplar of mind cure and New Thought. Gandhi may also have been influenced by Fletcher, at least in terms of his views on digestion: he is frequently quoted as having advised his followers to "Chew your water and drink your food."

183 *With royalties earned from* The Jungle: Lawrence Kaplan, "A Utopia during the Progressive Era: The Helicon Home Colony, 1906–1907," *American Studies* 25, no. 2 (1984): 63, https://journals.ku.edu/amsj/article/view/2567.

183 *a spa in Michigan founded by John Harvey Kellogg*: Kellogg's enterprise was called Battle Creek Sanitarium, "sanitarium" was a word Kellogg had made up, which he preferred to the original "sanatorium" because of the emphasis on "sanitary." A fervent Grahamite as well, Kellogg also gave the world cornflakes, in an attempt to help tamp down Americans' overactive sex drives; he had wanted a healthy "predigested" food for his clients. The cereal only became a hit when his brother Will added sugar to the process. Vandereycken and Van Deth, *From Fasting Saints to Anorexic Girls*, 206.

183 *credited with coining the verb "to fletcherize"*: As cited in Whorton, "'Physiologic Optimism,'" 205.

184 *Obsession with foreign rot*: Sinclair, *The Fasting Cure*, 45.

185 *Sir John Hall, the chief English physician*: Stephanie J. Snow, *Blessed Days of Anesthesia* (Oxford, UK: Oxford University Press, 2013), 99.

186 *His given name was too ordinary*: Robert Lewis Taylor, "Physical Culture: Weakness Is a Crime," *New Yorker*, October 21, 1950, 44.

186 *"Medicine has had its day"*: Robert Ernst, *Weakness Is a Crime: The Life of Bernarr Macfadden* (Syracuse, NY: Syracuse University Press, 1990), 22.

186 *The enemies were numerous*: Ibid., 31.

187 *he wrote more than a hundred*: Mark Adams, *Mr. America: How Muscular Millionaire Bernarr Macfadden Transformed the Nation through Sex, Salad, and the Ultimate Starvation Diet* (New York: HarperCollins, 2009), 163.

187 *At the core of Macfadden's health empire*: Macfadden Communications Group developed into one of the largest magazine publishers in the United States, eventually owning and publishing magazines such as *True Story*, *True Romance*, and *True Detective*, breathless pulps that have their spawn in today's

reality television shows and *America's Most Wanted*. Naturally, Macfadden sought the Republican nomination for U.S. president, and subsequently tried and failed to win the Democratic primary for U.S. senator from Florida (while promising to protect Floridians from racial integration).

187 *recommended occasionally eating sand*: Adams, *Mr. America*, 91.

187 *"In his advocacy of fasting"*: Taylor, "Physical Culture," 50.

188 *Shelton contended that calories*: Herbert M. Shelton, *The Science and Fine Art of Fasting*, Kindle ed. (Naples, FL: Mockingbird Press, 1978), 336–37.

188 *One lawsuit detailed the death*: "A Health Clinic Was Ordered Friday to Pay $873,000," UPI, September 17, 1982, https://www.upi.com/Archives/1982/09/17/A-health-clinic-was-ordered-Friday-to-pay-873000/8663401083200/.

188 *in 1964, the president of the San Diego chapter*: "Victim's Dad Said Fasting 'Cured' Her," *Santa Cruz Sentinel*, May 1, 1964, 10.

DAY 7, SATURDAY

190 *the act of* sallekhana: Diane Mehta, "On Chanting and Consciousness," *Harvard Divinity Bulletin*, Spring/Summer 2021, https://bulletin.hds.harvard.edu/on-chanting-and-consciousness/. *Anekāntavāda*, or "many-sidedness," is central to Jainism. Similar to the Talmudic concept that there are as many ways to interpret the Torah as there were Jews who fled Egypt during the Exodus, many-sidedness holds that truth is a multilayered thing. While complete truth is accessible to everyone, only those few able to exalt themselves and cast off karmic ties, whether through Sallekhana or another means, can perceive it in its entirety.

191 *But in the Stoic tradition*: In Cicero's *On Ends*, Cato the Stoic says that "it is sometimes a proper function both for the wise man to depart from life, although he is happy, and for a fool to remain alive, although he is wretched." 3.60–61, *The Hellenistic Philosophers*, trans. A. A. Long and D. N. Sedley (Cambridge, UK: Cambridge University Press, 1987), 425.

191 *Six times as many Americans*: Schwartz, *Never Satisfied*, 71.

191 *A. R. Turnbull, the medical superintendent*: As quoted in Miller, *A History of Force Feeding: Hunger Strikes, Prisons and Medical Ethics, 1909–1974*, 37–38.

192 *While relatively rare*: According to the National Institute of Mental Health, eating disorders are close to 4 percent among adolescents, twice as high among women. The lifetime prevalence of anorexia is 0.6 percent in the

general population, but three times higher among females (0.9) than males (0.3). "Eating Disorders," National Institute of Mental Health, https://www.nimh.nih.gov/health/statistics/eating-disorders.

192 *"I have no needs; take care of me"*: Priscilla Becker, "Big Little," in *Going Hungry: Writers on Desire, Self-Denial, and Overcoming Anorexia*, ed. Kate M. Taylor (New York: Anchor Books, 2008), 145.

192 *the poet Antal, a fifteen-year-old*: Narayanan, "Renunciation and Gender Issues in the Sri Vaisnava Community," 444.

193 *"The Sacred Words of a Woman"*: As quoted in ibid., 447.

193 *"I can't say that everyone who fasts"*: Kristen Portland, interview with the author, January 24, 2022. The need for control, shared by anorexics and censors, is pervasive in times of a pandemic. Book bans and restrictions at school and public libraries are at a record high, according to the American Library Association's "State of America's Libraries Special Report, Pandemic Year Two" edition (2022). Book banning and anorexia, each a form of hyper-restriction, are fasting gone haywire. See Jessica Grose, "Book Banning Is All about the Illusion of Parental Control," *New York Times*, February 9, 2022.

194 *English doctor Sir William Gull*: Vandereycken and Van Deth, *From Fasting Saints to Anorexic Girls*, 154.

194 *In 1873, Gull and Lasègue*: The gruesome Gull-Lasègue competition to claim naming rights over what was seen as a women's malady is painstakingly detailed by the scholars Walter Vandereycken and Ron Van Deth in *From Fasting Saints to Anorexic Girls*. The *OED* gives the first recorded use of anorexia in English as 1598, when it appeared in Joshua Sylvester's "The Furies": "Then the Anorexie, then the Dog-Hunger or the Bradypepsie." It is unlikely this was the introduction of the term, but it was certainly used for centuries thereafter. For example, see Benjamin Granger's "On Unusual Cases of Anorexy" in the *Edinburgh Medical and Surgical Journal*, April 1813, cited in Brumberg, *Fasting Girls*, 296–97. Without detracting from the dangers of consumerism and the intolerable and constant pressures on women to be slim, to describe anorexia as a "modern ailment," as many have done, is an error.

194 *psychiatrist Hilde Bruch*: Hilde Bruch, *The Golden Cage: The Enigma of Anorexia Nervosa* (Cambridge, MA: Harvard University Press, 1978), xxii.

195 *Gull provided the medical establishment*: William Withey Gull, "Anorexia Nervosa," *Transactions of the Clinical Society*, vol. VII (London: Longmans Green, 1874), 26.

195 *For "most of these cases"*: William Gull, "Clinical Notes: Anorexia Nervosa," *Lancet*, March 16, 1888, 517.

195 *Lasègue had used exactly*: Charles Lasègue and Simon Duplay, *Archives Générales de Medicine*, vol. 1 (Paris: P. Asselin, 1873), 393.

196 *in 1869, New York physician George Beard*: In an 1868 feature about the "Brooklyn Enigma" Mollie Fancher, the *Brooklyn Eagle* wrote: "It has been said by many medical men, that the remarkable vigor which characterizes the present century, is a result of the preponderance of nervous energy in the races that people the earth. This would seem to hold good from the slowest to the most active race. Where nervous energy is clogged and embedded in flesh and bone it is less conspicuous in results . . ." (Daily, *Mollie Fancher*, 139.) The "fasting girls" were similarly the result of a sensitive reaction to the modern American environment.

196 *"In civilized lands"*: George M. Beard, *American Nervousness: Its Causes and Consequences* (New York: G. P. Putnam's Sons, 1881), 207.

196 *One of the recommended treatments*: Whorton, "'Physiologic Optimism,'" 150.

197 *only body-focused (somatic)*: Bell, *Holy Anorexia*, 14–15.

197 *suffering from pituitary insufficiency*: Mara Selvini Palazzoli, *Self-Starvation: From Individual to Family Therapy in the Treatment of Anorexia Nervosa* (Northvale, NJ: Jason Aronson, 1996), 16.

197 *Palazzoli, a famed psychiatrist*: Ibid., 233.

197 *Women suffering from the disease*: G. F. M. Russell and J. Treasure, "The Modern History of Anorexia Nervosa: An Interpretation of Why the Illness Has Changed," *Annals of the New York Academy of Sciences* 575, no. 1 (December 1989): 14.

197 *"morbid dread of fatness"*: Hendricks, *The Oldest Cure in the World*, 92.

198 *The culture of slenderness*: See Sabrina Strings, *Fearing the Black Body: The Racial Origins of Fat Phobia* (New York: New York University Press, 2019).

198 *cultural critic Anna Mirzayan*: Anna Mirzayan, "Why Does the Art World Hate Fat People?," *Hyperallergic*, October 19, 2022, https://hyperallergic.com/771042/why-does-the-art-world-hate-fat-people/.

198 *Prejudice against overweight people*: "The Economics of Thinness," *Economist*, December 20, 2022, https://www.economist.com/christmas-specials/2022/12/20/the-economics-of-thinness.

198 *A study of women's fashion magazines*: Russell and Treasure, "The Modern History of Anorexia Nervosa," 17.

198 *Endless brands touted slimming certainties*: Schwartz, *Never Satisfied*, 181.

199 *in 1939, British physician John Alfred Ryle*: Vandereycken and Van Deth, *From Fasting Saints to Anorexic Girls*, 182.

199 *In early January 1998*: "Tenth Anniversary of the Devastating 1998 Ice Storm in the Northeast," National Weather Service, January 5, 2008, https://www.weather.gov/media/btv/events/IceStorm1998.pdf.

199 *Five months after the storm*: A. St-Hilaire et al., "A Prospective Study of Effects of Prenatal Maternal Stress on Later Eating-Disorder Manifestations in Affected Offspring: Preliminary Indications Based on the Project Ice Storm Cohort," *International Journal of Eating Disorders* 48, no. 5 (July 2015): 512–16.

199 *"Genetic susceptibility can be activated"*: Dr. Howard Steiger, interview with the author, April 3, 2022. For more on this topic see, for example, Laramie Duncan et al., "Significant Locus and Metabolic Genetic Correlations Revealed in Genome-Wide Association Study of Anorexia Nervosa," *American Journal of Psychiatry* 174, no. 9 (September 2017): 850–58.

200 *writes Rudolph Bell*: Bell, *Holy Anorexia*, x.

200 *"ultimately to obliterate"*: Ibid., 11.

200 *"an abhorrence of being looked at by men"*: Russell and Treasure, "The Modern History of Anorexia Nervosa," 16.

201 *the notion of becoming food herself*: For more on this topic, see Esther Brownsmith, "To Serve Woman: Jezebel, Anat, and the Metaphor of Women as Food" in *Researching Metaphor in the Near East*, eds. Ludovico Portuese and Marta Pallavidini (Wiesbaden, Germany: Harrasowitz Verlag, 2020).

201 *As documented both by her confessor*: D. Rampling, "Ascetic Ideals and Anorexia Nervosa," *Journal of Psychiatric Research* 19, nos. 2–3 (1985): 91.

201 *"If so much as a bean"*: Bell, *Holy Anorexia*, 20.

201 *"make a supreme effort to root out"*: Rampling, "Ascetic Ideals and Anorexia Nervosa," 91.

201 *"when Catherine advanced to receive"*: C. M. Antony, *Saint Catherine of Siena: Her Life and Times* (London: Burns & Oates, 1915), 63.

202 *"eating would kill her anyway"*: Bell, *Holy Anorexia*, 24.

202 *Beginning in the early sixteenth century*: Many examples are provided in Bell, *Holy Anorexia*; Bynum, *Holy Feast and Holy Fast*; Vandereycken and Van Deth, *From Fasting Saints to Anorexic Girls*.

202 *Paulus Lentulus, a prominent Swiss doctor*: Morgenthaler, "Eine Hysterika zu Beginn des 17. Jahrhunderts," 197.

202 *Richard Morton, a doctor*: Russell and Treasure, "The Modern History of Anorexia Nervosa," 16.

203 *Therese Neumann von Konnersreuth*: Father Richard Kunst, "September 18,

1962, the Death of Venerable Therese Neumann," *Papal Artifacts* blog, September 17, 2022, https://www.papalartifacts.com/december-18-1962-the-death-of-venerable-therese-neumann/.

203 *Alexandrina Maria da Costa*: "Alexandrina Maria da Costa (1904–1955)," Holy See, https://www.vatican.va/news_services/liturgy/saints/ns_lit_doc_20040425_da-costa_en.html.

204 *It now appears to be a complex*: See many studies, for example, H. J. Watson et al., "Genome-Wide Association Study Identifies Eight Risk Loci and Implicates Metabo-Psychiatric Origins for Anorexia Nervosa," *Nature Genetics* 51, no. 8 (August 2019): 1207–14.

EPILOGUE

205 *"Desire destroys its object"*: Sartre, *Being and Nothingness*, 751.

205 *"All our desires are contradictory"*: Weil, *Gravity and Grace*, 201.

206 *President George W. Bush famously*: Transcript of President George W. Bush speech, *CNN Saturday Morning News*, October 6, 2001, https://transcripts.cnn.com/show/smn/date/2001-10-06/segment/26.

206 *President Woodrow Wilson demanded*: Woodrow Wilson, "Address to the Salesmanship Congress in Detroit, Michigan, July 10, 1916," American Presidency Project, https://www.presidency.ucsb.edu/documents/address-the-salesmanship-congress-detroit-michigan.

206 *"the deadening and cheapening influences"*: Peter H. Van Ness, "Asceticism in Philosophical and Cultural-Critical Perspective," in *Asceticism*, eds. Wimbush and Valantasis (New York: Oxford University Press, 1995), 593.

206 *the body's primary function*: Jamsheed K. Choksy, "Fasting," *Encyclopaedia Iranica*, 394–96, https://www.iranicaonline.org/articles/fasting.

207 *in a famous incident in 1914*: John Mackie, "A Century Ago, the Komagata Maru Arrived in Vancouver and Challenged Racist Policies," *Vancouver Sun*, May 21, 2014, https://vancouversun.com/news/metro/a-century-ago-the-komagata-maru-arrived-in-vancouver-and-challenged-racist-policies.

207 *Cuong Lu, a friend*: Cuong Lu, interview with the author, March 27, 2021.

208 *His Most Reverend Excellency Cornelius "Connie" Lucey*: Fintan O'Toole, *We Don't Know Ourselves: A Personal History of Modern Ireland* (New York: Liveright, 2022), 169.

208 *"Transformation and destruction"*: Prem Krishnamurthy, interview with the author, April 9, 2021.

A SAMPLING OF FAMOUS FASTERS

215 *Byron*: Wilma Paterson, "Was Byron Anorexic?," *World Medicine* 17, no. 16 (May 15, 1982): 35–38, was the first essay to make this case, and it has since been widely accepted.

215 *Emily Dickinson*: See Heather Kirk Thomas's convincing "Emily Dickinson's 'Renunciation' and Anorexia Nervosa," *American Literature* 60, no. 2 (May 1988): 205–25.

Bibliography

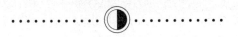

BOOKS

Ancient Laws of Ireland: Introduction to Senchus Mor, or, Law of Distress as Contained in the Harleian Manuscripts, vol 1. Published Under the Direction of the Commissioners for Publishing the Ancient Laws and Institutes of Ireland. Dublin: Alexander Thom, 1865.

The Qur'an. Translated by M. A. S. Abdel Haleem. Oxford, UK: Oxford University Press, 2004.

Adams, Mark. *Mr. America: How Muscular Millionaire Bernarr Macfadden Transformed the Nation through Sex, Salad, and the Ultimate Starvation Diet.* New York: HarperCollins, 2009.

Ajour, Ashjan. *Reclaiming Humanity in Palestinian Hunger Strikes: Revolutionary Subjectivity and Decolonizing the Body.* New York: Springer, 2021.

Albala, Ken, and Trudy Eden, eds. *Food and Faith in Christian Culture.* New York: Columbia University Press, 2011.

Alexander-Mott, LeeAnn, and Lumsden, D. Barry, eds. *Understanding Eating Disorders: Anorexia Nervosa, Bulimia Nervosa, and Obesity.* New York: Taylor and Francis, 1994.

Al-Ghazali. *The Mysteries of Charity and the Mysteries of Fasting: Books 5 and 6 of Ihya' 'ulum al-din, the Revival of the Religious Sciences.* Translated by M. Abdurrahman Fitzgerald. Louisville: Fons Vitae, 2019.

Anderson, Helen Arndt. *Breakfast: A History.* Lanham, MD: AltaMira Press, 2013.

Antony, C. M. *Saint Catherine of Siena: Her Life and Times.* London: Burns & Oates, 1915.

Apple, Sam. *Ravenous: Otto Warburg, the Nazis, and the Search for the Cancer-Diet Connection.* New York: Liveright, 2021.

Aquinas, Thomas. *Summa Theologica.* Claremont, CA: Coyote Canyon Press, 2018.

Aristotle. *Eudemian Ethics*. Edited and translated by Brad Inwood and Rachel Woolf. Cambridge, UK: Cambridge University Press, 2013.

Armbruster-Sandoval, Ralph. *Starving for Justice: Hunger Strikes, Spectacular Speech and the Struggle for Dignity*. Tucson: University of Arizona Press, 2017.

Athenaeus. *The Learned Banqueters: Books 12–13.594b*. Edited and translated by S. Douglas Olson. Cambridge, MA: Harvard University Press, 2006.

Beard, George M. *American Nervousness: Its Causes and Consequences*. New York: G. P. Putnam's Sons, 1881.

Bell, Rudolph M. *Holy Anorexia*. Chicago: University of Chicago Press, 1985.

Beresford, David. *Ten Men Dead: The Story of the 1981 Irish Hunger Strike*. New York: Atlantic Monthly Press, 1987.

Bordo, Susan. *Unbearable Weight: Feminism, Western Culture and the Body*. Oakland: University of California Press, 2004.

Boyarin, Daniel. *Socrates and the Fat Rabbis*. Chicago: University of Chicago Press, 2009.

———. *Unheroic Conduct: The Rise of Heterosexuality and the Invention of the Jewish Man*. Berkeley: University of California Press, 1997.

Bruch, Hilde. *Eating Disorders: Anorexia Nervosa, and the Person Within*. New York: Basic Books, 1979.

———. *The Golden Cage: The Enigma of Anorexia Nervosa*. Cambridge, MA: Harvard University Press, 1978.

Brumberg, Joan Jacobs. *Fasting Girls: The History of Anorexia Nervosa*. New York: Vintage, 2000.

Buchinger, Otto. *Das Heilfasten*. Stuttgart: Hippokrates-Verlag Marquardt & Cie., 1942.

Bukovsky, Vladimir, and Michael Scammell, trans. *To Build a Castle: My Life as a Dissenter*. New York: Viking, 1979.

Bynum, Caroline Walker. *Holy Feast and Holy Fast: The Religious Significance of Food to Medieval Women*. Berkeley: University of California Press, 1988.

Cage, John. *Silence: Lectures and Writings*. Middletown, CT: Wesleyan University Press, 1961.

Cargill, Kima. *The Psychology of Overeating: Food and the Culture of Consumerism*. London: Bloomsbury Academic, 2015.

Carroll, Abigail. *Three Squares: The Invention of the American Meal*. New York: Basic Books, 2013.

Cassian, John. "Conference I: First Conference of Abba Moses on the Monk's Goal," 193–289. In *Western Asceticism*. Edited by Owen Chadwic. London: SCM Press, 1958.

Chernin, Kim. *Reflections on the Tyranny of Slenderness*. New York: Harper Perennial, 1994.

Childs, Lydia Maria Francis. *Appeal in Favor of That Class of Americans Called Africans*. New York: John S. Taylor, 1836.

Corbin, Alain. *A History of Silence*. Cambridge, UK: Polity, 2018.

Cornaro, Lewis. *Discourses on a Sober and Temperate Life*. Translated and with an introduction by Sylvester Graham. New York: Mahlon Day, 1833.

Corrington-Streete, Gail P. "Trajectories of Ascetic Behavior." In *Asceticism*. Edited by Vincent L. Wimbush and Richard Valantasis. New York: Oxford University Press, 1995.

Daily, Abram H. *Mollie Fancher: The Brooklyn Enigma, the Psychological Marvel of the Nineteenth Century*. New York: Abram H. Daily, 1894.

Deleuze, Gilles. *Essays Critical and Clinical*. Translated by Daniel W. Smith and Michael A. Greco. Minneapolis: University of Minnesota Press, 1997.

Derrida, Jacques. *Of Grammatology*. Translated by Gayatri Chakravorty Spivak. Baltimore: Johns Hopkins University Press, 2016.

Deutsch, Leo. *Sixteen Years in Siberia: Some Experiences of a Russian Revolutionist*. New York: E. P. Dutton, 1904.

Devji, Faisal. *The Impossible Indian: Gandhi and the Temptation of Violence*. Cambridge, MA: Harvard University Press, 2012.

Diamond, Eliezer. *Holy Men and Hunger Artists: Fasting and Asceticism in Rabbinic Culture*. Oxford, UK: Oxford University Press, 2003.

Diogenes Laërtius. *Lives of the Eminent Philosophers*. Translated by Pamela Mensch. Oxford, UK: Oxford University Press, 2020.

Dupont-Sommer, André. *The Essene Writings from Qumran*. Translated by G. Vermes. Cleveland: Meridian Books, 1962.

Eckhart, Meister. *Meister Eckhart: The Essential Sermons, Commentaries, Treatises and Defense*. Translated by Edmund Colledge and Bernard McGinn. Mahwah, NJ: Paulist Press, 1981.

Edwards, Catherine. *The Politics of Immorality in Ancient Rome*. Cambridge, UK: Cambridge University Press, 1993.

Ellis, Peter Berresford. *A History of the Irish Working Class*. New York: George Braziller, 1973.

Ellmann, Maud. *The Hunger Artists*. London: Virago Press, 1993.

Elm, Susanna. *Virgins of God: The Making of Asceticism in Late Antiquity*. Oxford, UK: Oxford University Press, 1994.

Fasano, Alessio, and Susan Flaherty. *Gut Feelings: The Microbiome and Our Health*. Cambridge, MA: MIT Press, 2021.

Foster, Richard J. *Celebration of Discipline: The Path to Spiritual Growth*. New York: HarperCollins, 1998.

Foy, George Michelsen. *Zero Decibels: The Quest for Absolute Silence*. New York: Scribner, 2010.

Fuchs, Martin, et al. *Religious Individualisation: Historical Dimensions and Comparative Perspectives*, vol. 1. Berlin: De Gruyter, 2019.

Gardner, Martin. *Fads and Fallacies in the Name of Science*. New York: Dover, 1957.

Grant, Kevin. *Hunger Strikes and Fasts in the British Empire, 1890–1948*. Oakland: University of California Press, 2019.

Grimm, Veronika E. *From Feasting to Fasting: The Evolution of a Sin*. London: Routledge, 1996.

Gunn, Robert A. *Forty Days without Food!: A Biography of Henry S. Tanner, M.D., Including a Complete and Accurate History of His Wonderful Fasts with Valuable Deductions*. New York: A. Metz, 1880.

Hammond, William. *Fasting Girls: Their Physiology and Pathology*. New York: G. P. Putnam's Sons, 1879.

Harpham, Geoffrey Galt. *The Ascetic Imperative in Culture and Criticism*. Chicago: University of Chicago Press, 1987.

Hamsun, Knut. *Hunger*. Translated by Robert Bly. New York: Farrar, Straus and Giroux, 1986.

Hayward, Jeremy W. *Perceiving Ordinary Magic: Science and Intuitive Wisdom*. Boston: Shambhala, 1984.

Hendricks, Steve. *The Oldest Cure in the World: Adventures in the Art and Science of Fasting*. New York: Abrams, 2022.

Hersey, Tricia. *Rest Is Resistance: A Manifesto*. New York: Little, Brown, 2022.

Heywood, Leslie. *Dedication to Hunger: The Anorexic Aesthetic in Modern Culture*. Berkeley: University of California Press, 1996.

Hileman, Sharon. "'Yes I Can': Empowerment and Voice in Women's Prison Narratives," 58–70. In *No Small World: Visions and Revisions of World Literature*. Edited by Michael Thomas Carroll. Urbana, IL: National Council of Teachers of English, 1996.

Holmes, Brooke, and William V. Harris, eds. *Aelius Aristides between Greece, Rome, and the Gods*. New York: Columbia University Press, 2009.

Homer. *The Iliad*. Translated by Samuel Butler. London: Longmans, Green & Co., 1898.

Hooper, Finley, and Matthew Schwartz. *Roman Letters: History from a Personal Point of View*. Detroit: Wayne State University Press, 1991.

Kafka, Franz. *The Diaries of Franz Kafka*. Translated by Ross Benjamin. New York: Schocken, 2022.

———. *Investigations of a Dog and Other Stories*. Translated by Michael Hofmann. New York: New Directions, 2017.

———. *Letters to Felice*. Edited by Erich Heller and Jürgen Born, and translated by James Stern and Elisabeth Duckworth. New York: Schocken Books, 2016.

Keizer, Garret. *The Unwanted Sound of Everything We Want*. New York: Public Affairs, 2010.

Khawaja, Noreen. *The Religion of Existence: Asceticism in Philosophy from Kierkegaard to Sartre*. Chicago: University of Chicago Press, 2016.

Kimpel, Ben. *Philosophies of Life of the Ancient Greeks and Israelites*. New York: Philosophical Library, 1981.

Lasègue, Charles, and Simon Duplay. *Archives Générales de Medicine*, vol. 1. Paris: P. Asselin, 1873.

Lerat, Eva, and Sébastien Charbonnier. *Le jeûne: Une expérience philosophique*. Paris: Éditions le Pommier, 2022.

Lobel, Diana. *Philosophies of Happiness*. New York: Columbia University Press, 2017.

Ó Lúing, Seán. *I Die in a Good Cause*. Cork, Ireland: Mercier Press, 2017.

Maimonides, Mishneh. Torah, Fasts 4 and 5. Translated by Eliyahu Touger. Moznaim Publishing. https://www.sefaria.org/Mishneh_Torah%2C_Fasts.4.18?lang=bi&with=all&lang2=en.

Matthiessen, Peter. *Sal Si Puedes*. Berkeley: University of California Press, 2014.

McKitterick, Rosamund, and David Dumville, eds. *Ireland in Early Medieval Europe: Studies in Memory of Kathleen Hughes*. Cambridge, UK: Cambridge University Press, 1982.

Miller, Ian. *A History of Force Feeding: Hunger Strikes, Prisons and Medical Ethics, 1909–1974*. London: Palgrave Macmillan, 2016.

Minuchin, Salvador, Bernice L. Rosman, and Lester Baker. *Psychosomatic Families: Anorexia Nervosa in Context*. Cambridge, MA: Harvard University Press, 1978.

Moloney, Ed. *Voices from the Grave: Two Men's War in Ireland*. London: Faber & Faber, 2010.

Morales, Helen. *Antigone Rising: The Subversive Power of the Ancient Myths*. New York: Hachette, 2020.

Morton, Richard. *Phthisologia, or, a Treatise on Consumptions*, rev. ed. London: W. and J. Innys, 1720.

Moxon, Frank. *What Forcible Feeding Means*. London: Woman's Press, 1914.

Narayanan, Vasudha. "Renunciation and Gender Issues in the Sri Vaisnava

Community." In *Asceticism*. Edited by Vincent L. Wimbush and Richard Valantasis. New York: Oxford University Press, 1995.

O'Kelly, John Joseph. *Ireland: Elements of Her Early Story*. Dublin: M. H. Gill and Son, 1921.

O'Malley, Padraig. *Biting at the Grave: The Irish Hunger Strikes and the Politics of Despair*. Boston: Beacon Press, 1990.

O'Toole, Fintan. *We Don't Know Ourselves: A Personal History of Modern Ireland*. New York: Liveright, 2022.

Palazzoli, Mara Selvini. *Self-Starvation: From Individual to Family Therapy in the Treatment of Anorexia Nervosa*. Northvale, NJ: Jason Aronson, 1996.

Plato. *Phaedo*. In *The Dialogues of Plato*, vol. 2. Translated by Benjamin Jowett. New York: Macmillan, 1892.

Prochnik, George. *In Pursuit of Silence: Listening for Meaning in a World of Noise*. New York: Doubleday, 2010.

Rappoport, Leon. *How We Eat: Appetite, Culture, and the Psychology of Food*. Toronto: ECW Press, 2011.

Rist, J. M. *Epicurus: An Introduction*. Cambridge, UK: Cambridge University Press, 1972.

Rovelli, Carlo. *The Order of Time*. New York: Riverhead, 2019.

Russell, Sharman Apt. *Hunger: An Unnatural History*. New York: Basic Books, 2005.

Sartre, Jean-Paul. *Being and Nothingness*. Translated by Sarah Richmond. Abingdon, UK: Routledge, 2018.

Schopenhauer, Arthur. *The World as Will and Idea*, vol. 1. London: Kegan, Paul, Trench, Trübner, and Co., 1891.

Schwartz, Hillel. *Making Noise: From Babel to the Big Bang and Beyond*. New York: Zone Books, 2011.

———. *Never Satisfied: A Cultural History of Diets, Fantasies, and Fat*. New York: Anchor Books, 1990.

Sebald, W. G. *The Rings of Saturn*. New York: New Directions, 1998.

Shah, Nayan. *Refusal to Eat: A Century of Prison Strikes*. Oakland: University of California Press, 2022.

Sharp, Gene. *The Politics of Nonviolent Action, Part Two: The Methods of Nonviolent Action*. Boston: Porter Sargent, 1973.

Shelton, Herbert M. *The Science and Fine Art of Fasting*. Kindle ed. Naples, FL: Mockingbird Press, 1978.

Sinclair, Upton. *The Fasting Cure*. 1911; Carlisle, MA: Applewood Books, 2022.

Snow, Stephanie J. *Blessed Days of Anesthesia*. Oxford, UK: Oxford University Press, 2013.

Stevens, Doris. *Jailed for Freedom: American Women Win the Vote*. New York: Liveright, 1920.

Stokes, George T. *Ireland and the Celtic Church*. London: Society for Promoting Christian Knowledge, 1907.

Taylor, Kate M., ed. *Going Hungry: Writers on Desire, Self-Denial, and Overcoming Anorexia*. New York: Anchor Books, 2008.

Thorsteinsson, Runar M. *Roman Christianity and Roman Stoicism*. Oxford, UK: Oxford University Press, 2010.

Thurman, Robert A. F. "Tibetan Buddhist Perspectives on Asceticism." In *Asceticism*. Edited by Vincent L. Wimbush and Richard Valantasis. New York: Oxford University Press, 1995.

Trigg, Joseph W. *Origen*. London: Routledge, 1998.

Trigger, Bruce. *The Children of Aataentsic: A History of the Huron People to 1660*. Kingston, ON: McGill-Queens's University Press, 1987.

Tsing, Anna Lowenhaupt. *The Mushroom at the End of the World: On the Possibility of Life in Capitalist Ruins*. Princeton, NJ: Princeton University Press, 2015.

Tucker, Todd. *The Great Starvation Experiment: Ancel Keys and the Men Who Starved for Science*, rev. ed. Minneapolis: University of Minnesota Press, 2007.

Twain, Mark. *The Man that Corrupted Hadleyburg, and Other Essays and Stories*. New York: Harper and Brothers, 1898.

———. *A Tramp Abroad*. Hartford, CT: American Publishing Company, 1880.

Vandereycken, Walter, and Ron Van Deth. *From Fasting Saints to Anorexic Girls*. London: Athlone Press, 1994.

Wagtendonk, K. *Fasting in the Koran*. Leiden, Netherlands: E. J. Brill, 1968.

Wanley, Nathaniel. *The Wonders of the Little World: Or, A General History of Man. In Six Books. Wherein by Many Thousands of Examples Is Shewed What Man Hath Been from the First Ages of the World to These Times*. London: T. Bassett, 1678.

Ward, Harry M. *The War for Independence and the Transformation of American Society*. London: UCL Press, 1999.

Weil, Simone. *First and Last Notebooks*. Translated by Richard Rees. Eugene, OR: Wipf and Stock, 2015.

———. *Gravity and Grace*. Translated by Arthur Wills. Lincoln: University of Nebraska Press, 1997.

Whorton, James. *Crusaders for Fitness: The History of American Health Reformers*. Princeton, NJ: Princeton University Press, 1982.

Winick, Myron. *Hunger Disease: Studies by the Jewish Physicians in the Warsaw Ghetto*. New York: John Wiley & Sons, 1979.

Young, Sarah, ed. and trans. *Writing Resistance: Revolutionary Memoirs of Shlis-sel'burg Prison, 1884–1906*. London: UCL Press, 2021.

Zhuangzi. *The Complete Works of Zhuangzi*. Translated by Burton Watson. New York: Columbia University Press, 2013.

ARTICLES, ESSAYS, PODCASTS, AND VIDEOS

Ainsworth, Clare. "Growing Younger: Radical Insights into Ageing Could Help Us Reverse It." *New Scientist*, April 27, 2022. https://www.newscientist.com/article/mg25433843-000-growing-younger-radical-insights-into-ageing-could-help-us-reverse-it/.

Alexander, Shawn L. "Vengeance without Justice, Injustice without Retribution: The Afro-American Council's Struggle against Racial Violence." *Great Plains Quarterly* 27, no. 2 (Spring 2007): 117–33.

Almeneessier, A. S., et al. "The Effects of Diurnal Intermittent Fasting on the Wake-Promoting Neurotransmitter Orexin-A." *Annals of Thoracic Medicine* 13, no. 1 (January–March 2018): 48–54.

Anderson, Mark. "Anorexia and Modernism, or How I Learned to Diet in All Directions." *Discourse* 11, no. 1 (1988): 28–41. http://www.jstor.org/stable/41389106.

Appel, Jacob M. "Beyond Guantánamo." *Huffington Post*, March 18, 2010. https://www.huffpost.com/entry/beyond-guantanamo-torture_b_360082.

Arendt, Hannah. "Thinking and Moral Considerations: A Lecture." *Social Research* 38, no. 3 (Autumn 1971): 417–46.

Asbury, Herbert. "That Was New York: Forty Days and Forty Nights." *New Yorker*, April 27, 1934, 70–79.

Associated Press. "Man Indicted in Girl's Death of Malnutrition." *Hartford Courant*, October 3, 1963, 39A.

Avramova, Nina. "The Dark Side of Music: Using Sound in Torture." CNN, February 20, 2019. https://edition.cnn.com/2019/02/08/health/music-in-torture-intl/index.html.

Ball, Molly. "'What More Do We Need To Do To Win?' A Controversial Climate Group Rethinks Its Strategy." *Time*, March 17, 2022. https://time.com/6158322/sunrise-movement-climate-activism-struggles/.

Barry, Robert. "The Development of the Roman Catholic Teachings on Suicide." *Notre Dame Journal of Law, Ethics & Public Policy* 9, no. 449 (1995): 454. http://scholarship.law.nd.edu/ndjlepp/vol9/iss2/4.

Bastani, Abdolhossein, et al. "The Effects of Fasting during Ramadan on the Concentration of Serotonin, Dopamine, Brain-Derived Neurotrophic Factor and Nerve Growth Factor." *Neurology International* 9, no. 2 (June 23, 2017): 7043.

Bernardi L., et al. "Cardiovascular, Cerebrovascular, and Respiratory Changes Induced by Different Types of Music in Musicians and Non-Musicians: The Importance of Silence." *Heart* 92, no. 4 (April 2006): 445–52.

Bezuglov, Eduard, et al. "Running Performance during the Holy Month of Ramadan in Elite Professional Adult Soccer Players in Russia." *International Journal of Environmental Research and Public Health* 18, no. 21 (November 2021): 11731.

Bianchi, Giovanna, et al. "Fasting Induces Anti-Warburg Effect That Increases Respiration but Reduces ATP-Synthesis to Promote Apoptosis in Colon Cancer Models." *Oncotarget* 6, no. 14 (May 20, 2015): 11806–19.

Biggs, Michael. "The Rationality of Self-Inflicted Suffering: Hunger Strikes by Irish Republicans, 1916–1923." *Sociology Working Papers*, no. 3 (2007), 1–24.

Bigotti, F., D. Taylor, and J. Welsman. "Recreating the Pulsilogium of Santorio: Outlines for a Historically-Engaged Endeavour." *Bulletin of the Scientific Instrument Society* 133 (June 30, 2017): 30–35.

Bistrian, Bruce R. "Clinical Use of a Protein-Sparing Modified Fast." *Journal of the American Medical Association* 240, no. 21 (November 17, 1978): 2299–2302.

Black, R. D. Collison. "Economic Policy in Ireland and India in the Time of J. S. Mill." *Economic History Review* 21, no. 3 (August 1968): 321–36.

Blake, John B. "The Inoculation Controversy in Boston: 1721–1722." *New England Quarterly* 25, no. 4 (December 1952): 489–506.

Bly, Antonio T. "Crossing the Lake of Fire: Slave Resistance during the Middle Passage, 1720–1842." *Journal of Negro History* 83, no. 3 (Summer 1998): 178–86.

Bouchard, Claude. "Genetics of Obesity: What We Have Learned over Decades of Research." *Obesity* 29, no. 5 (May 2021): 802–20. https://onlinelibrary.wiley.com/doi/10.1002/oby.23116.

Bowerbank, Chloe. "'How Long Will It Go On?'—Sylvia Pankhurst and the Hunger Strike." UKVote100, September 27, 2017. https://ukvote100.org/2017/09/27/how-long-will-it-go-on-sylvia-pankhurst/.

Brooks, Svevo, et al. "A Guide to Political Fasting." Eugene, OR: Nonviolent Tactics Development Project, June 1981. https://nonviolence.rutgers.edu/files/original/2cdc488c7f145abccdb2a220c27d57d33b7f1374.pdf.

Brown, Andrew J. "Low-Carb Diets, Fasting and Euphoria: Is There a Link between Ketosis and Gamma-Hydroxybutyrate (GHB)?" *Medical Hypotheses* 68, no. 2 (2007): 268–71.

Brown, Ryan Lenora. "Guantánamo Hunger Strike: How Others Have Han-
    dled Such Protests." *Christian Science Monitor*, May 3, 2013. https://www
    .csmonitor.com/World/Global-Issues/2013/0503/Guantanamo-hunger
    -strike-How-others-have-handled-such-protests.

Bugeja, Lino. "Agostino Levanzin: Man for All Reasons." *Times of Malta*, July 14,
    2012. https://timesofmalta.com/articles/view/Agostino-Levanzin-man
    -for-all-reasons.428703.

Che, Chang, and Amy Chang Chien. "Memes, Puns and Blank Sheets of Paper:
    China's Creative Acts of Protest." *New York Times*, November 28, 2022.
    https://www.nytimes.com/2022/11/28/world/asia/china-protests-blank
    -sheets.html.

Choksy, Jamsheed K. "Fasting." *Encyclopaedia Iranica*. https://www.iranicaonline
    .org/articles/fasting.

Christopher, Roy. "The Science of Sound and Silence." *Roy Christopher* blog,
    no. 50. https://buttondown.email/roychristopher/archive/the-science-
    of-sound-and-silence/.

Cowen, P. J., and M. Browning. "What Has Serotonin to Do with Depression?"
    World Psychiatry 14, no. 2 (June 2015): 158–60.

Cuccolo, K., et al. "Intermittent Fasting Implementation and Association with
    Eating Disorder Symptomatology." *Eating Disorders: The Journal of Treatment
    and Prevention* 30, no. 5 (September–October 2022): 471–91.

Deadwyler, S. A., et al. "Systemic and Nasal Delivery of Orexin-A (Hypocretin-1)
    Reduces the Effects of Sleep Deprivation on Cognitive Performance in
    Nonhuman Primates." *Journal of Neuroscience* 27, no. 52 (December 26,
    2007): 14239–47.

Deal, William. "The Lotus Sūtra and the Rhetoric of Legitimization in
    Eleventh-Century Japanese Buddhism."*Japanese Journal of Religious
    Studies* 20, no. 4 (December 1993): 261–95.

De Cabo, Rafael, and Mark P. Mattson. "Effects of Intermittent Fasting on
    Health, Aging, and Disease." *New England Journal of Medicine* 381, no. 26
    (December 26, 2019): 2541–51.

Dehejia, Vidya. "Aniconism and the Multivalence of Emblems." *Ars Orientalis*
    21 (1991): 45–66.

Di Francesco, Andrea, et al. "A Time to Fast." *Science* 362, no. 6416 (November 16,
    2018): 770–75.

Duncan, Laramie, et al. "Significant Locus and Metabolic Genetic Correlations
    Revealed in Genome-Wide Association Study of Anorexia Nervosa." *Amer-
    ican Journal of Psychiatry* 174, no. 9 (September 1, 2017): 850–58.

Eckert, Elke, et al. "A 57-Year Follow-Up Investigation and Review of the Min-

nesota Study on Human Starvation and Its Relevance to Eating Disorders."
Archives of Psychology 2, no. 3 (March 2018). https://www.researchgate
.net/publication/324507398.

Ehrenreich, Barbara. "Welcome to Cancerland." *Harper's*, November 2001, 45.

Erlanger, Stephen. "Jailed Palestinians End Strike Meant to Win Concessions." *New York Times*, September 3, 2004. https://www.nytimes.com/2004/09/03/world/mid dleeast/jailed-palestinians-end-fast-meant-to-win-concessions.html.

———. "Palestinians on Fast in Israeli Jails Struggle for Attention." *New York Times*, August 28, 2004. https://www.nytimes.com/2004/08/28/world/ palestinians-on-fast-in-israeli-jails-struggle-for-attention.html.

Falk, Candace. "Emma Goldman." Shalvi/Hyman Encyclopedia of Jewish Women. Jewish Women's Archive. https://jwa.org/encyclopedia/article/ goldman-emma.

Fell, Robin. "Marion Wallace-Dunlop: The First Suffragette Hunger Striker." UKVote100, September 22, 2017. https://ukvote100.org/2017/09/22/ marion-wallace-dunlop-the-first-suffragette-hunger-striker/.

Fenneni, Mohamed, et al. "Effects of Ramadan on Physical Capacities of Boys Fasting for the First Time." *Libyan Journal of Medicine* 9, no. 1 (September 24, 2014): 25391.

Ferretti, Ennio. "Giovanni Succi, il digiunatore di Cesenatico che ispirò Kafka." Giannella Channel. https://www.giannellachannel.info/giovanni -succi-il-digiunatore-di-cesenatico-che-ispiro-kafka/.

Finch, Martha L. "Pinched with Hunger: Partaking of Plenty." In *Eating in Eden: Food and American Utopias*. Edited by Martha L. Finch and Etta Madden. Lincoln: University of Nebraska Press, 2006.

Fink, H. R. "The Hindu Custom of 'Sitting Dharna.'" *Calcutta Review*, vol. LXII. Edited by E. Lethbridge. Calcutta: Thomas S. Smith, 1876, 37–52.

Fischer, Molly. "Milking It." *New Yorker*, March 13, 2023, 28–33.

Foley, Helene P. "The 'Female Intruder' Reconsidered: Women in Aristophanes' Lysistrata and Ecclesiazusae." *Classical Philology* 77, no. 1 (1982): 1–21. http://www.jstor.org/stable/269802.

Fontana, Luigi. "The Scientific Basis of Caloric Restriction Leading to Longer Life." *Current Opinion in Gastroenterology* 25, no. 2 (March 2009): 144–50.

Forcen, Fernando Espi. "Anorexia Mirabilis: The Practice of Fasting by Saint Catherine of Siena in the Late Middle Ages." *American Journal of Psychiatry* 170, no. 4 (April 2013): 370–71.

Friend, Tad. "The Hard Sell." *New Yorker*, August 8, 2022, 30–41.

Fuller, P. M., et al. "Differential Rescue of Light- and Food-Entrainable Circadian Rhythms." *Science* 320, no. 5879 (May 23, 2008): 1074–77.

Gertner, Jon. "The Calorie-Restriction Experiment." *New York Times*, October 7, 2009. https://www.nytimes.com/2009/10/11/magazine/11Calories-t.html.

Girotto, Eleonora. "Russian Police Arrest Demonstrator Protesting with Blank Sign." *Independent*, May 13, 2022. https://www.independent.co.uk/tv /news/russia-protest-war-blank-sign-ve9882053.

Gooldin, Sigal. "Fasting Women, Living Skeletons and Hunger Artists: Spectacles of Body and Miracles at the Turn of a Century." *Body and Society* 9, no. 2 (June 2003): 27–53.

Grabowska, Wioleta, et al. "Sirtuins, a Promising Target in Slowing Down the Ageing Process." *Biogerontology* 18, no. 4 (2017): 447–76.

Grant, Kevin. "British Suffragettes and the Russian Method of Hunger Strike." *Comparative Studies in Society and History* 53, no. 1 (2011): 113–43.

Griffith, R. Marie. "Apostles of Abstinence: Fasting and Masculinity during the Progressive Era." *American Quarterly* 52, no. 4 (December 2000): 599–638.

Gudden, Jip, et al. "The Effects of Intermittent Fasting on Brain and Cognitive Function." *Nutrients* 13, no. 9 (September 2021): 3166.

Gull, William Withey. "Anorexia Nervosa." *Transactions of the Clinical Society,* vol. VII. London: Longmans Green, 1874, 22–27.

———. "Clinical Notes: Anorexia Nervosa." *Lancet*, March 16, 1888, 516–17.

Halonen, Jaana I. "Road Traffic Noise Is Associated with Increased Cardiovascular Morbidity and Mortality and All-Cause Mortality in London." *European Heart Journal* 36, no. 39 (October 2015): 2653–61.

Hamilton J. P., et al. "Default-Mode and Task-Positive Network Activity in Major Depressive Disorder: Implications for Adaptive and Maladaptive Rumination." *Biological Psychiatry* 70, no. 4 (August 15, 2011): 327–33.

Harrison, D. E., and J. R. Archer. "Natural Selection for Extended Longevity from Food Restriction." *Growth, Development, and Aging Journal* 53, nos. 1–2 (Spring–Summer 1989): 3.

Herring, Tiana. "The Research Is Clear: Solitary Confinement Causes Long-Lasting Harm." Prison Policy Initiative, December 8, 2020. https://www .prisonpolicy.org/blog/2020/12/08/solitary_symposium/.

Hoffman, Benjamin U., and Ellen A. Lumpkin. "A Gut Feeling." *Science* 361, no. 6408 (September 21, 2018): 1203.

Hopkins, E. Washburn. "On the Hindu Custom of Dying to Redress a Grievance." *Journal of the American Oriental Society* 21 (1900): 146–59.

Hoshur, Shohret. English version by Roseanne Gerin. "Chinese Officials Restrict Number of Uyghurs Observing Ramadan." Radio Free Asia, April 1, 2022. https://www.rfa.org/english/news/uyghur/ramadan -restrictions-04012022173039.html.

Jerome. "Letter CVII to Laeta." Umilta. http://www.umilta.net/jerome.html.

Jungkuntz, Richard P. "Christian Approval of Epicureanism." *Church History* 31, no. 3 (September 1962): 279–93.

Kaplan, Lawrence. "A Utopia during the Progressive Era: The Helicon Home Colony, 1906–1907." *American Studies* 25, no. 2 (1984): 59–73. https://journals.ku.edu/amsj/article/view/2567.

Kirste, Imke, et al. "Is Silence Golden? Effects of Auditory Stimuli and Their Absence on Adult Hippocampal Neurogenesis." *Brain Structure & Function* 220, no. 2 (2015): 1221–28. https://www.ncbi.nlm.nih.gov/pmc/articles/PMC4087081/.

Komaki, G., et al. "Orexin-A and Leptin Change Inversely in Fasting Non-Obese Subjects." *European Journal of Endocrinology* 144, no. 6 (June 2001): 645–51.

Korbonits, Márta, et al. "Refeeding David Blaine—Studies after a 44-Day Fast." *New England Journal of Medicine* 353 (November 24, 2005): 2306–07.

Kristeva, Julia. "Stabat Mater." Translated by Arthur Goldhammer. *Poetics Today* 6, nos. 1– 2 (1985): 133–52.

Lacertosa, M. "Sense Perception in the *Zhuangzi* 莊子." *Philosophy Compass* 17, no. 1 (January 2022): e12798.

Lennon, Joseph. "Fasting for the Public: Irish and Indian Sources of Marion Wallace Dunlop's 1909 Hunger Strike," 20–39. In *Enemies of Empire: New Perspectives on Imperialism, Literature and History*. Edited by Eóin Flannery and Angus Mitchell. Dublin: Four Courts Press, 2007.

Lev, Dov. "The Rabbinic Fast Days." Aish. https://aish.com/41-rabbinic-fast-days-2/.

Levine, Nathan H. "Barlaam and Josaphat." *Brill's Encyclopedia of Buddhism*, vol. 2. Leiden, Netherlands: Koninklijke Brill NV, 2019, 43.

Lincoln, Abraham. "A Proclamation for a National Day of Humiliation, Fasting, and Prayer!" Library of Congress. https://www.loc.gov/resource/lprbscsm.scsm0265/.

Liu, Deying, et al. "Calorie Restriction with or without Time-Restricted Eating in Weight Loss." *New England Journal of Medicine* 386 (April 2022): 1495–1504. https://www.nejm.org/doi/full/10.1056/NEJMoa2114833.

Lowe, D. A., et al. "Effects of Time-Restricted Eating on Weight Loss and Other Metabolic Parameters in Women and Men with Overweight and Obesity: The TREAT Randomized Clinical Trial." *JAMA Internal Medicine* 180, no. 11 (November 1, 2020): 1491–99.

Mackie, John. "A Century Ago, the Komagata Maru Arrived in Vancouver and Challenged Racist Policies." *Vancouver Sun*, May 21, 2014. https://

vancouversun.com/news/metro/a-century-ago-the-komagata-maru-ar
rived-in-vancouver-and-challenged-racist-policies.

Maclean, P. S., et al. "Biology's Response to Dieting: The Impetus for Weight
Regain." *American Journal of Physiology* 301, no. 3 (September 2011):
R581–600. https://www.ncbi.nlm.nih.gov/pmc/articles/PMC3174765/.

Manchishi, Stephen Malunga, et al. "Effect of Caloric Restriction on Depression."
Journal of Cellular and Molecular Medicine 22, no. 5 (May 2018): 2528–35.
https://pubmed.ncbi.nlm.nih.gov/29465826/.

Mann, Traci, et al. "Medicare's Search for Effective Obesity Treatments: Diets
Are Not the Answer." *American Psychology* 62, no. 3 (April 2007): 220–33.

Manon, Mathias. "Autointoxication and Historical Precursors of the
Microbiome-Gut-Brain Axis." *Microbial Ecology in Health and Disease* 29,
no. 2 (November 27, 2018): 1548249.

Marlow, Shelly. "Why Eileen Myles Spent a Week Living on the Streets of New
York." *Hyperallergic*, September 23, 2016. https://hyperallergic.com/324819
/why-eileen-myles-spent-a-week-living-on-the-streets-of-new-york/.

Martin, Michel. "NYC Taxi Drivers Enter Day 11 of Hunger Strike for Medallion Debt Relief." *All Things Considered*, NPR, October 30, 2021. https://
www.npr.org/2021/10/30/1050850701/nyc-taxi-drivers-enter-day-11-of
-hunger-strike-for-medallion-debt-relief.

Matias, I., et al. "Endocannabinoids Measurement in Human Saliva as Potential
Biomarker of Obesity." *PLoS One* 7, no. 7 (2012): e42399.

McDonald, Roger B., and Jon J. Ramsey. "Honoring Clive McKay and 75 Years
of Calorie Restriction Research." *Journal of Nutrition* 140, no. 7 (July 2010):
1205–10. https://www.ncbi.nlm.nih.gov/pmc/articles/PMC2884327/.

McGrath, Elena. "Housewives against Dictatorship: The Bolivian Hunger
Strike of 1978." Nursing Clio, December 29, 2016. https://nursingclio
.org/2016/12/29/housewives-against-dictatorship-the-bolivian-hunger-
strike-of-1978/.

McGregor, Steve. "Argonne Anti-Jet-Lag Diet Helps Summer Travelers Beat
Jet Lag." Argonne National Laboratory, May 16, 2008. https://www.anl
.gov/article/argonne-antijetlag-diet-helps-summer-travelers-beat-jet-lag.

Mehanna, H. M., et al. "Refeeding Syndrome: What It Is, and How to Prevent
and Treat It." *BMJ* 336, no. 7659 (June 28, 2008): 1495–98.

Mehta, Diane. "On Chanting and Consciousness." *Harvard Divinity Bulletin*, Spring/Summer 2021. https://bulletin.hds.harvard.edu/on-chant
ing-and-consciousness/.

Michiaki, Iwahana. "'Sokushinbutsu': Japan's Buddhist Mummies." Nippon.com,
January 26, 2022. https://www.nippon.com/en/japan-topics/g02008/.

Miller, Stephen. "Charles F. Ehret (1923–2007): Scientist Offered Solution to Victims of Jet Lag." *Wall Street Journal*, March 10, 2007. https://www.wsj com/articles/SB117349084761632907.

Minardi, Margot. "The Boston Inoculation Controversy of 1721–1722: An Incident in the History of Race." *William and Mary Quarterly* 61, no. 1 (January 2004): 47–76.

Mirzayan, Anna. "Why Does the Art World Hate Fat People?" *Hyperallergic*, October 19, 2022. https://hyperallergic.com/771042/why-does-the-art -world-hate-fat-people/.

Mishan, Ligaya. "In a Starving World, Is Eating Well Unethical?" *T: The New York Times Style Magazine*, March 18, 2022. https://www.nytimes .com/2022/03/18/t-magazine/indulgence-starvation-food-inequality .html.

Mogelson, Luke. "Everyone Is a Target." *New Yorker*, July 23, 2022. https:// www.newyorker.com/magazine/2022/08/01/the-desperate-lives-inside -ukraines-dead-cities.

Moncrieff, J., et al. "The Serotonin Theory of Depression: A Systematic Umbrella Review of the Evidence." *Molecular Psychiatry* 381 (July 2022): 1–14.

Morgenthaler, Von W. "Eine Hysterika zu Beginn des 17. Jahrhunderts." *Archiv für Geschichte der Medizin* 18, no. 2 (June 15, 1926): 196–201.

Moyer, Johanna B. "The Food Police: Sumptuary Prohibitions on Food in the Reformation." In *Food and Faith in Christian Culture*. Edited by Ken Albala and Trudy Ede. New York: Columbia University Press, 2011.

Neal, E. G., et al. "The Ketogenic Diet for the Treatment of Childhood Epilepsy: A Randomised Controlled Trial." *Lancet Neurology* 7, no. 6 (June 2008): 500–506.

Nemec, John. "Dying to Redress the Grievance of Another: On Prāya/Prāyopa-veśa(na) in Kalhaṇa's Rājataraṅgiṇī." *Journal of the American Oriental Society* 137, no. 1 (January–March 2017): 43–61.

Neuringer, Alan, and Walter Englert. "Epicurus and B. F. Skinner: In Search of the Good Life." *Journal of the Experimental Analysis of Behavior* 107, no. 1 (January 2017): 21–33.

Nussbaum, Martha. "Man Overboard." *New Republic*, June 22, 2006. https:// newrepublic.com/article/64199/man-overboard.

Owen, Tess. "Hundreds of Immigrants Detained in a Private Prison Have Gone on Hunger Strike." *Vice*, April 14, 2017. https://www.vice.com/en /article/5958m5/hundreds-of-immigrants-detained-in-a-private-prison -have-gone-on-hunger-strike.

Perrone, Anna, et al. "Advanced Glycation End Products (AGEs): Biochemistry,

Signaling, Analytical Methods, and Epigenetic Effects." *Oxidative Medicine and Cellular Activity* 2020, no. 3 (March 2020): 1–18.

Pieslak, Jonathan. "Cranking Up the Volume: Music as a Tool of Torture." *Global Dialogue (Online)* 12, no. 1 (Winter, 2010): 1–11.

Poulain, Alexandra. "*The King's Threshold, Calvary, The Death of Cuchulain*: Yeats's Passion Plays." *Yeats's Mask: Yeats Annual*, no. 19. Edited by Margaret Mills Harper and Warwick Gould. Cambridge, UK: Open Book, 2013, 49–63. http://books.openedition.org/obp/1412.

Power, Camilla. "Lysistrata: The Ritual Logic of the Sex-Strike," Academia, 2000. https://www.academia.edu/24291698/Lysistrata_the_Ritual_Logic_of_the_Sex-strike.

Prescott, Bonnie. "Study Identifies Food-Related Clock in the Brain." *Harvard Gazette*, May 19 2008. https://news.harvard.edu/gazette/story/2008/05/study-identifies-food-related-clock-in-the-brain.

Quinn, James. "Boycott, Charles Cunningham." *Dictionary of Irish Biography*. Last revised October 2009. https://www.dib.ie/biography/boycott-charles-cunningham-a0825.

Rampling, D. "Ascetic Ideals and Anorexia Nervosa." *Journal of Psychiatric Research* 19, nos. 2–3 (1985): 89–94.

Redman, Leanne M. "Caloric Restriction in Humans: Impact on Physiological, Psychological, and Behavioral Outcomes." *Antioxidants and Redox Signaling* 14, no. 2 (January 2011): 275–87.

Redman, L. M., et al. "Metabolic Slowing and Reduced Oxidative Damage with Sustained Caloric Restriction Support the Rate of Living and Oxidative Damage Theories of Aging." *Cell Metabolism* 27, no. 4 (April 3, 2018): 805–15.e4.

Reed, Robert Charles. "Decreation as Substitution: Reading Simone Weil through Levinas." *Journal of Religion* 93, no. 1 (January 2013): 25–40.

Reiter, Russel J., et al. "Anti-Warburg Effect of Melatonin: A Proposed Mechanism to Explain Its Inhibition of Multiple Diseases." *International Journal of Molecular Sciences* 22, no. 2 (January 2021): 764.

Rigaud, D., et al. "A Paradoxical Increase in Resting Energy Expenditure in Malnourished Patients Near Death: The King Penguin Syndrome." *American Journal of Clinical Nutrition* 72, no. 2 (August 2000): 355–60.

Rogal, Samuel J. "Pills for the Poor: John Wesley's Primitive Physick." *Yale Journal of Biological Medicine* 51, no. 1 (January–February 1978): 81–90.

Rollins, Hyder E. "Notes on Some English Accounts of Miraculous Fasts." *Journal of American Folklore* 34, no. 134 (October–December 1921): 357–76.

Rosenberg, Carol. "Doctor Describes and Denounces C.I.A. Practice of 'Rectal Feeding' of Prisoners." *New York Times*, February 24, 2023. https://www .nytimes.com/2023/02/24/us/politics/cia-torture-guantanamo-nashiri -doctor.html.

Ross, Jack L. "Anorexia Nervosa: An Overview." *Bulletin of the Menninger Clinic* 41, no. 5 (September 1, 1977): 418–36.

Russell, G. F. M., and J. Treasure. "The Modern History of Anorexia Nervosa: An Interpretation of Why the Illness Has Changed." *Annals of the New York Academy of Sciences* 575, no. 1 (December 1989): 13–30.

Safi, Michael. "How Love and a Taste of Honey Brought One Indian Woman's 16-Year Hunger Strike to an End." *Guardian*, November 11, 2018. https:// www.theguardian.com/world/2018/nov/11/irom-sharmila-love-story -worlds-longest-hunger-strike.

Sanidopoulos, John. "Saint Theodora of Alexandria, Who Struggled in the Guise of a Man." Orthodox Christianity Then and Now, September 11, 2015. https://www.johnsanidopoulos.com/2015/09/saint-theodora-of -alexandria-who.html.

Semmes, Clovis E. "Entrepreneur of Health: Dick Gregory, Black Consciousness, and the Human Potential Movement." *Journal of African American Studies* 16, no. 3 (2012): 537–49.

Shapin Steven. "Was Luigi Cornaro a Dietary Expert?" *Journal of the History of Medicine and Allied Sciences* 73, no. 2 (April 1, 2018): 135–49.

Shaw, Teresa M. "Practical, Theoretical and Cultural Tracings in Late Ancient Asceticism." In *Asceticism*. Edited by Vincent L. Wimbush and Richard Valantasis. New York: Oxford University Press, 1995), 75–79.

Shen, Chun, et al. "Associations of Social Isolation and Loneliness with Later Dementia." *Neurology* 99, no. 2 (July 2022): e164–e175.

Shindyapina, Anastasia V., et al. "Rapamycin Treatment during Development Extends Lifespan and Healthspan of Male Mice and Daphnia Magna." *Science Advances* 8, no. 37 (September 2022): https://doi .org/10.1101/2022.02.18.481092.

Snyder, Allan. "Explaining and Inducing Savant Skills: Privileged Access to Lower Level, Less-Processed Information." *Philosophical Transactions of the Royal Society* 364, no. 1522 (May 27, 2009): 1399–1405.

Srivastava, M., et al. "The Trichoplax Genome and the Nature of Placozoans." *Nature* 454 (August 2008): 955–60.

St-Hilaire, A., et al. "A Prospective Study of Effects of Prenatal Maternal Stress on Later Eating-Disorder Manifestations in Affected Offspring: Preliminary

Indications Based on the Project Ice Storm Cohort." *International Journal of Eating Disorders* 48, no. 5 (July 2015): 512–16.

Stewart, William K., and L. W. Fleming. "Features of a Successful Therapeutic Fast of 382 Days' Duration." *Postgraduate Medical Journal* 49, no. 569 (March 1973): 203–9.

Sukel, Kayt. "The Power of Quiet: The Mental and Physical Health Benefits of Silence." *New Scientist*, August 10, 2022. https://www.newscientist.com/article/mg25533990-700-the-power-of-quiet-the-mental-and-physical-health-benefits-of-silence/.

Tamney, Joseph. "Fasting and Modernization." *Journal for the Scientific Study of Religion* 19, no. 2 (June 1980): 129–37.

Taylor, Peter. "Bobby Sands: The Hunger Strike That Changed the Course of N Ireland's Conflict." BBC News, May 1, 2021. https://www.bbc.com/news/stories-56937259.

Taylor, Robert Lewis. "Physical Culture: Weakness Is a Crime." *New Yorker*, October 21, 1950, 39–52.

Thornton, Mark. "What Caused the Irish Potato Famine?" *Free Market* 16, no. 4, April 1998. https://mises.org/library/what-caused-irish-potato-famine.

Tillet, Salamishah, and Elizabeth Paton. "A Hunger Strike Makes Headlines before Milan Fashion Week Begins." *New York Times*, February 13, 2023. https://www.nytimes.com/2023/02/13/fashion/stella-jean-diversity-milan-fashion-week.html/.

U.S. Senate Select Committee on Intelligence. "Committee Study of the Central Intelligence Agency's Detention and Interrogation Program." Executive Summary. Approved December 13, 2021.

Watson, Bruce. "The Strange Tale of a World-Changing Fitness and Sleaze Titan." *Esquire*, September 9, 2013. https://www.esquire.com/news-politics/news/a23610/strange-tale-historic-fitness-guru-bernarr-macfadden/.

Weindruch, Richard. "Calorie Restriction and Aging." *Scientific American*, December 1, 2006. https://www.scientificamerican.com/article/calorie-restriction-and-aging/.

Whorton, James C. "'Physiologic Optimism': Horace Fletcher and Hygienic Ideology in Progressive America." *Bulletin of the History of Medicine* 55, no. 1 (Spring 1981): 59–87.

Willcox, D. C., et al. "Caloric Restriction and Human Longevity: What Can We Learn from the Okinawans?" *Biogerontology* 7 (2006): 174–75.

Wilson, Timothy D., et al. "Just Think: The Challenges of a Disengaged Mind." *Science* 345, no. 6192 (July 4, 2014): 75–77.

Wilson, Woodrow. "Address to the Salesmanship Conference, Detroit, Michigan." American Presidency Project, July 10, 1916. https://www.presidency.ucsb.edu/documents/address-the-salesmanship-congress-detroit-michigan.

Wimalaratana, Bellanwila Thera. "Buddhism and the Brahma Concept." Buddha-Sasana, August 31, 2005. https://www.budsas.org/ebud/ebdha321.htm.

Witte, Jessica. "The Welsh 'Fasting Girls' and Anorexia Nervosa in the Victorian Medical Imagination." *Journal of Literature and Science* 13, no. 2 (December 2020): 20–37.

Wu, Susanne. "Fasting Triggers Stem Cell Regeneration of Damaged, Old Immune System." USC News, June 5, 2014. https://news.usc.edu/63669/fasting-triggers-stem-cell-regeneration-of-damaged-old-immune-system/.

Xiaobo, Liu, et al. "Tiananmen Square Hunger Strike Declaration." Translated by Chong-Pin Lin. *World Affairs* 152, no. 3 (Winter 1989–90): 148–50.

Xing, Fan, et al. "The Anti-Warburg Effect Elicited by the cAMP-PGC1α Pathway Drives Differentiation of Glioblastoma Cells into Astrocytes." *Cell Reports* 18, no. 2 (January 10, 2017): 468–81.

Zhang, Yifan, et al. "The Effects of Calorie Restriction in Depression and Potential Mechanisms." *Current Neuropharmacology* 13, no. 4 (July 2015): 536–42. https://www.ncbi.nlm.nih.gov/pmc/articles/PMC4790398/.

Zhu, Y., et al. "Metabolic Regulation of Sirtuins upon Fasting and the Implication for Cancer." *Current Opinion in Oncology* 25, no. 6 (November 2013): 630–36.

NO LISTED AUTHOR

"A Health Clinic Was Ordered Friday to Pay $873,000." UPI, September 17, 1982. https://www.upi.com/Archives/1982/09/17/A-health-clinic-was-ordered-Friday-to-pay-873000/8663401083200/.

"Alexandrina Maria da Costa (1904–1955)." Holy See. https://www.vatican.va/news_services/liturgy/saints/ns_lit_doc_20040425_da-costa_en.html.

"Alice Paul Describes Force Feeding." Miller NAWSA Suffrage Scrapbooks, 1897–1911. Library of Congress. https://www.loc.gov/resource/rbcmil.scrp6014301/.

"AT 81 STARTS 80-DAY FAST; Dr. Tanner Says People Eat Too Much, and Essays to Prove It." *New York Times*, February 9, 1911. https://www.nytimes.com/1911/02/09/archives/at-81-starts-80day-fast-dr-tanner-says-people-eat-too-much-and.html.

"Blaring Music Used to Abuse War Prisoners." CBS News, December 9, 2008. https://www.cbsnews.com/news/blaring-music-used-to-abuse-war-prisoners/.

"Breaks 31 Days' Fast." *New York Times*, May 15, 1912. https://www.nytimes
    .com/1912/05/16/archives/breaks-31-days-fast-levanzin-lost-weight
    -but-felt-better-mentally.html.

"British Ban IRA Remarks from TV, Radio." *Chicago Tribune*, October 20, 1988.
    https://www.chicagotribune.com/news/ct-xpm-1988-10-20-8802080976
    -story.html.

*Burden of Disease from Environmental Noise: Quantification of Healthy Life Years
    Lost in Europe.* Copenhagen: World Health Organization, 2011.

"Eating Disorders." National Institute of Mental Health. https://www.nimh.nih
    .gov/health/statistics/eating-disorders.

"Emergency Department Visits for Suspected Suicide Attempts among Persons
    Aged 12–25 Years before and during the COVID-19 Pandemic—United
    States, January 2019–May 2021." Centers for Disease Control, June 18,
    2021. https://www.cdc.gov/mmwr/volumes/70/wr/mm7024e1.htm?s
    _cid=mm7024e1_w.

"Five Things to Know about How Orexin Affects Stress Resilience." Children's
    Hospital of Philadelphia, June 18, 2021. https://www.research.chop.edu
    /cornerstone-blog/five-things-to-know-about-how-orexin-affects-stress
    -resilience/.

"Japanese Monk Completes Feat of Extreme Fasting, First in Eight Years." *San
    Diego Union Tribune*, October 21, 2015. https://www.sandiegouniontri
    bune.com/en-espanol/sdhoy-japanese-monk-completes-feat-of-extreme
    -fasting-2015oct21-story.html#:~:text=A%2041yearold%20Japanese%20
    Buddhist%20monk,and%20sleep%20for%20nine%20days.

"Levanzin's New Charges." *New York Times*, May 21, 1912. https://www.nytimes
    .com/1912/05/22/archives/levanzins-new-charges-fasting-professor-says
    -he-was-nearly-killed.html. See also "Torture in Starving Test." *New York
    Times*, May 20, 1912. https://www.nytimes.com/1912/05/21/archives
    /torture-in-starving-test-levanzin-complains-of-treatment-at.html.

"Provisional Drug Overdose Death Counts." National Center for Health Sta-
    tistics, CDC, December 5, 2021. https://www.cdc.gov/nchs/nvss/vsrr
    /drug-overdose-data.htm.

"Roy Walford, 79; Eccentric UCLA Scientist Touted Food Restriction." *Los
    Angeles Times*, May 1, 2004. https://www.latimes.com/archives/la-xpm
    -2004-may-01-me-walford1-story.html.

"Succi, the Fasting Man." *Scientific American*, June 16, 1888, 377. https://
    archive.org/details/scientific-american-1888-06-16/page/n10
    /mode/1up?view=theater&q=giovanni+succi.

"Sustainable Management of Food Basics." United States Environmental Pro-

tection Agency. https://www.epa.gov/sustainable-management-food
/sustainable-management-food-basics.

"Tenth Anniversary of the Devastating 1998 Ice Storm in the Northeast." National
Weather Service, January 5, 2008. https://www.weather.gov/media/btv
/events/IceStorm1998.pdf.

"The Economics of Thinness." *Economist*, December 20, 2022. https://www.econ
omist.com/christmas-specials/2022/12/20/the-economics-of-thinness.

"Turkish Lawyer Dies after 238-Day Hunger Strike." Agence France Presse,
August 28, 2020. https://www.france24.com/en/20200828-turkish-law
yer-dies-after-238-day-hunger-strike.

"Wanting a New Prophet: Somebody to Truly Fix the Day of Tanner's Death."
New York Times, July 13, 1880. https://timesmachine.nytimes.com/times
machine/1880/07/13/109301031.html?pageNumber=8.

"Werkzeuge." Inspirationist Archive. https://inspirationistarchive.org/zeu
gnisse-testimonies/who-were-the-werkzeuge/.

"Yo-Yo Dieting May Increase Women's Heart Disease Risk." American Heart Association, March 7, 2019. https://newsroom.heart.org
/news/yo-yo-dieting-may-increase-womens-heart-disease-risk. Also
in ScienceDaily, March 7, 2019. https://www.sciencedaily.com/re
leases/2019/03/190307161902.htm.

INTERVIEWS

Bos, Dr. Michael, reverend of the Marble Collegiate Church of New York City,
June 15, 2021.

Campion, Paul, activist, Sunrise Movement, February 26, 2021.

Díaz, Dr. Luz Marina, director of religious education, Church of St. Francis
Xavier, New York City, and director of the Spiritual Direction Practicum
at Fordham University's Graduate School of Religion and Religious Education, November 16, 2021.

Devji, Faisal, professor of Indian History at the University of Oxford, May 12,
2021.

Francis, Sahar, director of Addameer, August 21, 2022.

Hermes, Dr. Britt Marie, March 24, 2023.

Holmes, Brooke, the Robert F. Goheen Professor in the Humanities and professor of classics at Princeton University, April 20, 2022.

Krishnamurthy, Prem, designer, author, and curator, April 9, 2021.

Lancaster, Wendell, senior pastor, the Greater Hood Memorial A.M.E. Zion
Church of New York City, May 18, 2022.

Lu, Cuong, Buddhist teacher and author based in the Netherlands, founder of the Mind-Only Institute, March 27, 2021.

Novella, Dr. Steven, associate professor of neurology at Yale School of Medicine, October 26, 2022.

Orfield, Steve, of Orfield Labs, Minneapolis, October 19, 2021.

Portland, Kristen, executive director of the National Association of Anorexia Nervosa and Associated Disorders, January 24, 2022.

Restrepo, Sandy, Esq., Colectiva Legal del Pueblo, May 2, 2023.

San-Chez, André, activist and educator, June 29, 2022.

Sheehan, Pat, Sinn Féin legislative representative for West Belfast, August 17, 2022.

Skolnik, Heidi, MS, CDN, FACSM, nutritionist and exercise physiologist, April 29, 2021.

Slahi, Mohamedou Ould, former prisoner at Guantánamo Bay, November 18, 2021.

Steiger, Dr. Howard, director of the Eating Disorders Program at Douglas Mental Health University Institute, and professor of psychiatry at McGill University, April 3, 2022.

Strassfeld, Rabbi Michael, of the Society for the Advancement of Judaism, May 26, 2021.

Webb, Shaykh Suhaib, former imam of the Islamic Society of Boston Cultural Center, May 25, 2021.

Zalmanov, Rabbi Eliezer, codirector of Chabad of Northwest Indiana, April 30, 2021.

Index

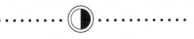

Page numbers in *italics* refer to images.

Abd El Fattah, Alaa, 155
absence, 2, 3, 11, 15, 19, 23, 29, 33, 84, 113
acetone, 49
Achilles, 25, 79
acidosis, 55
Adnan, Khader, 144–45
Afro-American Council, 108
AGEs (advanced glycation end products), 54
Aggarwal, Brooke, 60
aging, 51, 64, 66, 72–74
Ahmed, Ruhal, 18
air, living on (breatharianism), 177–79, 188
Albala, Ken, 89
Alcott, Louisa May, 165
Alcott, William Andrus, 165
alternative medicine, 166, 179, 185
Alvars, 192–93
anechoic chambers, 3–5, 7–10, 15–16
anorexia, viii, 53, 109, 160, 163, 192–204
    mirabilis, viii, 200–204
Antal, 192–93, 201
Anthony, St., 90–91
Antisthenes, 33–35
apoptosis, 74
Appel, Jacob M., 150
Aquinas, Thomas, 98
Aristides, Aelius, 44–45
Aristophanes, 33
Aristotle, 11, 36, 45, 177
Armed Forces Special Powers Act (AFSPA),
    118–19
Asbury, Herbert, 171
asceticism, ix, 18–21, 23–42, 75–109, 135
    in Buddhism, 20, 28–31, 34
    in Christianity, 77–82, 87–109, 116, 157
    in Greece, 24–27, 32–37, 96
    in Islam, 77, 101–4
    in Judaism, 76–87, 96, 102, 103
    women's practices of, 91–95, 97, 99–100
Ashe, Thomas, 132–33, *133*
Ashoka, Emperor, 31
askēsis, 24–25, 41
    see also asceticism
Asquith, Herbert, 130
Athenaeus of Naucratis, 37
Athens, 33, 35, 38
Atkins, Humphrey, 138–39
Atlantic, 5
atoms, 37–40, 208
ATP (adenosine triphosphate), 62–64
Augustine, St., 11, 95–96, 98
automaticity, 16–17, 19

Bacon, Roger, 177–78
Bakunin, Mikhail, 125
Balfour, Arthur, 125
Banerjee, Mamata, 119
Barker, Elizabeth "Lizzie," 130
Barlaam and Josaphat, 31–32
Barnum, P. T., 172, 185
"Bartleby, the Scrivener" (Melville), xi, 110,
    135–36
Basil of Caesarea, St., 92
Bauer, Felice, 177
BDNF (brain-derived neurotropic factor),
    52–53
Beard, George, 196
Beirão, Luaty, 153

Bell, Rudolph M., 100, 200, 201
Benedict, St., 98
Bentham, Jeremy, 40
Bernard, St., 11
BHB (beta-hydroxybutyrate), 52, 55, 80
Bible, 78–84, 90, 117
  Leviticus, 102
  Proverbs, 76, 101
  Song of Solomon, 94
Biden, Joe, 143
bigotry, 182
Biosphere 2, 71, 166
Black August, 140
Blaesilla, 95
Blaine, David, 174
blood pressure, 17–18, 55, 59, 71
blood sugar, 17, 49, 54, 55, 71
Bloody Sunday, 138
body temperature, 54, 55
Bogdanov, Alexander, 111
Bolivia, 152–53
Book of Five Rings, The (Miyamoto), xiii–xiv
Bos, Michael, 109
botulism, 184
Bownde, Nicholas, 106
Boyarin, Daniel, 77–78, 94
Boycott, Charles, 121
boycotts, 121, 137
  California grape, 149
brain, 18, 47–49, 53, 56
  automatization in, 16–17
  default mode network in, 6
  gray matter in, 12
brain-derived neurotropic factor (BDNF),
  52–53
breatharianism, 177–79, 188
Brief History of Time, A (Hawking), 111
Brillat-Savarin, Jean Anthelme, 2
Brod, Max, 176
Brooklyn, 5
Browne, Thomas, 10
Bruch, Hilde, 194–95, 197
Buchinger, Otto, 180
Buchinger Wilhelmi clinics, 180
Buddha, xii, 19, 28–32, 37, 38, 93, 113, 115,
  136, 207
  Brahmavihārā of, 29–30
  middle path of, 28–29, 93, 207
Buddhism, xii, xv, 13, 19–20, 25, 32, 113,
  149, 209–10
  asceticism in, 20, 28–31, 34

Theravāda, 30
Zen, 13, 29, 96
Bukovsky, Vladimir, 111, 145–46
Bush, George W., 206
Bynum, Caroline Walker, 99

cachexia, 55
cadaverine, 184
Cage, John, 9–11, 15, 71
CALERIE studies, 72–73
calorie restriction (CR), 51, 54, 57, 66,
  70–73
calories, 56, 188
Calvin, John, 105
Calvinism, 166
Campbell, Joseph, 4
Campion, Paul, 143–44
cancer, 62–63, 192
capitalism, xiv, 6–7, 41, 135, 166, 192
carbohydrates, 48, 54
cardiovascular disease, 17–18, 51, 54, 60, 62
Cargill, Kima, 61
Cartwright, Thomas, 105–6
Cassian, John, 96–97
Cat and Mouse Act, 130
Catherine of Siena, St., 100, 200–202, 201
Catherine of Veltlin, 163
Catholicism, 40, 100, 105, 106, 134, 149,
  200, 208
Catholic Worker Movement, 141
Cato, 76
Charbonnier, Sébastien, xiii, 16, 80
Chavez, Cesar, 54, 143, 146–50, 148, 155
Chernin, Kim, 157
China, 3
  Muslims in, 103–4
  Tiananmen Square demonstrations in,
    122–23
Christianity, xiii, 11, 19, 27, 31–32, 34,
    39–40, 112, 113, 116, 117, 165, 169,
    185
  asceticism in, 77–82, 87–109, 116, 157
  Catholicism, 40, 100, 105, 106, 134, 149,
    200, 208
  Lent in, xv, 58, 98, 102, 103, 124, 208
  Protestantism, 41, 105–7, 109, 162, 165,
    178
  Puritanism, 40, 41, 86, 105–7, 166
  Reformation in, 104–5
Christopher, Roy, 5, 7
Churchill, Winston, 126

CIA, 18, 150
Cicero, 39
circadian rhythms, 46–47
civil rights, 140–41
Collins, Michael, 132
concentration camp inmates, 128–29
Confucius, Confucians, 13–14, 18, 21,
   33–34
consciousness, 12, 111
Constantine, Emperor, 93
consumption and consumerism, ix, xi, xiii,
   33, 34, 41, 72, 76, 97, 109, 157, 164,
   205–7, 210
Coptic Christians, xiii
Cordus, Aulus Cremutius, 115
Cornaro, Luigi, 157–59, 161–62, 164–65,
   168, 180
Cornwallis, Lord, 120
cortisol, 17
COVID-19 pandemic, 12, 194
Crosby, Sondra, 150–51
Crossan, John Dominic, 81
Cynics, 33–36

da Costa, Alexandrina Maria, 203–4
Daily Mail, 125
Daniel, 79–80
Dante Alighieri, 39
Daoism, 13
Davis, Angela, 140
Day, Dorothy, 141
death, xiv, 37, 39
   suicide, xiv, 12, 101, 113, 134, 190, 191,
      209
death from fasting, 19, 56, 85, 98, 164, 179,
   188, 202, 209
   as choice in the elderly and sick, 190–91
   in hunger strikes, 115, 122, 123, 129,
      131–34, 138, 139, 145
   in prāya, 112–14, 116, 118
   in sallekhana, 190
de Cabo, Rafael, 50, 57
decreation, 82–83
de Flores, Angélica, 152–53
de Gaulle, Charles, 83
degrowth, 83
Deleuze, Gilles, 135–36
de Lora, Aurora, 152–53
Democritus, 37
de Paniagua, Nelly, 152–53
de Pimentel, Luzmila, 152–53

Derrida, Jacques, 29
Desai, Bhairavi, x
desire, 37, 38, 78
Despard, Charlotte, 132
Devji, Faisal, 135, 137
Dewey, Edward Hooker, 168–69, 169, 180
dharna, 118–19, 152
Diamond, Eliezer, 41, 77
dieting, 60, 160, 166, 198
digestion, 23, 27
diseases, 44, 50, 51, 53, 54, 72, 192
   cancer, 62–63, 192
   heart disease, 17–18, 51, 54, 60, 62
   naturopathy and, 179
Diogenes Laërtius, 33, 34, 37, 39, 40
Diogenes of Sinope, xiii, 34–35
dissipation, 23
doiri, 20

eating disorders, 59–60, 199–200
   see also anorexia
Eckhart, Meister, 11, 98–99
Edward VII, King, 194
Edward VIII, King, 199
Egypt, 44, 85, 97, 155
Ehrenreich, Barbara, 63
Ehret, Charles F., 46
Eid al-Fitr, 103
Ekadashi, xv
electrolytes, 58
Ellmann, Maud, 11, 166
Elm, Susanna, 92, 93
emptiness, 2, 12–14, 17, 22, 29, 44, 82, 90,
   98–99, 113, 210
endocannabinoids, 52
Enlightenment, 41, 78, 128
entropy, 13, 14, 23
Epictetus, 39
Epicurus, Epicureans, 18, 24, 36–41, 76, 87,
   88, 92, 208
epilepsy, 49–50
Erasmus, 40
Erne, John Crichton, 3rd Earl, 121
Essenes, 86–88
Ethiopia, xiii
Extinction Rebellion, 153

Fabry von Hilden, Wilhelm, 161
famine, viii, xiii, 27, 33
Fancher, Mollie, 109, 170–72, 196
farmworkers, 146–49

fashion industry and the culture of
    slenderness, 157, 198–99
fasting
    bodily effects of, ix, 43–74
    breaking a fast, 57–58, 171–72, 175
    famous fasters, x, 215
    fraudulent claims of, 156, 161–64, 170,
        172, 178–79
    intermittent, 50, 58–60
    voluntary nature of, viii, 208
Fasting Cure, The (Sinclair), 181, 184
fat, body, 49
    obesity, 60–62, 198
fat people, prejudice against, 198–99
Feynman, Richard, 70
Finch, Martha L., 106
First World War, 206
Fleigen, Eve, 160–61, *161*, 163, 170, 177
Fletcher, Horace, 182–83
focus, 19
Fontana, Luigi, 72–73
food poisoning, 184
force-feeding, 192
    of hunger strikers, 127–29, *128*, 132–33,
        136, 141, 142, 145–46, 150–51
    of slaves, 122
Foster, Richard J., 108–9
Foy, George Michelsen, 15
Francis, Sahar, 144
Francis of Assisi, St., 200
Franklin, Benjamin, 15, 158
fraud, 156, 161–64, 170, 172, 178–79
free radicals, 64, 73
French Revolution, 35–36
From Dictatorship to Democracy (Sharp), 153
fullness, 2, 12, 99

Galen, 27, 88–89, 157, 165, 177, 186
Galileo, 159
gamma hydroxybutyrate (GHB), 52
Gamson, William, 112
Gandhi, Mahatma, ix–x, 118, 120, 121, 133,
    135–37, 143, 148–49, 155
Gardner, Martin, 179
genes, 64, 73
George III, 107
Germany
    Nazi, 62–63, 128–29, 176, 180
    Weimar, 180–81
GHB (gamma hydroxybutyrate), 52
ghrelin, 47

Girma, Kidus, x
glucose, 48–50, 54, 55, 57, 59, 62
gluttony, 26, 88, 89, 96–98, 158, 165
glycogen, 49
God, 15, 29, 40, 41, 77, 78, 80–85, 88, 91,
    96, 97, 99–103, 105, 108, 109, 117,
    185, 201, 204
Goldman, Emma, 79
golodovka, 124
Gonzalez, Xochitl, 5
Graham, Sylvester, 164–65
Gray, Francine du Plessix, 83
Great Ice Storm, 199
Greece, ancient, 72, 76
    asceticism in, 24–27, 32–37, 96
    Epicureans in, 18, 24, 36–41, 76, 87, 88,
        92, 208
Greek Orthodox Church, 92
Gregory, Dick, 152
Gregory XI, Pope, 100
Grimm, Veronika E., 86
Group of 193, 124
Guantánamo Bay, 18, 150–51
Gull, Sir William, 194–96
gut, 44–46, 48, 52
Güven, Leyla, 153–54
Guyenet, Stephan, 61
Guzmán, Luis de, 19

Haggadah, 77–78
Hakewill, George, 202
Hall, Sir John, 185
Hammond, William A., 170–71, 196
Hamsun, Knut, 176
Hancock, John, 107
Harper, Stephen, 153
Harrison, William Henry, 108
Hawking, Stephen, 111
heart disease, 17–18, 51, 54, 60, 62
hedonism, 36, 39, 52
Heisenberg, Werner, 29
Hercules, 34
Hermes, Britt Marie, 179
Herodotus, 26
Hersey, Tricia, 7
Herzen, Alexander, 125
Hesychasm, 31
Hibbs, Albert, 70–71
Hildegard of Bingen, 99, 190
Hinduism, xii, xv, 29–30, 112, 113, 134–35,
    137, 149, 192, 207, 208

Hippocrates, 44, 45, 88
hitbodedut, xii
Hitler, Adolf, 63
Hobbes, Thomas, 40
Ho Chi Minh, 133–34
Holloway Prison, 126, *127*
Holmes, Brooke, 45
Horace, 40–41
hormones, 47–49, 52, 54, 55
Hornet, 166–68, *168*
Hoshur, Shohret, 104
Housewives Committee, 152–53
Hume, David, 40
humors, four, 88–89
hunger, viii, xiii, 11, 47, 48, 165
Hunger (Hamsun), 176
"Hunger Artist, A" (Kafka), 110, 173, 176
hunger artists, 169–70, 173–75, 180–81, 204
hunger strikes, ix, x, 11, 56, 114–55, 204,
    205, 207
  deaths from, 115, 122, 123, 129, 131–34,
    138, 139, 145
  force-feeding in, 127–29, *128*, 132–33,
    136, 141, 142, 145–46, 150–51
Hu Yaobang, 122
hygienic movement, 162, 165, 169, 181–82,
    187, 188

Ibn Ajibba, Ahmad, 103
Ibn Gabirol, Solomon, 99
Iliad (Homer), 25
immigrants, 142, 182, 183, 207
immune system, 62
India, xi, xiii, 112, 118–21, 135, 190, 207
inedia (breatharianism), 177–79, 188
industrialization, 135, 164, 177
Industrial Workers of the World (IWW),
    130
Inspirationist Awakening, 178
insulin, 58, 59
Ireland, xi, xiii, 116–17, 119–21, 130–34,
    137–40
Irish Republican Army (IRA), 133, 137–40
Irish Volunteers, 132
Islam, xv, 31, 103
  asceticism in, 77, 101–4
  in China, 103–4
  Eid al-Fitr in, 103
  Ramadan in, xv, 53, 58–59, 101–4, 151,
    207
Israel, 144–45

Jackson, George, 140
Jackson, Michael, 152
Jacob, Sarah, 109, 164, 170
Jainism, 190
James, Henry, 183
James, William, 183
Japan, 112
Jarry, Alfred, 186
Jefferson, Thomas, 107
Jennings, Isaac, 165–66
Jerome of Stridon, xii, 93–95, 100, 210
Jesuits, 19, 32
Jesus, 78–82, 88, 95, 99, 105, 117, 201
jet lag, 46–47
John the Baptist, 81, 82, 87
Josaphat, 31–32
Josephus, 86
Judaism, xii, xv, 31, 112, 191
  asceticism in, 76–87, 96, 102, 103
  Yom Kippur in, xv, 79, 85, 102, 103
Judas Iscariot, 89
Jung, Carl, 178
Jungle, The (Sinclair), 181, 183, 184
Justinian I, 90

Kafka, Franz, 110, 173, 176–77, 180, 181
kaihōgyō, 20
Kellogg, John Harvey, 183
Kennan, George, 124
Kennan, George F., 124
Kennedy, Robert F., 147, *148*
kenosis, 82
ketoacidosis, 55
ketones, ketosis, 49–50, 52–55, 68, 80
Keys, Ancel B., 65–69
Kimbrough, Mary Craig, 184
King Lear (Shakespeare), 46, 210
king penguin syndrome, 55
King's Threshold, The (Yeats), 111, 133
Klein bottle, xiv, *xiv*
Knights Templar, 112
knowledge, 90–91
Kratzer, Christina, 178
Kravchinsky, Sergius, 124
Krishnamurthy, Prem, 208
Kristeva, Julia, 11
Kussmaul, Adolf, 128

Lasègue, Ernest-Charles, 194–96
Lavoisier, Antoine, 178
Law, Bonar, 134

Learned Banqueters, The (Athenaeus of
    Naucratis), 37
Leary, Timothy, 70
Lebensreform movement, 177, 180
Leigh, Mary, 130
Lenin, Vladimir, 111, 125
Lent, xv, 58, 98, 102, 103, 124, 208
Lentulus, Paulus, 202
leptin, 47
Lerat, Eva, xiii, 16, 80
Levanzin, Agostino, 174–75, 191
Leviathan (Hobbes), 40
Leviticus, 102
life span, 64–66, 72–73
Lincoln, Abraham, 108
literacy, 90–91
Liu Xiaobo, 123
Lives of Eminent Philosophers (Diogenes
    Laërtius), 34
Loyola, Ignatius, 18–19
Lu, Cuong, 207
Lucey, Cornelius "Connie," 208
Lucretius, 39
Luria, Isaac, 15, 208
Luther, Martin, 105, 158
Lutheranism, 158, 161–62
luxury, 33–34
Lynch, Liam, 134
lynching, 108
Lysistrata (Aristophanes), 33

Macarius of Alexandria, 91
Macfadden, Bernarr, 184–88, *185*
MacSwiney, Terence, 133–34, 138, 208
Madison, James, 108
Máel Ruain, 117
Maimonides, 85
Maine, Sir Henry, 118
Manichaeanism, 96
Marx, Karl, 125
Mather, Cotton, 107
Mather, Increase, 107
Matthiessen, Peter, 54, 147
Mattson, Mark, 50
maya, 30
McCay, Clive M., 65–68, 70–72
meditation, 2, 4, 31
metabolism, 54, 55, 58, 64, 66, 73, 159
metaxu, xii, 15
Methodism, 162
Mezentsev, Nikolai, 124, 139

Michelangelo, 21
Microsoft, 5
migrant workers, 146–49
Mill, John Stuart, 120
Minnesota Starvation Experiment, 67–70
Mirzayan, Anna, 198
Mishan, Ligaya, 56
Mishneh Torah, 85
mitochondria, 53, 63–65
Miyamoto Musashi, xiii–xiv
Moore, Ann, 163–64, 170
More, Thomas, 40
Morton, Richard, 202–3
Moses, 78, 79, 81, 88, 117
Murphy, Joseph, 134, 138
Muslims, *see* Islam
Mussolini, Benito, 187, 210

Nataraja, 208
national days of fasting, xi, 107–8
Native Americans, 52, 166
natural hygiene movement, 162, 165, 169,
    181–82, 187, 188
naturopathy, 171, 179, 182, 184–86
Navalny, Aleksei, 154
Nazi Germany, 62–63, 128–29, 176, 180
Nehru, Jawaharlal, 120
Nemec, John, 113
Nerva, Marcus Cocceius, 115
Neumann von Konnersreuth, Therese, 203
neurasthenia, 196
neurons, 47, 53
neurotransmitters, 48
    serotonin, 52, 55, 60–61
New Scientist, 6
Newton, Isaac, 40
New York City
    Brooklyn, 5
    cabdrivers in, x
New Yorker, 171, 186
Nicholas of Flüe, St., 100, 170, 178
9/11 attacks, 205–6, 209–10
nirvana, 113
noise, 4, 6, 7, 17–18
nonviolence, ix, 121, 135, 146, 148–49,
    148, 153
Northwest Detention Center, 141–42

Obama, Barack, 142
obesity, 60–62, 198
Öcalan, Abdullah, 153–54

Odin, x
Odysseus, 25, 46
Of Grammatology (Derrida), 29
Okinawa Centenarian Study, 50–51
On Abstinence from Eating Animals
    (Porphyry), 26
Order of Time, The (Rovelli), 12
orexin-A, 53
Orfield, Steve, 4–5, 7–8, 10, 16, 19
Orfield Labs, 3–5, 7–10, 15–16
Origen, 89–90, 94, 99
Osho, 25
O'Toole, Fintan, 208
oxidative stress, 73

pain, 36, 37, 96, 97
Paine, Thomas, 15
Palamas, Gregory, 31
Palazzoli, Mara Selvini, 197
Palestinians, 144–45
Palladius, 91
Pankhurst, Emmeline, 173
Pankhurst, Sylvia, 125, 129, 173
Parmenides, 26
Parnell, Charles Stewart, 121
Patrick, St., 116–17
Paul, Alice, 129, 130
Paul, St., xii
Peacemakers, 141
Pelagius, 117
Peloponnesian War, 33
peristalsis, 45, 52
Pharisees, 87
Phillips, Nathan, 154
Physical Culture, 186
Pinel, Philippe, 128
pituitary gland, 197
Plato, xii, 15, 32–33, 35, 36, 38
pleasure, 36–39, 96
Pliny the Elder, 86, 87, 177
Porphyry, 26–27
Portland, Kristen, 193–94
Pound, Ezra, 210
prāya, 112–14, 116, 118
Priestley, Joseph, 178
proteins, 54–58, 64, 65
Protestantism, 41, 105–7, 109, 162, 165, 178
Proverbs, 76, 101
ptomaines, 184
Puritanism, 40, 41, 86, 105–7, 166
putrescine, 184

Pythagorean cup, 27, *28*
Pythagoras, Pythagoreans, 26–28

quarantine, 79
Quran, 102, 151

Ramadan, xv, 53, 58–59, 101–4, 151, 207
Rājataranginī, (*The River of Kings*),
    112–14
Reagan, Ronald, 149
Redmond, John, 130
refeeding syndrome, 57–58, 172, 175
Reik, Wolf, 74
religions, ix, 31, 41, 206–7
    see also specific religions
repentance (*teshuva*), 84, 85
Republic, The (Plato), 36
Rest Is Resistance (Hersey), 7
Restore Hyper Wellness, 157
Restrepo, Sandy, 142
Rings of Saturn, The (Sebald), 10
River of Kings, The (*Rājataranginī*),
    112–14
Robinson, Eroseanna, 141
Rockefeller, John D., 183
Role, Mike, 8, 10, 16
Romans, 26, 39, 76, 81, 84, 93, 95, 114–15
Rosweyde, Heribert, 21
Rousseau, Jean-Jacques, 40
Rovelli, Carlo, 12, 22, 110–11
Rumi, xvi
Rushkoff, Douglas, 83
Russia, 3, 18, 123–25, 145–46
Russian Orthodox Church, 123–24
Ryle, John Alfred, 199

"Sacred Words of a Woman, The" (Antal),
    193
sallekhana, 190
salmonella, 184
Samut, Robert, 175
San-Chez, André, 155
sand mandala, 209–10
Sands, Bobby, 138, 139
sannyasi, 112, 134–35
Santorio, Santorio, 158–60, *159*
Saper, Clifford, 47
Sartre, Jean-Paul, 5, 38, 76, 205
satyagraha, 137
Sayings of the Fathers, The, 21–22
Scientific American, 173

Scheele, Carl, 178
Schopenhauer, Arthur, 82
Schreier, Apollonia, 202, 203
Schwartz, Hillel, 160
Sebald, W. G., 10, 83
Second World War, 65, 67–70, 83, 180
self-control, 41, 194
self-denial, ix, 96
self-obsession, xiv
senses, 26, 46, 53, 88
sensory deprivation, 4, 6
    in anechoic chamber, 3–5, 7–10, 15–16
serotonin, 52, 55, 60–61
Serval, Clare de, 174
sex, 26, 27, 33, 86, 88, 89, 93–95, 105, 192,
    200
Shakers, 86, 178
Sharmila, Irom, 118–19, 202
Sharp, Gene, 153
Sheehan, Pat, 137–39
Sheehy-Skeffington, Hanna, 132
Shelton, Herbert M., 188
Shiva, 208
shramanas, 28
Shugendō, 19
Sikhism, 206, 207
silence, 3–7, 9, 15, 17–19, 29
    vows of, 91
Simeon the Stylite, 91
Simmonds, Morris, 196–97
Simpson, Wallis, 199
Sinclair, Upton, 181, 183–84, 186
sirtuins, 64–65
Skinner, B. F., 42
Slahi, Mohamedou Ould, 151
slavery, 122, 141, 152, 154, 182
slenderness, culture of, 157, 198–99
sleep, 46–47, 52, 53, 60, 105
snacking, 61
Snyder, Allan, 16
social connection, 11–12, 44
Socrates, 26, 32, 33, 35
sokushinbutsu, 19
solitary confinement, 12
somatostatin, 54
Song of Solomon, 94
Sontag, Susan, xiv
sound, 9
    noise, 4, 6, 7, 17–18
Soviet Union, 145–46
Soyinka, Wole, 11

Sparta, 33
speculum oris, 122
speech, 2, 3, 91
Spence, Theresa, 153
Spinoza, Baruch, 78
stars, 39
starvation, xiii, 55–56
Steiger, Howard, 60–61, 200
Stella Jean, x
Stevens, Doris, 131
stillness, 2, 6, 9–10, 12, 13, 17
Stoics, 18, 35–37, 39, 96, 191
stomach, 45–48, 165
Strassfeld, Michael, 81–82, 84
Strassfeld, Sharon, 81
Strings, Sabrina, 60
Studio 80, 7
Succi, Giovanni, 173–74, 174, 191
Suetonius, 115
suffragists, 108, 119, 125–27, 127, 129–32,
    145
suicide, xiv, 12, 101, 113, 134, 190, 191, 209
Sunrise Movement, x, 143–44, 153

Tacitus, 115
Talmud, 79, 82, 84–86
Tanner, Henry S., 169–73, 191
taxi drivers, x
Taylor, Breonna, 154
Taylor, Zachary, 108
Taylorism, 182–83
Tertullian, 88
teshuva, 84, 85
Thanksgiving, 166
Thatcher, Margaret, 134, 139
Theodora of Alexandria, 92
Theodosius II, 91
Thermidorian Reaction, 36
thermogenesis, 48
Thomas Aquinas, 98
Tiananmen Square demonstrations, 122–23
Tiberius, 114–16
Timtik, Ebru, 56
Tírechán, 117
Tish'ah b'Av, 85
To Build a Castle (Bukovsky), 111
Torah, 76, 77, 79, 81, 85, 102
torture, 18, 128–30
Trevelyan, Charles, 120
Trían, King, 117
troscead, 116, 117, 124, 131, 152

Trotsky, Leon, 125
tryptophan, 55
Turnbull, A. R., 191–92
Twain, Mark, 166–68, *168*
tzimtzum, 15, 82, 208

Ukraine, 3, 18
Ulmer, Margaretha, 163
uncertainty principle, 29
United Farm Workers, 54, 146
United Nations, 12
University of Virginia, 5
Uposatha, xv
Utopia (More), 40
Uyghurs, 104

Vatican Sayings (Epicurus), 24
Victoria, Queen, 194
Vietnam War, 152
violence, 17

Walford, Roy, 70–72
Wallace, William, 126
Wallace-Dunlop, Marion, 126–27, *127*, 129
Wanley, Nathaniel, 160
Warburg, Otto, 62–63
Webb, Shaykh Suhaib, 103
Weber, Max, 41, 157
weight loss, 59–61, 182
Weil, Simone, viii, xii, 29, 82–83, 205, 208
Weimar Germany, 180–81
Weindruch, Richard, 66
wellness, xiv, 157
Wesley, John, 162

Wilson, Woodrow, 206
witches, 100–101, 107
women and girls
    anorexia in, *see* anorexia
    ascetics, 91–95, 97, 99–100
    fasting of, ix, 109, 160–61, *161*, 163–64,
        168, 170–71, 191–92, 196
    misogyny and, 93, 94
    nervous disorders diagnosed in, 195–96
    suffragists, 108, 119, 125–27, *127*,
        129–32, 145
    witches, 100–101, 107
Wong, Jan, 123
World as Will and Idea, The (Schopenhauer),
    82
World Health Organization, 17
World War I, 206
World War II, 65, 67–70, 83, 180

Xenophon, 33

yamabushi, 112
Yan Hui, 13–14, 21
Yeats, W. B., 111, 133
Yom Kippur, xv, 79, 85, 102, 103

Zeno of Citium, 35–36
Zero Decibels (Foy), 15
Zhuang, Master, 13, 20
Zhuangzi, 13–15, 18, 20–21, 78, 136,
    208
Zola, Rachelle, 154
Zoroastrianism, 206–7
Zwingli, Ulrich, 106

Image Credits

xiv Courtesy Professor John M. Sullivan

28 Nevit Dilmen, Wikimedia Commons

127 Heritage Image Partnership Ltd. / Alamy Stock Photo

128 Retro AdArchives / Alamy Stock Photo

133 AA Images / Alamy Stock Photo

148 Bettmann / via Getty Images

159 Courtesy the Wellcome Collection

161 Courtesy the Wellcome Collection

168 Wikimedia Commons

174 Peter Horry / Alamy Stock Photo

201 Brooklyn Museum, Frank L. Babbott Fund, Frank Sherman Benson Fund, Carll H. de Silver Fund, A. Augustus Healy Fund, Caroline A. L. Pratt Fund, Charles Stewart Smith Memorial Fund, and Ella C. Woodward Memorial Fund.

203 Courtesy the Wellcome Collection

About the Author

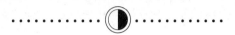

John Oakes is the publisher of *The Evergreen Review*. He is the editor at large for OR Books, which he cofounded in 2009. Oakes has written for a variety of publications, among them *The Oxford Handbook of Publishing, Publishers Weekly,* the *Review of Contemporary Fiction,* the Associated Press, and the *Journal of Electronic Publishing.* Oakes is a cum laude graduate of Princeton University, where he earned the English Department undergraduate thesis prize for an essay on Samuel Beckett. He was born and raised in New York City, where he lives, and is the father of three adult children. While working on *The Fast,* he was awarded residencies at Yaddo (New York) and Jentel (Wyoming). *The Fast* is his first book.

SMALLNESS

by Tukaram (first part of seventeenth century)
translated by Anand

लहानपण देगा देवा | मुंगी साखरेचा रवा ||
ऐरावत रत्न थोर | त्यासी अंकुशाचा मार ||
जया अंगी मोठेपण | तया यातना कठीण ||
तुका म्हणे बरवे जाण | व्हावे लहानाहून लहान ||
महापुरे झाडे जाती | तेथे लव्हाळे वाचती ||

O Lord, give me smallness | A granule of sugar that the ant gets ||
Airawat, Indra's jewel of a mount | Gets beaten by a mahout ||
Those who grow big and famous | Will suffer the blows of fate ||
Tuka says to know this is all | We must grow smaller than small ||
A flood sweeps trees away | Grasses find a way ||